PERSONAL +
COMMUNITY
HEALTH

FOURTH EDITION

DR. JONI BOYD + DR. SHELLEY HAMILL

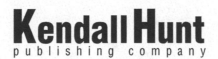

Kendall Hunt
publishing company

Cover image © Shutterstock.com

Kendall Hunt
publishing company

www.kendallhunt.com
Send all inquiries to:
4050 Westmark Drive
Dubuque, IA 52004-1840

Copyright © 2016, 2018, 2020, 2022 by Kendall Hunt Publishing Company

ISBN 979-8-7657-0665-7

Published in the United States of America

Contents

Acknowledgments

First and foremost, I want to thank my God for the opportunity to fulfill my goals and dreams. I want to thank my husband, Timothy; my children, Timmy Jr., JohnieMae, Grace, and Titus, for your motivation for me to continue, even when times are tough. Thank you to June, Sheila, and Courtney for your support throughout all my endeavors. Thank you to my mentor, co-author, and friend, Shelley. Your guidance and friendship only compliment the passion for excellence and collegiality that make you awesome to work with.

+ Joni M. Boyd

I am grateful for the opportunity to continue on this journey and am most thankful for the support of those behind the scenes and in front. Mom, thank you for the life lessons and providing the strong foundation. Dibbrell, as always, for the love and support. In addition, Joni, my co-author, friend, and colleague, it has been wonderful to continue our adventures in publishing together. You continue to amaze me with all that you have done and continue to do. I might not have started down this road without your encouragement and support, so thank you! I look forward to our future endeavors.

+ Shelley Hamill

As this is our fourth edition, we have again had the opportunity to update information to keep things current. We have hopefully fixed some typos (gosh I found a few), and we are proud of this next offering.

We would also like to thank the reviewers contacted by the publisher for their input. Your thoughts and comments were wonderful guides in some of the decisions we made during our revisions. Thank you for taking the time.

+ Joni & Shelley

We are extremely grateful for the contributions of the following individuals:

Dr. Kelly Boyd, Associate Professor, East Strausburg University
Dr. Irene Cucina, Professor, Plymouth State University
Karin Evans, MA, RD, Instructor, Winthrop University
Dr. Danne Kasparek, Emeriti faculty, Winthrop University
Bethann Rohaly, MS, Instructor, Winthrop University
Jennifer Vickery, MS, Instructor (retired), Winthrop University

And finally, Caylee King, Matthew Edwards, Katie Parker, Taylor Smith, Elizabeth Thrower, Demi Henschel and our wonderful graduate assistants who have been invaluable in the process. Not sure we could have done this without you. Thank you!

+ Joni & Shelley

Welcome to Personal and Community Health!

This course is designed as an introduction to personal health with a focus on what each of us can do to work towards achieving optimal health. Each chapter has a foundation of content information, possible strategies for us to utilize, and resources for students to consider accessing.

The authors, in collaboration with other faculty, staff, and students, created this text with the intent of making it student friendly, meaningful, and written in a conversational tone for easy comprehension. Each chapter opens with either an activity or pre-assessment for students to begin determining where they are in their journey towards optimal health. Additionally, we have designed chapter questions to provide application of skills and knowledge for students. While there may be a tremendous amount of information about each topic, this course is designed as an overview. If you wish to delve further into certain topics, we encourage you to take additional courses that specifically focus on that area of interest.

This is the fourth edition of this text. We initially started with foundational texts, which aided in our development and are grateful to those authors that were cited throughout and credited for their work. This text has been vastly re-written with current data, examples, and in our own voices. We have addressed feedback from reviewers the publisher invited and incorporated many of their suggestions. And, of course, we have incorporated lessons we have learned while teaching this course. We are truly proud of this latest edition and believe each improvement has made this text even better. We hope you agree.

Dr. Joni Boyd ✛ Dr. Shelley Hamill

About the Authors

Shelley Hamill, PhD, MCHES is a professor at Winthrop University. She is a Master Certified Health Education Specialist and has more than 30 years of combined teaching experience at the elementary, middle, and college levels. Dr. Hamill teaches courses in personal health, human sexuality, women's health, and teaching methods, in addition to activity courses including aerobic walking and tennis. Dr. Hamill has been recognized for her contributions to health education receiving numerous awards throughout her career. Additionally, she was recognized by Dr. David Satcher, US Surgeon General for her work with tribal communities dealing with HIV/AIDS, STDs, and substance abuse.

Joni Boyd, PhD CSCS*D, is an Associate Professor of Exercise Science and the Advisor to the Coaching Minor at Winthrop University. She has a PhD in Health Aspects of Physical Activity from University of South Carolina, where her research focused on locus of control, health behaviors, and religion. She has served as the National Strength & Conditioning Association State Director for South Carolina and a Master Instructor for Athletics and Fitness Association of America. Dr. Boyd has a vast range of research interests and topics, including functional-based movements, strength and conditioning, coaching styles, warm-up protocols, group exercise cohesion, nutrition-driven athletic and academic performance, and general health and well-being of college students. Dr. Boyd holds over 20 certifications and credentials within the health, exercise science, and nutrition fields. Ultimately, Dr. Boyd works to help students find where they belong in the worlds of health, exercise, and sports.

Chapter 1

Foundations +

OBJECTIVES

Students will be able to:

- Identify dimensions of wellness;
- Discuss which dimensions they are strongest in;
- Discuss which dimensions they might need to improve;
- Define Health Literacy
- Discuss the role they have as a consumer in their own wellness.

PERSONAL OBSERVATIONS

Directions: As you begin this journey in exploring personal health, use Figure 1.1 on page 5 and answer the following questions:

1. In which dimensions of life are you most well?
2. In which dimensions are you least well?
3. Comment on the pattern you see in your inventory.
4. How do you feel about what you see?
5. What improvements, if any, would you like to see?
6. List two or three immediate steps you could take to make your wheel more round and make these improvements.
7. What is health literacy?
8. What role do you play as a consumer in your wellness?

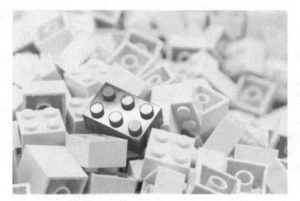

© ThamKC/Shutterstock.com

What is health? Have you thought about what it means to be healthy? Perhaps it just means not being sick or maybe having the energy to do what you want to do. Maybe, it includes more than just the physical aspects and includes other areas like mental health or social health. Many sources have defined health as being of sound mind and body. The World Health Organization defines **health** as a "state of complete physical, mental, and social well-being and not merely the absence of disease or infirmity". Yet, as comprehensive as that may sound, the definition of health today has evolved to include not just the physical and mental aspects, but also emotional, spiritual, and environmental components as well. Instead of looking at what health is, we have moved the focus on what is **wellness**. Wellness is seen as a life philosophy about making informed healthy choices, which can lead, over time to a healthy lifestyle. So how do we learn to make those healthy choices towards a healthier lifestyle? We learn by becoming health literate.

Health Literacy

"Health literacy is the degree to which individuals have the capacity to obtain, process, and understand basic health information and services needed to make appropriate health decisions." (NNLM). In order to make healthy choices, we need to have the knowledge about what those choices are. We also need to have the skills that help us deal with the pressures associated with making the healthier choice rather than the choices our peers might make. Becoming health literate individuals is one of the goals we should all strive to achieve.

Consider this: According to the World Health Organization (2022) since the emergence of the corona virus and it's many variants (COVID), there have been over five million deaths world wide attribute to the virus. In the United States alone, there have been over 900 thousand deaths. How do you, as a health literate person, navigate the many sources of information, and in some cases disinformation, to make informed decisions about your health as well as the health of your family? That is what it means to be health literate. Learning to recognize options and evaluate information to make the healthiest choices. It is a learned skill and again, one we should all strive to achieve.

DIMENSIONS OF WELLNESS

To a large degree, each of us is responsible for our behavioral choices that may directly impact our health. Sometimes we make better choices than others which can put us either at risk for potential negative consequences or support more positive health outcomes. The goal is for each of us to consistently focus on health-enhancing behaviors and to work towards adopting a wellness lifestyle that allows us to reach our full potential.

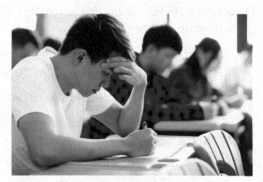
© Tom Wang/Shutterstock.com

It is the complex interaction of each of the eight dimensions of wellness, (see Figure 1.1), that will lead us, over time, to a higher quality of life and better overall health and well-being. Constant, ongoing assessment of our behaviors in the following dimensions is key to living a balanced life.

Emotional

What does it mean to be emotionally healthy? Are you able to express your emotions in a positive healthy way or do you keep them bottled up? Are you able to cope with unexpected life changes or challenges? Are

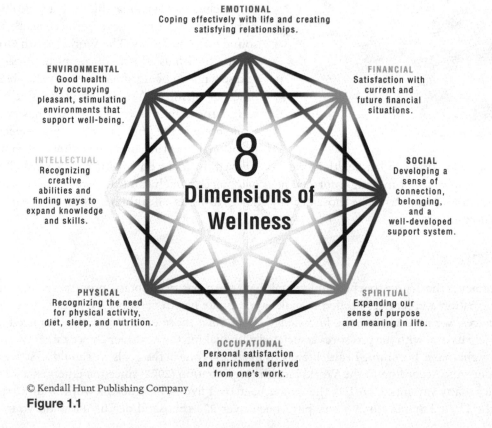

© Kendall Hunt Publishing Company

Figure 1.1

you aware of what your emotions actually are at given moments? A person who is emotionally healthy has the ability to do all of those things. Keeping your emotions buried inside can actually affect you immune system in a negative way. It can lead to chronic stress which can elevate your blood pressure and even make you more susceptible to passing pathogens such as cold and flu viruses.

Intellectual

People who are intellectually healthy are always looking to learn new things, explore new ideas, and engage on on-going learning experiences. When you are intellectually healthy, you want to find out why things are the way they are. How do things work?

Social

Are you an introvert (someone who isn't a fan of social interaction, which can leave you drained)? Or perhaps you are an extrovert (someone who gets energy from interacting with others)? Perhaps you are somewhere in between depending on the situation. A socially healthy person is someone, no matter their personality, who can relate and interact with others. We need to be connected to others in some sense as it is important to our overall wellbeing.

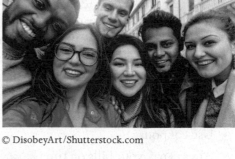
© DisobeyArt/Shutterstock.com

Spiritual

Where do you find your foundation? What gives you inner strength, inner peace, even confidence? Spiritual health is that space that helps us find those things. It is where our sense of beliefs, ethics, morals, and values originates. And, it can be found in many places, whether organized religion, nature, whatever provides that meaning and purpose for life.

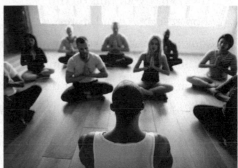
© Rawpixel.com/Shutterstock.com

Physical

When we think about health and wellness, most people immediately focus on physical health. What does that really mean? It actually covers many things including muscular strength and endurance, cardiovascular fitness, flexibility, even body composition. And, let's not forget we need enough sleep, proper nutrition and we need to avoid risky behaviors like texting and driving, drinking and driving, and engaging in unprotected sex just to name a few. Being physically healthy, just like all the rest, takes work, effort, and time.

Occupational

Do you like your job? Wait, you are in college so maybe you aren't in the job you hope to have but rather getting the education so you can. Occupational wellness is finding that profession that is fulfilling. Are you in it for the money or is it your passion. Maybe your career will help pay for your outside fun but remember, work life balance are important!

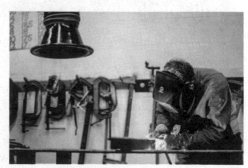
© Winthrop University

Environmental

The environment we live in plays a pivotal role in our overall health and wellbeing. Having access to clean water, healthy food, clear air and adequate shelter are essential. Additionally, safety is another important component, not just physical safety, but emotional safety as well. What role do you play in maintaining a healthy environment?

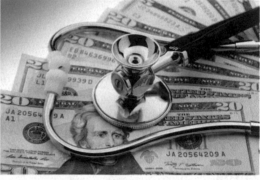

Courtesy of Shelley Hamill

FINANCIAL WELLNESS

We all hope to achieve financial wellness. We want to have enough to pay for what we need with a little left over for what we want (and let's not forget savings). The first step in the process towards financial wellness is to work towards being financially responsible. There are several things you can do towards that end. Here are just a few:

- Have a budget and stick to it
- Avoid having too many credit cards and pay the balance(s) off each month if you can
- Use coupons
- Always pay your bills on time
- Shop at second hand stores
- Look for items to go on sale and avoid impulse buys.
- Eat out less and cook at home more.
- Prepare your lunch rather than having to go out each day.
- Again, just a few items to help with good money management.

© Christian Delbert/Shutterstock.com

We have a wide range of lifestyle choices when it comes to wellness. What we choose to do and the decisions we make in each of the eight dimensions of wellness will have an impact on our overall quality of life. Making an active effort to combine and try to balance each of the eight dimensions is key to a long and fulfilling life.

Did you know . . .

There are all kinds of tests in college—beyond those you take for a grade.

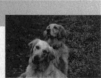

Courtesy of Shelley Hamill

Examples include:

- Time management
- Getting enough sleep
- Social pressures
- Possibly pressures to engage in sex
- Finding a school life balance between friends, classes, work, and extracurricular activities.

10 Leading Causes of Death by Age Group, United States – 2018

Rank	<1	1-4	5-9	10-14	15-24	25-34	35-44	45-54	55-64	65+	Total
					Age Groups						
1	Congenital Anomalies 4,473	Unintentional Injury 1,226	Unintentional Injury 734	Unintentional Injury 692	Unintentional Injury 12,044	Unintentional Injury 24,614	Unintentional Injury 22,667	Malignant Neoplasms 37,301	Malignant Neoplasms 113,947	Heart Disease 526,509	Heart Disease 655,381
2	Short Gestation 3,679	Congenital Anomalies 384	Malignant Neoplasms 393	Suicide 596	Suicide 6,211	Suicide 8,020	Malignant Neoplasms 10,640	Heart Disease 32,220	Heart Disease 81,042	Malignant Neoplasms 431,102	Malignant Neoplasms 599,274
3	Maternal Pregnancy Comp. 1,358	Homicide 353	Congenital Anomalies 201	Malignant Neoplasms 450	Homicide 4,607	Homicide 5,234	Heart Disease 10,532	Unintentional Injury 23,056	Unintentional Injury 23,693	Chronic Low. Respiratory Disease 135,560	Unintentional Injury 167,127
4	SIDS 1,334	Malignant Neoplasms 326	Homicide 121	Congenital Anomalies 172	Malignant Neoplasms 1,371	Malignant Neoplasms 3,684	Suicide 7,521	Suicide 8,345	Chronic Low. Respiratory Disease 18,804	Cerebro-vascular 127,244	Chronic Low. Respiratory Disease 159,486
5	Unintentional Injury 1,168	Influenza & Pneumonia 122	Influenza & Pneumonia 71	Homicide 168	Heart Disease 905	Heart Disease 3,561	Homicide 3,304	Liver Disease 8,157	Diabetes Mellitus 14,941	Alzheimer's Disease 120,658	Cerebro-vascular 147,810
6	Placenta Cord. Membranes 724	Heart Disease 115	Chronic Low. Respiratory Disease 68	Heart Disease 101	Congenital Anomalies 354	Liver Disease 1,008	Liver Disease 3,108	Diabetes Mellitus 6,414	Liver Disease 13,945	Diabetes Mellitus 60,182	Alzheimer's Disease 122,019
7	Bacterial Sepsis 579	Perinatal Period 62	Heart Disease 68	Chronic Low Respiratory Disease 64	Diabetes Mellitus 246	Diabetes Mellitus 837	Diabetes Mellitus 2,282	Cerebro-vascular 5,128	Cerebro-vascular 12,789	Unintentional Injury 57,213	Diabetes Mellitus 84,946
8	Circulatory System Disease 428	Septicemia 54	Cerebro-vascular 34	Cerebro-vascular 54	Influenza & Pneumonia 200	Cerebro-vascular 567	Cerebro-vascular 1,704	Chronic Low. Respiratory Disease 3,807	Suicide 8,540	Influenza & Pneumonia 48,888	Influenza & Pneumonia 59,120
9	Respiratory Distress 390	Chronic Low. Respiratory Disease 50	Septicemia 34	Influenza & Pneumonia 51	Chronic Low. Respiratory Disease 165	HIV 482	Influenza & Pneumonia 956	Septicemia 2,380	Septicemia 5,956	Nephritis 42,232	Nephritis 51,386
10	Neonatal Hemorrhage 375	Cerebro-vascular 43	Benign Neoplasms 19	Benign Neoplasms 30	Complicated Pregnancy 151	Influenza & Pneumonia 457	Septicemia 829	Influenza & Pneumonia 2,339	Influenza & Pneumonia 5,858	Parkinson's Disease 32,988	Suicide 48,344

Data Source: National Vital Statistics System, National Center for Health Statistics, CDC.
Produced by: National Center for Injury Prevention and Control, CDC using WISQARS™.

Centers for Disease Control and Prevention National Center for Injury Prevention and Control

Figure 1.2 Courtesy of the CDC

The leading causes of death for all age groups are listed in figure 1.2 (CDC). While unintentional injury is clearly a significant concern for ages 1-44, it is also important to note the changes that begin to occur in leading causes of death starting with age 45. Many of these health issues are related to lifelong health risk behaviors.

Factors That Influence Health and Wellness

Lifestyle choices, including dietary behaviors, activity levels, tobacco use and alcohol consumption, all play a role in our overall health. While you may not see an immediate impact unless you have an acute reaction to something, you will see the consequences long term as you age. The following chart identifies the leading causes of death, but note what the contributing factors actually are. Additionally, pay attention to some of the things you can do to help reduce the risks for preventable diseases. Some of these involve things you can do on a daily basis.

Another way to look at our dietary decisions can be seen in Figure 1.3 identifying complications from obesity. Our food choices matter long term as does our activity level or lack thereof.

Top 5 Leading Causes of Death:	Ways to Prevent Leading Causes of Death
Cancer	• Screenings and vaccines • Getting Tested for Hepatitis C • Avoid tobacco use • Protect your skin from sun exposure • Maintaining a healthy weight
Heart disease	• Eating a healthy diet • Maintaining a healthy weight • Getting enough physical activity • Not smoking or using other forms of tobacco • Limiting alcohol use

Stroke
Stroke
HELP!
	• Eating a healthy diet
	• Maintaining healthy weight
	• Not smoking or using other forms of tobacco
	• Control Medical Conditions:
	  o Check Cholesterol, Blood Pressure and Diabetes
	  o Treat your heart disease and take your medication

Chronic lower respiratory diseases (CLRD)	• Avoiding exposure to tobacco smoke • Avoid home and workplace air pollutants • Avoid respiratory infections by washing your hands regularly with soap and water o It is estimated that hands spread 80 percent of common infectious respiratory diseases like colds and flu.

Unintentional Injuries	• Depending on the setting be mindful of:
	  o Distractions
	  o Your surroundings
	  o The people around you

Courtesy of Caylee King. Copyright © Kendall Hunt Publishing Company.

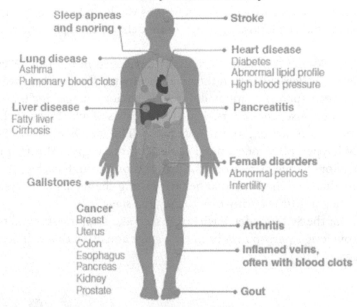

Figure 1.3 Adapted from Yale University Rudd Center for Food Policy and Obesity

A WELLNESS PROFILE

How do you know if you are working towards wellness? Are you paying attention to the choices you are making? Achieving and maintaining wellness requires effort and evaluation. The evaluation is examining what we are doing and if it is working. There are many behaviors and choices that would be beneficial in our daily routines that could contribute to our wellness. The following are just samples of what we could do:

- Don't smoke or vape (really not good for you)
- Be mindful of alcohol consumption (if you drink)
- Make healthy choices when it comes to food (at least most of the time.
- Exercise regularly
- Maintain a healthy weight
- Stay hydrated
- Get enough sleep
- Have a plan for dealing with stress
- Know the facts when it comes to protection from cardiovascular disease, infections, sexually transmitted infections, etc.
- These are just a few of the many daily habits we should practice for wellness.

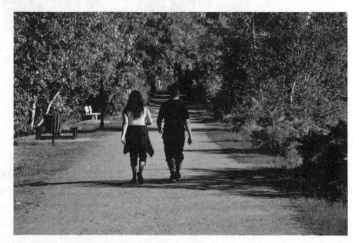

© Lester Balajadia/Shutterstock.com

The Stages of Change

There are many models that discuss why we act or behave as we do and what occurs when we are looking to change a particular behavior. The following behavior models are examples and may be applied across a wide range of behaviors.

"The Stages of Change Model (SCM) was originally developed in the late 1970s and early 1980s by James Prochaska and Carlo DiClemente when they were studying how smokers were able to quit smoking. The SCM model has been applied to many different behavior changes including weight loss, injury prevention, alcohol use, drug abuse, and others. The SCM consists of five stages of change: precontemplation, contemplation, preparation, action, and maintenance. The idea behind the SCM is that behavior change does not usually happen all at one time. People tend to progress through the stages until they achieve a successful behavior change or relapse. The progression through each of these stages is different depending upon the individual and the particular behavior being changed. Each person must decide when a stage is complete and when it is time to move on to the next stage."[1]

Below are the stages for the SCM model. Each one is seen as a stepping stone to the next. Again, there is no set time limit for how long a person may be in each stage and often this will depend on how difficult the behavior is to change.

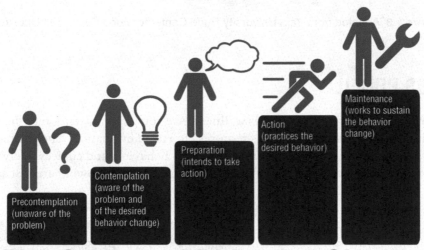

The Stages of Behavior Change

© Kendall Hunt Publishing Company

Precontemplation

"Precontemplation is the stage at which there is no intention to change a specific behavior in the foreseeable future. Many individuals in this stage are unaware of their unhealthy behavior. They are not thinking about change and are not interested in any help. People in this stage tend to defend their current behavior and do not feel it is a problem. They may resent efforts to help them change."[1]

Contemplation

"Contemplation is the stage at which people are more aware of the consequences of their unhealthy behavior and have spent time thinking about the behavior but have not yet made a commitment to take action.

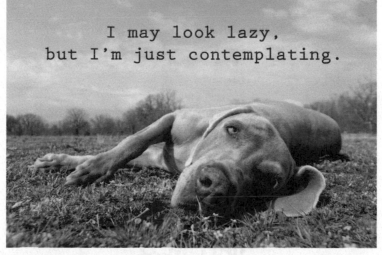

© Sari ONeal/Shutterstock.com

They consider the possibility of changing, but tend to be ambivalent about change. In this stage, people straddle the fence, weighing the pros and cons of changing or modifying their behavior."[1]

Preparation

"The stage that combines intention and behavioral criteria is called preparation. In this stage, people have made a commitment to make a change. This can be a research phase where people are taking small steps toward change. They gather information about what they will need to do to change their behavior. Sometimes, people skip this stage and try to move directly from contemplation to action. Many times, this can result in failure because they did not research or accept what it was going to take to make a major lifestyle change."[1]

Action

"The stage at which individuals actually modify their behavior is the action stage. This requires a considerable commitment of time and energy. The amount of time people spend in the action stage varies. On average, it generally lasts about six months. In this stage, unhealthy people depend on their own willpower. They are making efforts to change the unhealthy behavior and are at greatest risk for relapse. During this stage, support from friends and family can be very helpful.

"Along the way to a permanent behavior change, most people experience a relapse. In fact, it is much more common to have at least one setback than not. Relapse is often accompanied by feelings of discouragement. While relapse can be frustrating, the majority of people who successfully change their behavior do not follow a straight path to a lifetime free of unwanted behaviors. Rather, they cycle through the five stages several times before achieving a consistent behavior change. Therefore, the SCM considers relapse to be normal. Relapses can be important opportunities for learning and becoming stronger. This is where a behavior change journal and weekly reflections can help an individual see how much progress has been made, as well as what may trigger relapses. The main thing to remember is that the goal is getting closer. Do not get upset by life or setbacks, but keep moving forward and get closer to the end goal."[1]

Maintenance

"Maintenance is the stage in which people work to prevent relapse and focus on the gains attained during the action stage. Maintenance involves being able to successfully avoid temptations to return to the

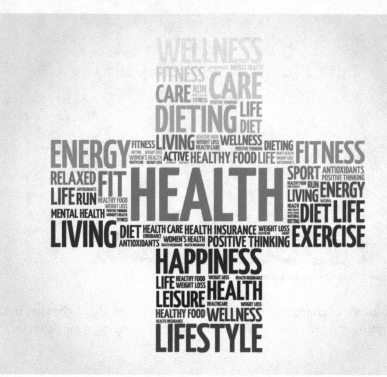

previous behavior. The goal of the maintenance stage is to continue the new behavior or lack thereof without relapse. People are more able to successfully anticipate situations in which a relapse could occur and prepare coping or avoidance strategies in advance."[1]

Cognitive Dissonance Theory

"Cognitive Dissonance refers to situations involving conflicting attitudes, beliefs or behaviors" (Simply psychology). In 1957, Leon Festinger proposed cognitive dissonance theory, which states that a powerful motive to maintain cognitive consistency can give rise to irrational behavior. He focused on the principle of cognitive consistency, which means we want consistency in our beliefs and want to avoid disharmony.

For example, a person who smokes knows that smoking causes lung cancer. There is an underlying dissonance if they do not change that behavior. If we want to reduce dissonance, we either change our behavior, acquire new information about the behavior, (research is inconclusive about lung cancer and tobacco), or we reduce the importance of that behavior (live for today).

Another way to look at this is that as humans, we see ourselves as we want to be, our ideal selves. If there is a difference in who we really are and our ideal, there is dissonance. By utilizing the same step mentioned above, we can work towards that goal and reduce our dissonance.

Self-Efficacy Theory

Self-efficacy centers the belief in your ability to reach goals and complete tasks. If you have a strong sense of self, and believe you can succeed, you are more likely to challenge yourself. The higher your sense of self-efficacy, the less likely you are to blame others if you do not succeed at something and are quicker to rebound from those setbacks. Your resiliency, the ability to adapt to adversity and stress, allows you to come back stronger and to continue moving forward.

Theory of Planned Behavior

Lastly, this theory suggests that your attitude about a behavior may affect your intention to engage in that behavior. Behavioral intention is generally established by attitude towards the behavior, (either good or bad), subjective norms (social pressures), and perceived behavioral control (perception of ease or difficulty to perform). For example, the likelihood you would start an exercise program is guided by your belief that you really need to get in shape, your friends support, and your belief that you can actually motivate yourself to get started.

BEHAVIOR CHANGE AND GOAL SETTING

So, how do you get started? What is the first step towards changing a behavior?

Choose a behavior that you are really invested in. Think about what you do, or don't do, on a daily or weekly basis. Is there something you want to change? How about your relationships? Is there something you could do to make things better? Ideas for behavior change include: increasing exercise, quitting smoking, decreasing procrastination, decreasing or eliminating sodas, eating more fruits and/or vegetables, getting more sleep, drinking more water, every day, stretching, and so on.

Only change one behavior at a time. After reviewing your habits or behaviors you would like to change, select one to focus on. People tend to get excited and want to change several different behaviors. Even if the behaviors are related, it is best to choose only one to focus on at a time. After a specific behavior has become a habit (at least six months in the maintenance stage) you can consider working on another behavior.

Once you have identified the behavior you wish to change, you need to set a goal. Your goal should be **specific**, **measurable**, **attainable**, **relevant** or **realistic**, and **time-bound**, otherwise known as a **SMART** goal. There are two other parts that have been added to the model and they are **evaluate** (see if your plan is working) and **revise** (if needed). The "r" could also stand for "**reward**" is things are going well and you want to **reward** yourself for the progress. Hence your goal will actually be **SMARTER**.

The goal should be specific and measurable. The more specific the goal and the plan to achieve this goal are, the more likely the behavior change will be successful. If you want to increase fitness, it would be best to be very specific about the short- and long-term goals. For example, you should consider your baseline (where you are right now). If you are not exercising at all, you should not begin working out five times per week the following week. During the first week you may want to exercise two times for fifteen minutes each exercise session. The following week the goal could be three times at twenty minutes each exercise session. The final goal may be five days per week for thirty minutes each time. This particular goal should take at least a month or two to achieve. The Behavior Change and Goal Setting notebook activity at the end of the chapter can help outline a plan of change.

Any behavior change target should be realistic. Often, behavior change goals include weight loss. To increase the long-term success rate, the most a person should lose is two pounds per week. One pound is equal to 3,500 calories. In order to lose two pounds per week the caloric deficit would need to be 7,000 calories. This translates to a deficit of

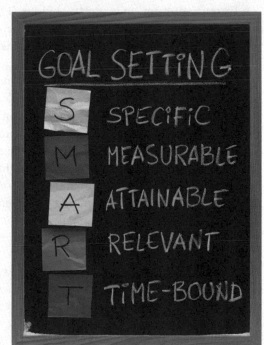

© marekuliasz/Shutterstock.com

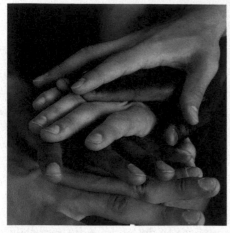

© Martin Allinger/Shutterstock.com

1,000 calories per day, which is not easy to achieve. The best way to achieve this caloric deficit is to include both exercise and limit caloric consumption. For example, you could expend part of the needed caloric deficit with exercise (approximately 500 calories per day) as well as consume fewer (approximately 500) calories per day for a total daily caloric deficit of 1,000. Remember, this is the most a person should lose per week.

Have a reward system. It is nice to have short- and long-term goals that have a small reward when a goal is reached. These rewards should never be counterproductive. For example, if you are trying to lose weight, the worst type of reward would be to have a dessert. Some constructive reward ideas could be to go to a movie, go for a specific hike, buy a little something you have been wanting or just give yourself time to hang out with friends.

Keep a journal. Some people love to journal. It is especially helpful if you are trying to change a behavior. It is a way to hold yourself accountable and to track what you have been doing along the way. You can see if you have met your weekly goals and perhaps even identify what steps are working and which ones are not.

Have a support group. When you are working towards changing a behavior, it is important to have people who are supporting your efforts and not, unknowingly sabotaging what you are trying to do. For example, if you are trying to lose weight, your friends might need to know so that they don't bring you those fresh baked brownies! And, friends can not only support you, but can hold you accountable as well

Prevention

Part of the reason for changing unhealthy behaviors is to avoid short term or long term health consequences. We all know the best way to avoid injuries and certain diseases is through prevention, right? There are actually three levels of prevention: primary, secondary, and tertiary.

Primary prevention is pretty obvious. The idea is to do things to avoid getting injured or developing disease. Getting your immunizations, exercising, proper nutrition, using sunscreen, are just a few of the ways we focus on primary prevention. As this is a personal health class, the focus is on primary prevention.

Secondary prevention focuses on screenings and early detection. While we may be working hard to avoid having any health issues, early detection and screenings can help us deal with things quickly should they arise. Having our blood pressure and blood sugar checked, mammograms, even mental health check-ins can all help minimize long term consequences of disease. Secondary prevention also focuses on preventing the spread of communicable disease. Regular screenings may detect a disease before symptoms might appear. For example, a person may have unknowingly contracted a sexually transmitted infection and not have any symptoms yet. A screening could detect the disease and be a secondary prevention strategy for the individual and a primary prevention strategy for anyone they might engage with in the future.

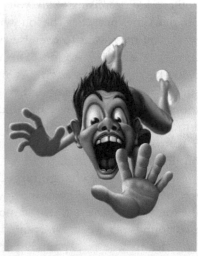

Sometimes, despite our best efforts, diseases may develop whether chronic or acute. **Tertiary prevention** focuses on improving the quality of life for individuals with varying diseases. Whether restoring function, limiting complications, or slowing and/or stopping progression, tertiary prevention works to make the quality of life for people dealing with disease better.

© Aidar/Shutterstock.com

HEALTHY PEOPLE 2030: IMPROVING THE HEALTH OF AMERICANS

While we have been focused on individual goals for behavior change, there are agencies and organizations that look at goals and objectives for behavior changes for society as a whole. Not only do these goals address specific deficits in policy or access to care, but they also identify behaviors that need to be encouraged or discouraged. Additionally, there are many **health disparities** within our society. Whether associated through race, ethnicity, gender, age, sexual identity or other variables, social determinants play a significant role in the health status of individuals. As such, agencies look at how to reduce or eliminate those disparities.

Healthy People 2030 is a 10-year agenda developed with the help of numerous agencies and individuals to improve the health of the Nation. There are 10 leading health indicators by life-stages. They are:

- Access to Health Services
- Clinical Prevention Services
- Nutrition, healthy eating, and obesity
- Drug and alcohol use
- Environmental Health
- Violence Prevention
- Social Determinants
- Vaccinations/Health Care
- Sexually Transmitted Infections and health care access
- Mental Health/Mental Disorders/Injury Prevention

© Harish Marnad/Shutterstock.com

There are four major factors that influence personal health:

1. personal behavior
2. heredity
3. environment
4. access to professional health care personnel

"The importance of prevention is made clear in *Healthy People 2030*. *Healthy People* was first developed in 1979 as a *Surgeon General's Report*. It has been reformulated since 1979 as *Healthy People 1990: Promoting Health/Preventing Disease*, *Healthy People 2000: National Health Promotion and Disease Prevention and Healthy People 2010; Objectives for Improving Health*. The original efforts of these programs were to establish national health objectives and to serve as a base of knowledge for the development of both state-level and community-level plans and programs to improve the nation's overall health. Much like the programs *Healthy People 2030* is based on, it was developed through broad consultation programs and the best and most current scientific knowledge in the public and private sectors. It is also designed in a way that will allow communities to measure the success rates, over time, of the programs they choose to implement.

As a set, Leading Health Indicators cover the life span. Based on the selection criteria, all LHIs:

- Are core objectives
- Focus on upstream measures, such as risk factors and behaviors, rather than disease outcomes

- Address issues of national importance
- Address high-priority public health issues that have a major impact on public health outcomes
- Are modifiable in the short term (through evidence-based interventions and strategies to motivate action at the national, state, local, and community level)
- Address social determinants of health, health disparities, and health equity
- Have new data available periodically, preferably annually

Healthy People 2030 has five overarching goals. The first goal is to attain high quality, longer lives free of preventable disease, disability, injury, and premature death. The second goal is to achieve health equity, eliminate disparities, and improve the health of all groups. The third goal is to create social and physical environments that promote good health for all. The fourth goal is to promote quality of life, healthy development and health behaviors across all life stages. Lastly, engage leadership, key constituents, and the public across multiple sectors to take action and design policies that improve the health and well-being of all.

Healthy Campus 2030 is a companion to Healthy People and focuses on specific issues that affect college students, faculty and staff. The intent is to provide a framework to help institutions identity priorities and develop action plans to meet individual campus needs.

Are You a Healthy Consumer?

We have identified many things in this chapter about wellness, health behaviors, behavior change and national health objectives. So what are you doing to foster a better health outcome? What are you, as a consumer, doing to contribute to not only your health, but the community as well? We discussed what it means to be health literate at the beginning of the chapter. What are you doing to build your health literacy and be a wise consumer? Things to think about as we continue this course.

"Health is 'a state of complete physical, mental, and social well-being and not merely the absence of disease or infirmity,' accord-

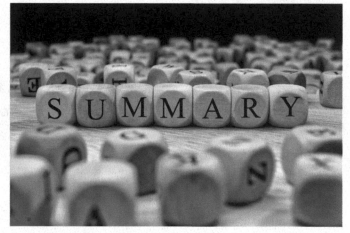

© Fabrik Bilder/Shutterstock.com

ing to the World Health Organization. By definition, health is a universal trait. Due to the fact that personal behaviors are one of the four major factors that influence a person's lifespan and quality of life, health also takes on a very individual and unique quality."

For the most part, wellness outcomes are based on individual choices and behaviors. By focusing on the eight dimensions of wellness – environmental, emotional, financial, intellectual, occupational, physical, social, and spiritual- and making good choices, you may be able to prevent, to some degree, disease and premature death.

Remember, in order to focus on changing a behavior, you have to set goals. Using one of the behavior change models listed in this chapter, along with setting SMARTER goals can guide you towards being successful in those behavior changes. And, of course, the earlier you get started the better!

Lastly, do not forget that prevention is the key in promoting wellness. Whether primary, secondary or tertiary, each plays a role in supporting our overall wellness. Clearly a focus on primary prevention is where we start but note that the other two are also important.

NOTES

PERSONAL REFLECTIONS . . . SO, WHAT HAVE YOU LEARNED?

1. In your own words, describe the concept of the "dimensions of wellness". How is it related to holistic health? Why is it important?

2. In which dimension would you consider yourself the most developed and why? Which one needs the most work and why?

3. Identify a behavior you might want to change. Select one of the models for behavior change and list the steps needed to make that change occur based on the model. Do not forget to make the goal "SMARTER".

4. Select two healthy objectives from Healthy People 2030 that you think are the most important and explain why.

NOTES

RESOURCES ON CAMPUS FOR YOU!

Every campus has health and counseling services available to students. Identify what services are available to you and be sure to utilize their services as needed.

STUDENT LIFE

The Division of Student Life's mission is providing opportunities and services to foster student development along cognitive, personal, and interpersonal dimensions. As educators, we work with our faculty colleagues to nurture and stimulate student learning and success within a pluralistic campus community. We accomplish this by delivering primary services that provide for the out-of-classroom caring for students, the foundation upon which classroom growth occurs. We enhance the quality of campus life, establish a sense of community and school spirit, and foster students' overall maturation and ethical development.

RECREATIONAL SERVICES

Recreational Services, offers spirited and competitive activities involving intramural and extramural sports, fitness activities, special events, and aquatics.

The Office of Recreational Services is a valuable resource for students, faculty and staff who wish to pursue a healthy lifestyle. Through participation in various programs, participants can gain a multitude of personal benefits including improved levels of physical fitness and wellness, opportunities for social interaction, time management skills, engagement in a group dynamic setting, a healthy means of stress relief, as well as the creation of a sense of ownership and belonging between students and the community.

REFERENCES

Center for Disease Control, Ten Leading Causes of Death by Age Group, United States-2018. Last reviewed June 24, 2020. cdc.gov/injury/images/lc-charts/leading_causes_of_death_by_age_group_2018_1100w850h.jpg

Corbin, C. B., Welk, G. J., Corbin, W. R. and Welk, K. A. (2010). *Concepts of Physical Fitness* (16th ed). McBrown.

Evans, R. & Sims, S. (2016). Health and Physical Education for Elementary Teachers: An integrated approach. Human Kinetics.

Floyd, P., Mims, S., and Yelding-Howard, C. (2007). *Personal Health: Perspectives and Lifestyles* (4th ed). Morton Publishing Co.

https://www.cdc.gov/cancer/dcpc/prevention/index.htm. Last reviewed August 3, 2021.

https://www.cdc.gov/cancer/dcpc/prevention/other.htm. Last reviewed June 3, 2019.

https://health.gov/healthypeople

http://www.m-w.com/dictionary.htm

https://nnlm.gov/outreach/consumer/hlthlit.html

http://www.wellnesswise.com/dimensions.htm

https://health.gov/healthypeople/about/healthy-pcoplc-2030-framework

https://health.gov/healthypeople/objectives-and-data/leading-health-indicators

Hyman, B., Oden, G., Bacharach, D., and Collins, R. (2006). *Fitness for living* (3rd ed). Kendall Hunt Publishing Company.

Insel, P. M. and Roth, W. T. *Core Concepts in Health* (12th ed). McGraw-Hill Publishing. 2009.

Payne, W. A., Hahn, D. B., and Lucas, E. B. (2008). *Understanding Your Health* (10th ed). McGraw-Hill Publishing.

Pruitt, B.E. and Stein, J. (1999). *Health Styles*. Allyn & Bacon.

www.simplypsychology.org/cognitive-dissonance.html

Chapter 2

Stress Management +

OBJECTIVES

Students will be able to:

- Define and identify types of stress, sources, and causes.
- Explain the body's response to eustress and distress, and the overall effect on health.
- Describe the impact of stress on physical health and disease risk.
- Explain the impact of stress on mental health, such as depression, anxiety, and suicidal behaviors.
- Discuss why sustainable and healthy stress-coping strategies are critical for positive health outcomes.
- Identify immediate, short-term, long-term strategies for stress coping and management.
- Describe the role of sleep and recommendations for effective stress management.
- Recognize and identify healthy consumer practices.

"ARE YOU UNDER STRESS?

I am physically tired.	Yes	No
I am emotionally tired.	Yes	No
I have headaches.	Yes	No
I have an upset stomach.	Yes	No
I have trouble sleeping.	Yes	No
I am irritable.	Yes	No
I am too tense.	Yes	No
I am angry.	Yes	No
I get into verbal/physical fights.	Yes	No
I have a hard time concentrating.	Yes	No
I am nervous.	Yes	No
I am worried.	Yes	No

Three or more 'yes' answers can indicate a high stress level."[7]

Critical Thinking . . .

What do you think are the major causes of stress in your life? Would you consider your stress as good stress or bad stress?

Do you think you have healthy, effective, stress-coping strategies?

How does your stress level affect physical activity, sleep, nutrition, or consumer behaviors?

TYPES OF STRESS

Stress is a natural part of life and exists in both positive and negative forms. Stress affects people in different ways. Especially in today's society, stress follows the fast-paced lifestyle of many Americans, as they attempt to meet various demands and expectations. Although stress is a natural part of life, the pressures of success often becomes overwhelming for many, and lack of effective stress management can lead to detrimental health.

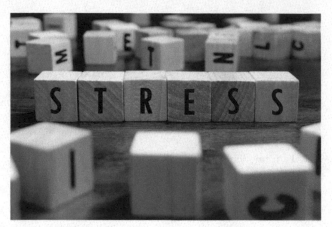

© schatzie/Shutterstock.com

Stress is the nonspecific response to demands placed on the body or basically how we respond to issues that arise in our lives. The body produces the same physiological reaction of a release in hormones to prepare itself for changes, which is why it is termed "nonspecific response." Specifically, when stress presents in our lives, the body releases adrenaline and cortisol. **Adrenaline** is a hormone secreted by the adrenal glands that increases rates of blood circulation and breathing and prepares muscles for exertion. Another hormone, **cortisol** is also released in response to stress, and it helps to control blood sugar levels and influence blood pressure.

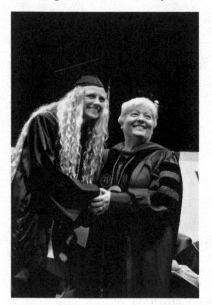

© Winthrop University

People vary on how they react to the stress response from a physical, emotional, mental, or behavioral perspective. A major stress to one person may not create the same level of response in another. Some people may perceive some stress or stressors as positive or motivational, where others can perceive the same stress as negative or threatening. There is a difference between positive and negative stress.

Eustress is a positive stress that produces a sense of well-being, and it is critical to the overall health of an individual. Eustress generally creates a sense of excitement and positive outcomes. Examples of eustress could be the feeling that accompanies big events, such as graduation, competition, weddings, or a ceremony. Eustress is a major component of positive health outcomes and overall well-being. Research has shown that individuals who are experiencing eustress had more positive social behavior, better health outcomes, and improved memory (Stauble et al., 2013; von Dawans et al., 2012). There is additional support for better immune system function and recovery with good stress, or eustress, (Dhabhar et al., 2012), and can enhance creativity and increase alertness (St. Lifer, 2013). Additionally, eustress can build emotional resilience through positive feelings of contentment, inspiration, improved self-efficacy and autonomy. It is important to note that nerves can still accompany events of eustress, which is what creates the stress response.

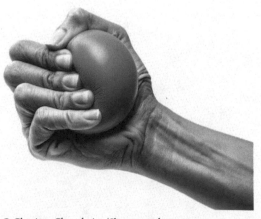

Distress is the response to negatively charged stress that results in a physiologically, physically, and mentally damaging response. Distress is often the result of events

© Chutima Chaochaiya/Shutterstock.com

perceived as negative or threatening. Examples of distress include relationship problems, poor academic performance, or legal troubles. Distress can also result from health-related events, such as illness, injuries, or death of a close friend or loved one. Distress is a normal response for individuals to experience because life holds difficult, hurtful, and negative events. The response to distress affects emotional, physical, mental, and physiological states. What is most important is how individuals respond to the impacts of distress. Short-term distress can produce changes that increase resistance and resilience and implement positive outcomes. Long-term distress, however, can create additional problems and concerns—such as feeling overwhelmed and emotionally and behaviorally stale—and even lead to burnout. It is important for individuals to find positive, healthy, and effective ways to cope with distressful events. Examples of coping could include meditation, religious beliefs, physical activities, counseling, and therapy. Finding an appropriate outlet is critical, and some options are discussed in this chapter.

Individuals considering certain careers should be aware of the stress events tied to those careers. Whereas most careers may include eustress in the concept of promotion and performance, it is also wise to consider the distress that may occur with some occupation responsibilities or environments. Students desiring to work in health care should be aware of the distress that can come with exposure to illnesses, disabilities, violence, and death. Students planning to become educators should prepare for exposure to poverty, disparities, and educational challenges that can affect some children. All careers and occupations can carry burdens of distress, and individuals should be prepared to cope with those challenges.

SOURCES AND CAUSES OF STRESS

Although there are many individual sources and causes of stress, they can generally be categorized into environmental, physiological, or psychosocial stressors. A **stressor** is any real or perceived event that pressures us to cope (Donatelle, 2014), or generally speaking, it is the source of a stress.

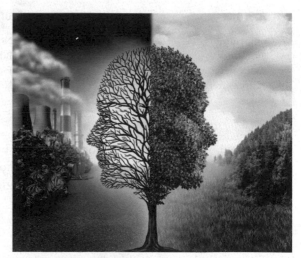

© Lightspring/Shutterstock.com

Environmental Stressors

Environmental stressors are situations or events that create stress within our environment. They can include day-to-day hassles and daily-life complexities. Examples include weather, noise, distractions, traffic, and even crowds. Environmental stressors can also originate from major external events, such as war, flood, or disaster.

Physiological Stressors

Physiological stressors can be very damaging to the overall health if they persist for a long time or if coping strategies are ineffective. These stressors tend to be more chronic in nature, such as a long-term illness or a difficult disability. Other sources might be an outcome that was very traumatic, such as the death of a loved one or a life-altering change. One physiological stressor can affect many members of a family.

Psychosocial Stressors

Psychosocial stressors include the wide variety of stressors that we encounter in our day-to-day life. Sources of psychosocial stress include the ebbs and flows of relationships with those closest to you and the range of feelings and emotions regarding these situations. Other examples can include losing your job, breaking up with someone you loved, ending a friendship, an unplanned pregnancy, a speeding ticket, car accident, missing class, or failing an exam.

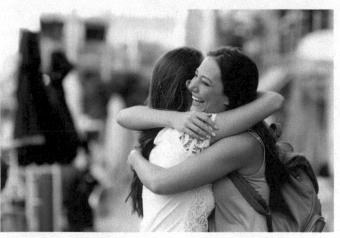
© Antonio Guillem/Shutterstock.com

Stress in College—What Are Stressors of College Students?

Stress in college is very real! College presents a new lifestyle, followed by changes in expectations, schedules, and/or living environments. The pressure to succeed can also be overwhelming. Table 2.1 provide a list of stressors reported by college students.

TABLE 2.1 The Commonly Reported Stressors of College Students

Academic	Time	Money	Self	Social
• Competition	• Deadlines	• Not enough	• Behavior	• Obligations
• Schoolwork	• Procrastination	• Bills/overspending	• Appearance	• Not dating
• Grades and exams	• Late for	• Job responsibilities	• Poor health	• Roommate
• Poor resources	appointments	• No job	• Weight	problems
• Professors	• No time to exercise		• Self-esteem	• STD concerns

STD, sexually transmitted disease.

Think about how these stressors affect your behaviors and overall health. What can you do to effectively cope with these stressors? We will discuss how the stress response can affect the college experience. Additionally, we will cover healthy coping strategies to help manage the effect of stress.

RESPONSES TO STRESS

The fight or flight response is the automatic response to stress. It is believed that the fight or flight response has been a human response to stress throughout history. Think of how an ancient human would respond.

In today's version, we still have a fight or flight response, but the stakes are different, although the physiological outcomes are still similar. When discussing the fight of flight response to stress, we need to look further at the physiological response the body has to the stressor. The **general adaptation syndrome (GAS)**, was originally developed by Hans Selye (considered to be the father of stress research) to describe a three-stage response to stress he was investigating. This response involves both the nervous system and hormonal systems of the human body. Following is a brief overview of the GAS.

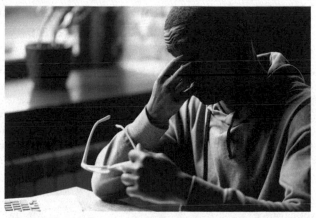

© fizkes/Shutterstock.com

Stage 1: This represents the **alarm stage,** which is the first response to a stressor, and it prepares the body for the fight or flight response. The body releases cortisol and adrenaline, which provide the energy to deal with the stressor. The alarm stage can create acute levels of fatigue.

Stage 2: In the **resistance stage**, the body reacts to the stressor or adapts to it if given enough time. The body is able to make changes that allow for management of the stressor, in order to control the negative effects that it may cause. This helps the body return to a balance, also called homeostasis. It is important that time is provided to allow the body to adjust. If not, then homeostasis cannot be reached and the body will move into Stage 3.

Stage 3: The **exhaustion stage** occurs when the body does not adapt or adjust to the stressor in order to reach homeostasis. This can lead to negative outcomes and consequences, beginning with exhaustion and fatigue. If the stressor persists into stage 3, the immune system becomes weaker and unable to resist toxins and pathogens. Finally, additional, more serious consequences can occur, including, illness, depression, or disability.

IMPACT OF STRESS
Symptoms of Stress

For many people, a negative stressful situation triggers an alarm and that person must decide how to deal with that stress. If the person successfully deals with or manages the stressful situation, then homeostasis returns and the body avoids negative outcomes of stress. If the person is unable to manage or cope with the stress or stressor, then the immune system weakens, increasing the likelihood of illness or disease. The illness could be as minor as a cold or allergic reaction, or as serious as a chronic disease. Heart disease, cancer, and diabetes are the leading causes of death in the United States and increase in high levels of negative stress. Other negative health consequences of unmanaged distress include high blood pressure, headaches, ulcers, and insomnia.

There are four areas where most people will show the effects of stress. These areas include our emotions, our behaviors, our physical appearance, or our mental state. Check out each of these areas in Table 2.2 below, and try to identify the area where stress likely surfaces for you. An important step of stress management is to understand when and how stress affects you, especially when the effect is negative. Where do you feel the greatest effect of your stress? Once you identify how it affects you, we can begin to process the impact and find strategies to reduce it.

TABLE 2.2 Stress Often Affects at Least One of Four Areas of Emotions, Behaviors, Physical Appearance, or Mental State

Emotions	Behaviors
• Do you always feel rushed or nervous? • Do you find it difficult to relax? • Are you irritable and moody, or easily angered? • Do you want to cry for no apparent reason? • Is it difficult for you to listen or pay attention? • Is it hard for you to fall or stay asleep?	• Has your appetite changed? • Have you gained or lost weight? • Are you neglecting yourself/your appearance? • Are you withdrawing from others or events? • Have you taken to substance abuse, such as cigarette smoking, drug use, or excessive alcohol or coffee intakes? • Are you participating in healthy behaviors?
Physical Appearance	**Mental State**
• Do you have a racing heart rate? • Are you out of breath or have tightness in your chest? • Do you have frequent headaches or muscle aches? • Is it difficult for you to digest food—leading to nausea or diarrhea? • Do you suffer from frequent infections? • Is it difficult to find energy for daily activities?	• Are you indecisive in many areas of your life? • Is it difficult for you to concentrate? • Do you regularly have bad dreams or nightmares? • Do you have negative or suicidal thoughts? • Do you think bad about yourself or others? • Is anger, anxiety, or depression affecting your decisions?

STRESS AND DISEASE

Stress has been linked to higher risk for diseases and illnesses, including heart disease, cancer, and some infections.

Heart Disease: Research has linked heart disease to high levels of distress, depression, and anxiety among multiple age groups and populations. In a study of 10,000 Israeli men, the risk of developing heart disease was up to three times greater in those that had high levels of stress than those that did not. In another study, depression was a significant predictor of heart disease in college graduates. Additionally, those with chronic mild anxiety and depression were more likely to develop heart disease than those who did not. As shown in Figure 2.1, high levels of stress increase risk for disease.

Cancer: The risk of cancer increases with high levels of distress, according to research. In fact, in 2,000 middle-aged men, the risk of death from cancer doubled for those with high levels of stress and depression. Cancer is a disease that affects the immune response, and a weakened immune system (from long-term distress) is more susceptible to the risk of cancer.

Viruses and Infections: Can you think of a stressful time that resulted in a sickness, illness, or infection? This is a common outcome of highly stressful events, especially negative stressful events. There is evidence that cold, flu, and other infections are four times more common following stressful life events. Other studies have shown that individuals who reported higher levels of stress also reported higher amounts of cold and flu-like symptoms. Many difficult life events can be a source of distress, including the loss of a family member, separation, or divorce. Marital disruption is a powerful predictor of stress-related physical illness, leading to greater numbers of illnesses and physician visits among individuals who got separated than those who remain married. For college students, the final exam period is highly stressful, and is also a likely time for a virus or infection. Students must make sure to take steps to reduce the level of stress during this time.

Mortality: Mortality can be both a direct and indirect effect of high levels of unmanaged stress. A study of 95,647 widows found more than double the normal mortality rate during the first week following

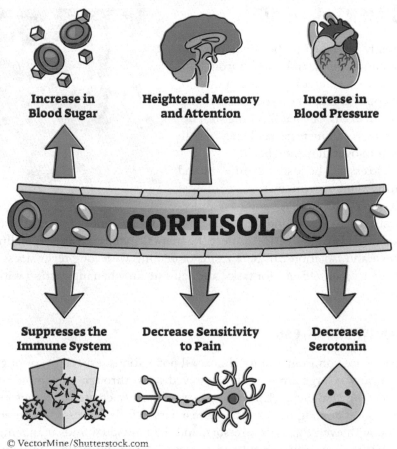

Increase in Blood Sugar

Heightened Memory and Attention

Increase in Blood Pressure

CORTISOL

Suppresses the Immune System

Decrease Sensitivity to Pain

Decrease Serotonin

© VectorMine/Shutterstock.com

Figure 2.1 The Effect of Stress and Increased Cortisol on Disease Risk

widowhood, primarily from cardiovascular disease, violent causes, and suicide. Another study showed the risk of dying from heart disease was four times greater in men who were isolated and reported high stress levels. Other studies have linked the lack of social health with an overall increase in mortality or death. Learning effective stress-management strategies can improve the quality of life and reduce mortality in all age groups.

Did you know . . .

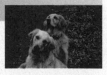

Courtesy of Shelley Hamill

Stress and the Immune System

- The immune system triggers chemicals to suppress the immune response increasing the susceptibility to illness.
- The immune system struggles to heal even minor issues during high levels of stress.
- The immune system can eventually become unable to fight toxins and pathogens, increasing infections.
- Over time, the risk of major disease increases owing to a suppressed immune function.

STRESS AND MENTAL HEALTH

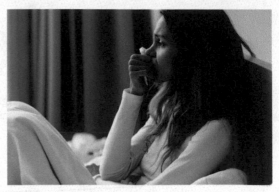

Mental health is greatly impacted by both eustress and distress. Eustress can improve mental health through increase in self-confidence, self-efficacy, and self-esteem. Think of how good you will feel when you accomplish a stressful task, such as an exam, or even finishing your degree. This type of eustress can increase resiliency and allow for improvements in overall mental health.

© fizkes/Shutterstock.com

    The impact of distress can be just as significant and potentially devastating. There are many types of mental health disorders; they range in severity and have different relationships to stress. Even if an individual does not have a diagnosed mental health disorder, high levels of unmanaged distress can negatively affect the mental state. Increases in feelings of anxiety, depression, nervousness, and isolation can be a result of dealing with long-term stress. Individuals may have lower self-confidence, self-efficacy for tasks, and self-esteem when interacting with others and completing daily tasks.

Depression, Anxiety, and Stress

Depression and anxiety are common among almost all populations, especially among college-aged students. Students often carry a large amount of unresolved stress through new-found responsibilities, expectations, and scheduling challenges. Unmanaged stress quickly creates a vicious cycle with anxiety, depression, or both as shown in Figure 2.2. The more a person feels depressed or anxious, the less likely that person is to cope with even the daily stressors, and the individual finds managing a big distress almost impossible, creating even more stress and anxiety. More information on depression is covered within the chapter on Psychological Health.

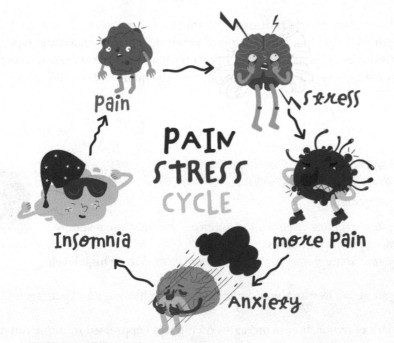

© Double Brain/Shutterstock.com

Figure 2.2 The Pain Stress Cycle Can Create a Variety of Health Problems

Suicidal Behavior and Stress

Stress is a big influence in suicidal thoughts and attempts. Each year, one in 10,000 college students commits suicide. Almost 12% of college students report thinking of suicide during their first four years in college, with 2.6% reporting persistent suicidal thoughts. More information on suicide is covered within the chapter on Psychological Health.

Disordered Eating and Stress

It is important to recognize that stress is related to the high prevalence of disordered eating in almost all populations. **Eating disorders** are characterized by unhealthy eating patterns that lead to diagnosable conditions that are life-threatening. However, individuals do not have to have a diagnosed eating disorder to have disordered eating habits. **Disordered eating** occurs when individuals use eating habits to cope with the stress they are feeling, leading to extreme levels of caloric restriction or caloric consumption. High levels of unmanaged stress can push individuals to unhealthy eating, especially if self-confidence and self-esteem have already been compromised. Individuals may choose to eat to cope

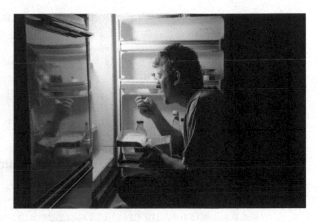

© Double Brain/Shutterstock.com

with stress, which leads to additional health problems. This is an example of unhealthy or disordered eating. More information on this is covered within the chapter on Psychological Health.

STRESS-COPING STRATEGIES

Once you recognize the type, source, and manifestation of stress in your life, you can begin to target the right strategy to address its impact. Understanding how stress is affecting you will allow you to cope with and manage the stress more effectively. Uncontrolled or unmanaged stress can lead to negative health consequences. There are many ways to cope with and manage stress. Stress coping is specific to individuals and to the type and source of stress. A stress-coping strategy that works for you may not work for someone else.

Here are a few strategies to help cope with and manage the different stressors in your life.

1. *Identify the Stressor:* Be honest with yourself and clearly identify what is causing the stress. Is the cause of stress environmental, physiological, or psychological? It is possible that the totality of the stress is multiple sources, which is common. Trying to pinpoint the greatest sources of your stress is the key to implementing a successful coping strategy.

2. *Determine How the Stress Affects You:* How does this stress affect your life? Does it surface through your emotions, behaviors, mental state, or physical appearance? Make a stress journal of when you notice these symptoms begin and their level of severity.

3. *Identify an Immediate Coping Strategy:* Not all stress-coping strategies work the same way. Some strategies provide an immediate method to cope in a healthy way. For example, one immediate way to cope when you feel stress mounting is to take deep breaths and keep the moment in perspective. Are you able to remove yourself from the situation? Or is it something you can accept in the moment? Having an immediate strategy for stress can allow you to gather your thoughts and consider more long-term coping methods. Other immediate strategies include pausing before reacting, grounding to what is priority, and taking a break!

Spotlight on . . .

Pets and Stress

Research shows that, unless you are someone who really dislikes animals or too busy to care for one properly, pets can provide excellent social support, stress relief, and other health benefits—perhaps more than people! The following are some health benefits pets can provide:

- Pets can improve your mood. Think how happy they are to see you and how playful they can be!

- Pets control blood pressure better than drugs. In a study on pets and blood pressure, groups of hypertensive New York stockbrokers who got dogs or cats were found to have lower blood pressure and heart rates than those who did not get pets.

- Pets encourage you to exercise. They need to be walked and played with, right?

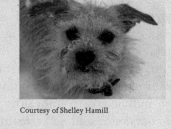

- Pets stave off loneliness and provide unconditional love. Pets can be there for you in ways that people cannot. They can offer love and companionship and can also enjoy comfortable silences and keep secrets and are excellent snugglers (Scott, 2015).

Courtesy of Shelley Hamill

4. *Identify a Short-term Strategy for Coping:* A short-term strategy will give you a strategy to manage the stressor or situation that is causing concern. An example of a short-term strategy is to plan and organize your priorities, schedule, and space. Having an organizational structure to your environment can help you tackle the stressors more effectively. For example, if an assignment is due, but you cannot find the charger for your laptop, then the stressor is not addressed and a new one is presented. Stay organized and plan your time wisely. Other short-term strategies include creating a comfort zone environment, taking a walk or nap break, and making healthy food and activity choices. For example, dealing with a stressor can be more acceptable when you feel good about yourself through healthy diet and physical activity.

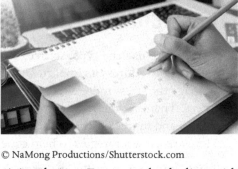

© NaMong Productions/Shutterstock.com

5. *Identify a Long-term Strategy for Coping:* Long-term strategies for stress coping are life-altering behaviors that allow you to maintain a homeostasis amid the stress and stressors. Examples of long-term strategies include nurturing your mind and body through self-care, resisting unhealthy and risky behavior, and developing and nourishing connections with others through healthy relationships. Other long-term strategies include practicing mindfulness, awareness, and sensitivity to others. **Mindfulness** refers to when we are aware of where our energy and thoughts are directed.

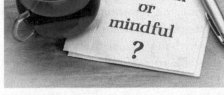

© marekuliasz/Shutterstock.com

6. *Seek Help When Necessary:* Sometimes, the stress in our lives is beyond our current coping strategies. That is okay, and it happens to all of us. In these moments, do not hesitate to seek social and emotional support systems—individuals who care, love, and will listen to you. Express feelings constructively. If you need professional help, reach out to someone. If you are a student, find the student support services on campus that can direct you to professional help. Often, this is free service to students. Many faculty know how to access this resource, so reach out to the one you trust.

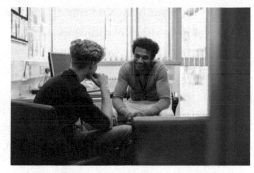

© Monkey Business Images/Shutterstock.com

Positive Self-talk: The constant interpretation of daily situations can affect the type of self-talk that an individual relies on. Positive self-talk is an effective strategy to keep the stress in perspective. Positive self-talk includes using positive statements like, "I can do this," or "I will continue to work hard." Negative self-talk, such as "I am going to fail my test" or "there is no way I can complete this task on time," can negatively affect the outcome of the situation. Thinking positively is a habit, and it has been shown to improve health outcomes. Work to improve your self-talk every day!

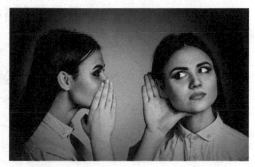

© pathdoc/Shutterstock.com

How Do You Manage Stress?

Some common stress-management strategies that are effective and efficient! These are categorized as immediate, short-term, and long-term, but they can be used anytime and anywhere!

Immediate Strategies

- Recognize and anticipate stress and symptoms of stress.
- Monitor and regulate emotional response from stress.
- Control immediate physical and behavioral response from stress.
- Be aware of your limitations to the stress (what you can and cannot do).
- Take a deep breath and find the positive in the situation.
- Practice positive self-talk.

Short-Term Strategies

- Prioritize time and energy to what is most important.
- Engage in regular physical activity, healthy diet, and sleep practices.
- Recognize warning signs and symptoms of chronic stress.
- Plan for time to reflect, relax, and recharge.
- Participate in activities that are fun and engaging.
- Practice positive self-talk.

Long-Term Strategies

- Strengthen belief in your control over the events that shape your life.
- Practice positive self-talk.

- Nurture your body and mind with healthy behaviors.
- Develop healthy relationships.
- Enjoy life as much as possible.
- Learn from mistakes, and give yourself grace when you fall short.

Take a few moments to think about how you manage stress. How many coping strategies on this chart (Figure 2.3) relate to you? Are there some that you did not consider to be a coping strategy? Circle the strategies you use on a regular basis. Then, think about which stress that strategy helps you to manage.

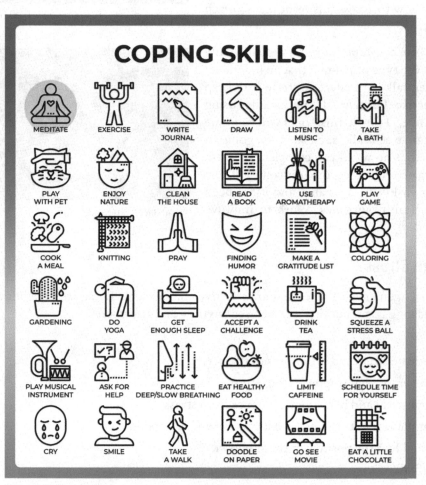

© Becris/Shutterstock.com

Figure 2.3 There Are Many Healthy and Effective Ways to Cope and Mange Stress

Spotlight on . . .

Academic Success

It is understandable that academic pressures of college can be a substantial source of different stressors for college students. Class times, professors, assignments, exams, and grades can be a challenge in achieving academic success. When these stressors are coupled with the many other demands and expectations of college life, many students can feel overwhelmed. When you feel this way, it is important to remember the priority of why you are here, which is to graduate! Putting your priorities in perspective is critical for stress management and, ultimately, success in college and throughout life. Your university has several resources available for you to manage stress, from counseling and meditation sessions to exercise classes and theatrical productions. The best and most efficient means of coping with stress is an individual task for each person. What works well for your friends may not work well for you! Check the information at the end of this chapter for more on resources.

STRESS AND SLEEP

Sleep quality relates strongly to overall health and well-being. Healthy sleep habits can boost your immune system, strengthen the heart, increase cognitive function, improve memory, and control weight. In addition, sleep is critical for the active population to recover, serving to repair muscle damage and to reduce soreness from exercise and training. For adolescents and young adults, sleep allows for healthy development of body and brain, assisting with learning and memory. Benefits of sleep are shown in Figure 2.4.

While the benefits of sleep are clear, a lack of sleep can cause complex issues. Problems can arise with lack of sleep for activities such as completing a task, concentrating, making decisions, working with and getting along with other people, and unsafe actions. Those who sleep less than 6 hours per night are at increased risk of injuries, accidents, and early death. Sleep deprivation is linked to approximately 100,000

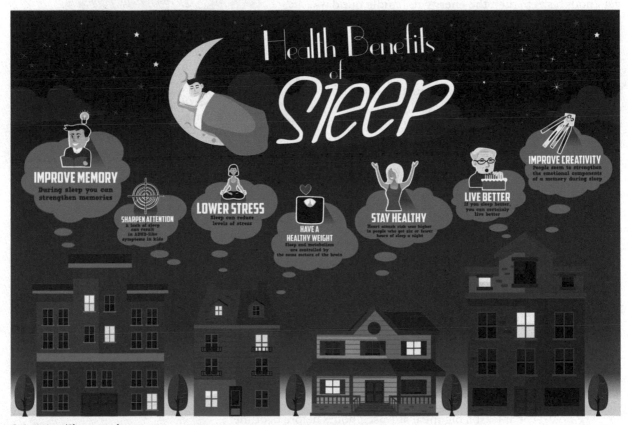

© Artisticco/Shutterstock.com

Figure 2.4 There Are Many Health Benefits to Healthy Sleep Patterns

vehicle crashes and 1,500 deaths each year. Stress levels can affect sleep patterns, and many individuals suffer from insomnia. **Insomnia** is the inability to have a regular sleep practice and can lead to many negative health outcomes, such as increased risk of depression, obesity, and heart disease. Some symptoms of insomnia include

- inability to fall or stay asleep
- disturbed and ineffective sleep
- irritability, inability to concentrate, and extreme daytime sleepiness

What Happens During Sleep?

Healthy sleep consists of four or five cycles of non-rapid eye movement (NREM) sleep and rapid eye movement (REM) sleep. The entire cycle of NREM and REM sleep takes about 90 minutes. The average adult sleeps about 7.5 hours, completing four to five full cycles, with 25% of that in REM. NREM refers to restful sleep, in which brain activity, heart rate, respiration, blood pressure, and metabolism (vital signs) slow down and the body temperature falls. Slow wave sleep usually terminates with the sleeper's changing position. The brain waves now reverse their course as the sleeper heads for the active REM stage.

The Connection of Sleep and Stress

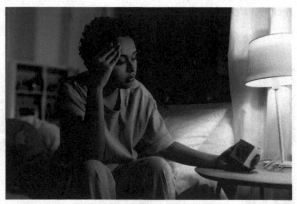

Sleep and stress level are closely related. If we do not get enough sleep, then the energy to handle our day-to-day stressors can become overwhelming. Conversely, when stress levels rise for many people, sleep quantity and quality are often adversely affected. Many Americans suffer from some kind of sleep problem, and the college-aged population is no different. The American College Health Association's (ACHA) research on college students' health showed that less than 12% of college students reported feeling well rested from their sleep patterns. Most (60%)

© Syda Productions/Shutterstock.com

reported that they feel sleepy, tired, or dragged out (ACHA, 2012). Other studies have shown that most college students who average between 6 and 6.9 hours of sleep per night feel sad, tired, and stressed.

Recommendations for Sleep

The National Sleep Foundation (NSF) recommends that college students aim for 7 to 8 hours of sleep each night (NSF, 2015). The NSF has published several guidelines for better sleep.

- Maintain a regular sleep schedule, including weekends and breaks from school or job.
- Establish a regular bedtime routine that generally starts at the same time each evening.
- Create an environment that is dark, quiet, comfortable, and cool.
- Try to remove other jobs from the bedroom. It is best to take work materials, computers, and televisions out of the sleeping environment.
- Try not to eat at least a big meal at least 2 hours before bedtime.
- Avoid alcohol, nicotine, and caffeine several hours before bedtime as they can disrupt sleep patterns.

STRESS AND YOU
Are You a Healthy Consumer?

Now that you know how stress can impact certain areas of your health, let us consider how it can impact another specific area: consumerism. How does stress affect your consumer behaviors? Research has identified four basic ways in which stress can influence consumer behaviors, according to Durante and Laran (2016).

1. Stress can lead to beneficial or impulsive consumer behaviors.
2. Stress can lead to increased spending on items we deem to be necessary.
3. Stress can lead to increased saving if we perceive low income could be possible.
4. Ultimately, stress pushes us to allocate our resources so that we feel we are in control.

We have identified many things in this chapter about stress, causes of stress, and impact of stress. If stress pushes you to be a healthy consumer, then you intake healthy consumption of coping strategies: healthy foods, healthy activities, tools to relieve stress in a positive way. Impulsive behavior under stress might push you to consume more negative coping strategies and increase long-term stress. Tobacco, unhealthy food, risky behaviors, or just relying on a quick gratification of material things can be impulsive consumer behavior. Thinking about how stress affects your consumer behaviors and answer the following questions:

Do you believe stress influences your consumer behavior? Does your response to stress create a positive, healthy, nurturing environment? Would you consider your response to stress as one that elicits impulsiveness and one that enables a more stressful, negative environment?

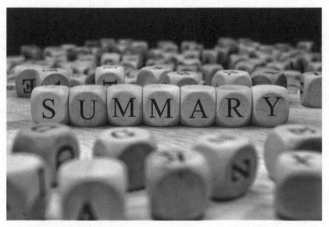

© Fabrik Bilder/Shutterstock.com

In this chapter, we have defined stress, identified stressors, and categorized stress as both positive and negative. We have compared the effects of both short-term and long-term stress and how they affect an individual's overall health. It is also critical to understand how coping strategies influence health. Unhealthy coping strategies essentially "double" the negative impact of stress because they add additional health concerns to your body. Identifying unhealthy coping strategies and working to change your behavior can better reduce stress, create a positive environment, and improve your overall health. Working to produce healthy stress-coping strategies is a critical step in managing stress and its impact on health. Finding immediate, short-term, and long-term strategies for stress coping is important for a healthy living. When the body is fully rested with quality sleep, the ability to cope with and handle stress is improved and the negative effects of stress are reduced.

PERSONAL REFLECTIONS . . . SO, WHAT HAVE YOU LEARNED?

1. Based on the questions from the beginning of this chapter, do you have a high stress level? What are your main sources of stress, and how much of your stress is eustress or distress?

2. What are three ways stress negatively affects your life or your health? What are three ways stress positively affects your life or your health?

3. What are three healthy coping strategies that you turn to in times of stress? What is at least one unhealthy coping strategy that you use to deal with stress? How can you change the negative strategy into a positive one?

4. How are sleep and stress related? How does the body use sleep to cope with stress? Does your sleep environment allow for restful, restorative sleep? What steps could you take to improve your sleep patterns?

5. How can stress impact consumerism? How can you turn any negative impulsive behavior into positive, healthy consumerism?

NOTES

RESOURCES ON CAMPUS FOR YOU!

Academic Services

- One-on-one consultations
- Interim grade consultations
- Individual and group study spaces
- Referrals to other university support services
- Personal assistance with academic questions or concerns
- Individual and group tutoring opportunities
- Academic skill development—time management, study skills, organization, etc.
- Development of academic action plans and success contracts
- Specialized services for students on academic probation and students with incompletes

Workshops/Seminars

Academic success workshops are offered on many college campuses. These sessions can be facilitated for classes, residence halls, organizations, or other events. Workshop topics include the following:

- Notemaking
- Study strategies
- Time and stress management
- Test taking
- Textbook reading
- Tutee seminars

Tutoring

Peer tutors are available at all colleges and universities through academic support. Student tutors are hired each semester to assist students in developing the skills to become independent learners. Check your university's academic service centers for more information.

REFERENCES

American College Health Association. (2012). *American College Health Association–National College Health Assessment II: Reference Group Data Report Fall 2011*. Author.

Dhabhar, F. S., Malarkey, W. B., Neri, E., & McEwen, B. S. (2012). Stress-induced redistribution of immune cells—from barracks to boulevards to battlefields: A tale of three hormones. *Psychoneuroendocrinology, 37*(9), 1345–1368.

Donatelle, R. J. (2014). *Access to health* (12th ed.). Benjamin Cummings.

Durante, K. M., & Laran, J. (2016). The effect of stress on consumer saving and spending. *Journal of Marketing Research, 53*(5), 814–828.

National Sleep Foundation. (2015). https://sleepfoundation.org/

Scott, E. (2015). How owning a dog or cat can reduce stress. http://stress.about.com/od/lowstresslifestyle/a/petsandstress.htm

Stauble, M. R., Thompson, L. A., & Morgan, G. (2013). Increases in cortisol are positively associated with gains in encoding and maintenance working memory performance in young men. *Stress, 16*(4), 402–410.

St. Lifer, H. (2013). 7 reasons (a little) stress can be good for you. http://www.goodhousekeeping.com/health/wellness/advice/a18528/stress/

von Dawans, B., Fischbacher, U., Kirschbaum, C., Fehr, E., & Heinrichs, M. (2012). The social dimension of stress reactivity: Acute stress increases prosocial behavior in humans. *Psychological Science, 23*(6), 651–660.

Chapter 3
Psychological Health +

OBJECTIVES

- Identify and define the different dimensions of psychological health, including mental, emotional, intellectual, and spiritual health.

- Describe the characteristics of those who are healthy within the mental, emotional, intellectual, and spiritual dimension.

- Explain how self-esteem, self-efficacy, and resilience can affect several dimensions of psychological health.

- Define emotional intelligence, and discuss how it relates to overall health.

- Differentiate between religion and spirituality, and describe how they can impact people differently.

- Identify several mental health disorders and their impact on life.

- Differentiate between depression, anxiety, panic attacks, and obsessive-compulsive disorder (OCD).

- Describe the services, options, and resources available to address mental health concerns.

"Are you Psychologically Healthy?   1 = Never   2 = Sometimes   3 = Always

	1	2	3
1. I sleep too much or too little, or I wake up constantly.	1	2	3
2. My mood swings from depression to happiness for no reason.	1	2	3
3. I eat more than I should.	1	2	3
4. I enjoy time playing video games more than I enjoy anything else.	1	2	3
5. People sometimes think that I am unstable or unreliable.	1	2	3
6. I have poor self-esteem.	1	2	3
7. I feel that I do not play any useful part in life.	1	2	3
8. I have thought about ending my life.	1	2	3
9. I am overwhelmed by thoughts I cannot seem to control.	1	2	3
10. I have disturbing dreams or recollections about my past.	1	2	3
11. I hate the way I look.	1	2	3
12. I cry or get very angry at times.	1	2	3
13. My feelings are interfering with work, school, and friendships.	1	2	3
14. I feel unhappy, sad, or worthless.	1	2	3
15. I feel out of control.	1	2	3
16. I feel empty or that my life has little meaning.	1	2	3
17. I find it difficult to cope with things.	1	2	3
18. I avoid making new friends.	1	2	3
19. I have trouble concentrating at work or school.	1	2	3

Sum your answers for a score. Scores range between 19–57, with high scores indicating higher levels of stress. Self-reflect on your score."

Critical Thinking . . .

How does your psychological health impact your overall health?

What are the different components of psychological health and how strong are you in each?

How do your behaviors impact your psychological health and overall well-being?

Introduction to Psychological Health

Psychological health is the day-to-day combination of our feelings, thoughts, and relationships as they exist in our lives and includes the mental, emotional, social, intellectual, and spiritual dimensions of health.

MENTAL HEALTH

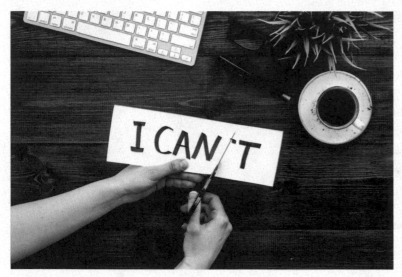

© 9dream studio/Shutterstock.com

Mental health refers to the general thoughts and feelings that you have on a day-to-day basis, specifically with regard to your overall well-being. Mental health includes components like self-confidence, self-esteem, self-efficacy, and resilience. Through a clear understanding of these terms, we can have meaningful discussions and experiences.

You have probably heard of self-confidence, self-esteem, and self-efficacy. Sometimes they are used interchangeably, but they do have different meanings. **Self-confidence** is the confidence or trust that you have in your abilities, qualities, or judgments. It influences your decision-making and how far outside of your comfort zone you will go when to you try new things. **Self-esteem** refers to your overall opinion of yourself, and it affects your level of acceptance of your abilities and limitations. **Self-efficacy** refers to the ability to complete a goal, task, or event. Self-efficacy is the determining factor for the success of a specific thing. For example, what is your self-efficacy to run a marathon today? How would your self-efficacy change after you have completed 6 weeks of marathon training? Right! It would increase! While all three of these terms are related and important to mental health, self-efficacy might be the most impactful, yet overlooked. Self-efficacy for each goal or responsibility is influenced by the setting and resources to complete the job. If you are intentional about how you address a goal, then you can increase the probability of success in achieving the goal.

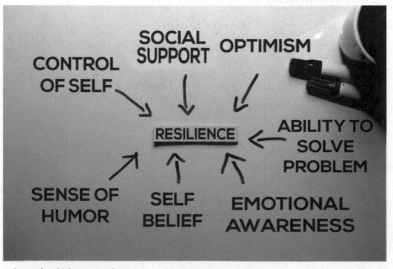

© bangoland/Shutterstock.com

When you experience bouts of success, it increases your self-efficacy for a new goal, which can significantly influence your self-esteem, self-confidence, and resilience, another popular term that is used quite often in the context of mental health. **Resilience** is the ability to recover quickly from difficulties and tough times.

Everyone faces times of loss, confusion, or frustration. Those who are resilient are able to bounce back from those difficult times. There are several factors that affect a person's resilience, including the previously mentioned terms of self-efficacy and self-confidence, as well as social support, emotional awareness, and optimism, which will be discussed later in this chapter.

When have you showed resilience? Have you experienced a very difficult period of emotions that you were able to overcome? Take a moment to reflect on a time that was challenging for you, but you were able to surmount the difficulties and push forward. What helped with your resilience? How were you able to "bounce back"? This is an optimal time to journal your experience with resilience. Once you see how you were able to be resilient in a difficult situation, you can apply self-efficacy to difficult times in the present or future. Focusing on nurturing your self-confidence, self-esteem, and self-efficacy can greatly influence your overall resilience. The next section on emotional health will provide details on steps that you can use to increase your feelings of self and, in essence, your resilience.

Spotlight on . . .

Body Image

Body image is how someone sees themselves in their mind. Although, a person's body may be healthy, their minds are full of negative thoughts about their body. Body image is psychological and is a person's opinion about himself or herself, which can be influenced by past experiences, other people, and the media. People compare themselves with others, which results in a negative body image. It is vital to have a good outlook and attitude about yourself. Everyone's body is different. Love and accept yourself for who you are.

Simple Steps to Increase Mental Health

There are ways to increase resilience, self-esteem, self-efficacy, and self-confidence. Here are a few practical ways to increase resilience in your thought processes of daily life.

1. **Be aware of your thoughts.** Focus on positivity, rejecting negative thoughts as they enter your mind. Train yourself to identify negativity and recognize the impact that it has on your overall thoughts and ideals. Do not let negative thoughts derail your energy.

2. **Focus to reframe the situation.** Step back and think about the situation and reframe your thoughts. Keep your perspective focused on the facts, and do not an over-analyze what you are unsure of or still do not know. Focus on keeping the positive in perspective.

3. **Learn from previous mistakes.** Use the knowledge you have gained in previous experiences to drive your future responses and behaviors. Mistakes and failures are an opportunity to try to regroup, refocus, and retry.

4. **Set short, achievable goals.** Each time you reach a goal that you have set (short or long; big or small), your self-confidence and self-efficacy will increase! You will feel better about yourself and begin to trust yourself in goal-setting situations. Just ask yourself, what is the next best step?

5. **Choose how you respond.** The best advice is to remember that you are in charge of how you respond and how you allow situations to affect you. This may seem difficult, but you can control how you think, feel, and behave. Think ahead to how your response may impact your future, and focus on behaviors with positive outcomes.

MENTAL HEALTH

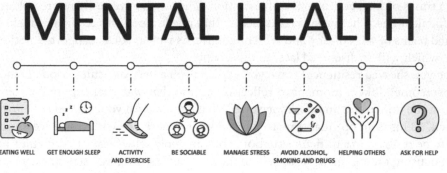

EATING WELL   GET ENOUGH SLEEP   ACTIVITY AND EXERCISE   BE SOCIABLE   MANAGE STRESS   AVOID ALCOHOL, SMOKING AND DRUGS   HELPING OTHERS   ASK FOR HELP

© limeart/Shutterstock.com

Figure 3.1 There Are Many Components that Balance Mental Health

Mental Health on Overall Wellness

Mental health is certainly a commonly discussed topic, and there is much attention on the overall concept of mental health. Those who are mentally healthy show strength and resilience within the dimension that supports overall health and well-being. Strong mental health provides a foundation for the other components of psychological health, such as the emotional, social, intellectual, and spiritual. Those who show strength in mental health are able to use healthy and sustainable strategies to cope with stress, increasing their resilience in difficult times. Mental health can impact the other dimensions of holistic health including physical, environmental, and occupational. Increasing the awareness of mental health should be a priority focus for everyone. As seen in Figure 3.1, many components lead to a balanced mental health status.

EMOTIONAL HEALTH

Emotions are the feelings we have about things that happen in our life. They alert us to the things that are most important, even if we did not always think so. The ability to read, nurture, and work with your emotions will provide a foundation of strength for your emotional health. Emotional health is critical, as it allows you to experience feelings and express empathy and sensibility. **Feelings** are defined as a response or reaction to your emotions. **Empathy** is the ability to understand and share the feelings of others. **Sensibility** refers to our responsiveness toward other things or persons, such as the feelings of another person or changes in the environment.

Happiness and Joy

How can you tell when you are happy? How do others see that you are happy? Is your grin bigger or your presence lighter? Do your family and friends think you are a happy person?

Happiness and joy are feelings derived from the same thought. Sometimes, they are used interchangeably, but happiness and joy are different levels of the same emotion. **Joy** can explain the excitement you feel when you are finally offered a job you have desired. **Happiness** explains the emotion that you feel when you are in a career you love. Think of joy as more of a dynamic, excitable moment, while happiness is a stable state of positivity and contentedness.

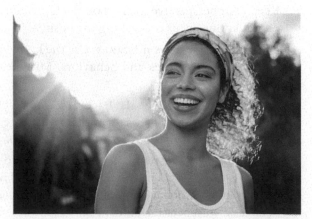

© Rido/Shutterstock.com

There are different ways to add joy and happiness into your everyday life. It could be spending time with your family and friends, participating in hobbies and adventures, listening to your favorite music, or loving what you do at work. Finding activities that make you feel joy and happiness makes life better.

Emotional Intelligence

Emotional intelligence is the ability to perceive, understand, manage, and handle your emotions, and use the information to guide their thoughts, decisions, and actions (Mayer & Salovey, 1993; Salovey & Mayer, 1990). Individuals who have high emotional intelligence are able to manage their emotions through a recognition of their own feelings as well as those of others, and use the emotional information to guide subsequent thoughts and behavior. They can also identify the different types of feelings and emotions they are feeling, and have an understanding of how those feelings affect them. For example, a student with high emotional intelligence understands

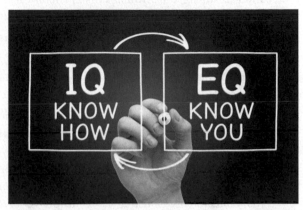

© Ivelin Radkov/Shutterstock.com

how an upcoming exam might make he/she feel more anxious and edgy. The student may refrain from situations where they would need to make major decisions or confront issues due to their level of anxiety about the upcoming exam. This recognition can reduce unpleasant encounters with others, since they are able to identify their emotions and focus on the management of their emotions for the upcoming exam. Someone that may lack emotional intelligence may not be as aware of their feelings or the source, therefore increasing the chance of thoughts and behaviors that may not be truly reflective of a situation. If you are interested in learning more about emotional intelligence, you should consider reading the best-seller by scientist and journalist Daniel Goleman, *Emotional Intelligence* (Goleman, 1995). Goleman expands on emotional intelligence as the array of skills and characteristics that drive leadership performance.

Steps to Increase Emotional Intelligence

Emotional intelligence is comprised of four aspects on which individuals should focus:

1. **Awareness of emotions:** This is the fundamental ability to recognize feelings and emotions, through the following:

   - Awareness of emotional clues in yourself and in people around you.
   - Ability to discern between different types of emotion.
   - Identify the level of intensity to which the emotion is present.
   - Determination of what these emotional clues mean.

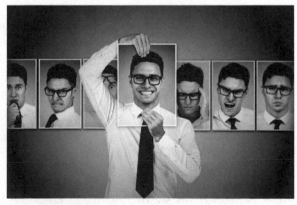

© FGC/Shutterstock.com

   People with this ability are better pilots of their lives because they have a sense of how they really feel about their personal decisions, from whom to marry to what job to take. They recognize the emotions of others and as a result have healthier and stronger relationships.

2. **Using or generating emotions:** This is the ability to know which emotions are best for different situations. People with this ability employ their feelings to enhance their thinking and endeavors. They realize that emotions, when rightly used, can help them solve problems, make better decisions, reason out situations, and be more creative. They will be more self-motivated and will prioritize their thinking process based on emotional input.

3. **Understanding emotions.** This is the ability to recognize and grasp emotional information, and it includes emotional comprehension and analysis.

   • **Emotional comprehension** is how emotions combine to form another emotion, progress or intensify, or transition from one emotion to another.

   • **Emotional analysis** is the ability to understand possible causes of emotions and predict what kind of emotions people will have in different situations.

   People with this ability have a solid grasp of emotional intelligence. They will tend to be more accurate in their interpretation of moods and emotional situations, and as a result will be more likely to deal correctly with such situations.

4. **Managing emotions:** This is the ability to regulate emotions in yourself and in other people. This involves monitoring and distinguishing differences and accurately labeling emotions as they happen. This concept uses strategies to improve or modify feelings and moods, without the denial or suppression of raw emotion. People with this ability are able to assess the effectiveness of how they recognize and handle emotions in various situations.

Emotional Health on Overall Wellness

It is critical that emotions are not confused with weakness, as this can lead to confusion, judgment, and emotional suppression. Emotional intelligence and emotional strengths are more difficult to nurture than mental intelligence or physical strength. However, emotions are the gateway to the overall life experience. Take time to nurture and grow your emotional intelligence. Listen to others through their emotions, and use your emotional strengths as a bridge to self-esteem and healthy relationships. Those with strengths in emotional wellness are able to cope with stress in healthy and sustainable ways, use resilience to bounce back from difficult situations, and build healthy relationships with others.

SOCIAL HEALTH

Social health includes the state of our relationships with other people, including our family, friends, and neighbors. Additionally, social health includes how much we are involved with our community, both large and small. Engagement with others extends outside of our comfort areas, reaching into how we interact with strangers or individuals we just meet. Social health also includes an individual's virtual and online presence in social media and technology platforms. It is safe to say that positive social health continues to evolve, as we become more accepting and tolerant of others' beliefs and social norms.

Support From Family and Friends

When talking about what makes up social health, we need to include all of the interactions and relationships we have made during our lives. The most important social connections start with families, who provide love, care, patience, and support. Our families can be those that are related to us by blood or through choice and know us better than anyone else. They have seen us grow up and know our personalities. They know when we are down, when we are happy, what makes our angry, and how to deal with these emotions without judgment. Family is capable of unconditional love no matter the circumstances.

Who are those you would consider "family"? Think of those that are closest to you who know you the best. Is your family big or small? This support from family can really help mold and shape us into the person we are, through their influence and our own experiences. Family can bring attention to the areas of character where we do well and not so well. Who are the individuals in your family that you feel influenced who you are today? How have they helped you develop in certain areas?

Introvert Versus Extrovert . . . and the Impact on Health

An **introvert** is someone who mentally "turns in," especially in certain environments. Introverts tend to shy away from large crowds or social interactions. They may also find energy in time spent alone or with one or two very close friends. An **extrovert** is someone who tends to find energy from interactions and time spent with others, often desiring to be around others.

Research has shown both positive and negative outcomes of both introversion and extroversion. Introverts tends to form stronger bonds, have better sleep outcomes, engage in less risky behaviors, and are not stressed by the "fear of missing out" on something. However, introverts may also be less happy, have a slower reaction time when driving, and hesitate to talk to their doctor about health concerns. Extroverts tend to report higher levels of happiness, have stronger immune systems, and are more proactive about health concerns with their physician. Some negative impacts of extroverts are higher levels of social-based stress, poorer sleep outcomes, and higher rates of risky behavior.

What can we do to bridge the gap between introverts and extroverts? While the college life tends to reward extroverts and their typical behavior, it is important to understand that both personalities can be acceptable and healthy. Introverts can try to better understand why they may feel awkward or uncomfortable in certain situations and incorporate strategies to effectively and healthily deal with their emotions. Extroverts can work to engage introverts in a respectful manner and learn to appreciate their comfort boundaries. Working together, we can understand, appreciate, and value the diversity of everyone!

The Power of Community

Think about your community, which consists of a group of people who interact with common interests within a larger society. Community starts with your immediate surroundings and then expands to take on various levels and spaces, and you probably are a member of multiple community groups. You may have a neighborhood community, a recreational community, and/or a church community. How would you rank your involvement and commitment to making your communities better? Each community is reliant upon the social engagement of its members. The individual members push the direction of their community toward its purpose, vision, and mission. Without intentional engagement, communities will not grow and thrive.

Most college campuses have clubs and organizations for student involvement and social interaction. Within the hierarchy of clubs and organizations, there are leadership opportunities, community service initiatives, and service learning projects for individuals to experience. These are especially valuable when you can feel a part of the group or team and relate to others with like-interests. The Social Determinant Theory states that

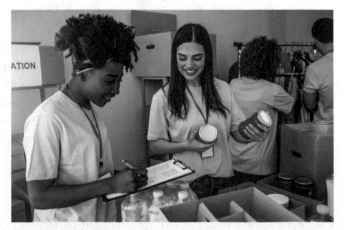

© Dragana Gordic/Shutterstock.com

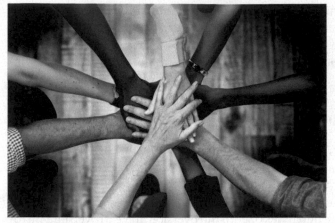
© Stefano Garau/Shutterstock.com

individuals are more likely to "buy in" to a group (community) if they feel a satisfactory level of autonomy, relatedness, and competence. **Autonomy** refers to a level of input that is valued in the group. Do your communities provide you with an opportunity to voice your thoughts or make a decision? Voting is an example of having autonomy in a community. **Relatedness** is the level of relation you have to the community. You are related to a neighborhood because you live there! You can choose to be a part of a community because you feel strongly about its mission, like a club or organization. **Competence** refers to the level of confidence you have about being able to contribute to the community in a positive way. You can complete certain tasks, like social engagement or fundraising. This is why it is important to contribute to the communities where you belong, work, or enjoy.

Steps to Improve Your Social Health

It is possible to improve your social health and wellness, which plays a huge role in the way we experience the world. Brain health is heavily influenced by social connections, and there is support for a connection between health relationships and long, happy lives. These steps can assist you in forming deeper connections with others and the larger world.

1. **Surround yourself with strong, positive influences.** Create a strong foundation by surrounding yourself with the right people. Those who are positive and encouraging will have the best influence on your overall well-being. Fill your inner circle with those that truly care about you in a supportive way.

2. **Practice self-care**. This is critical for all levels of health and wellness. Take care of yourself physically and mentally so you are in the right mindset for social engagement. Take time to assess, work hard, have fun, and relax. Give yourself grace when it is needed, and rely on healthy coping strategies.

3. **Do things you like!** Engaging in hobbies and fun activities help to reduces stress and increase enjoyment. Find ways to enjoy your hobby, and when possible, include others to strengthen relationships.

4. **Take your health seriously**. Practice healthy sleep, nutrition, and exercise habits. Maintain a normal weight, drink less alcohol, and do not smoke. Research shows that those who follow all five of these habits can live 10 years longer than those who do not.

5. **Improve communication skills.** By nurturing your communication skills, you are improving a life-long skill. Active listening skills can help you become a more positive influence on those around you and improve your role as a leader, spouse, employee, parent, and friend.

Social Health on Overall Wellness

Social health is the foundation to healthy relationships, which we will cover in another chapter. Those who have strong social health have exhibit better overall wellness and life experiences. Small steps can build communication skills that develop positive and healthy lifestyles. Building strengths within the social dimension has numerous long-term benefits for your physical, mental, and emotional well-being. To ensure a holistic balance of health, social involvement is critical. Being involved on campus and within your community can engage your social strengths, build relationships, and influence your expectations of the world. There are many opportunities for service and volunteering, both within the your college community and the community at large.

INTELLECTUAL HEALTH

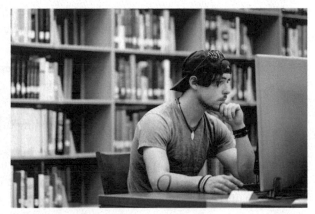

Intellectual refers to the dimension of "thinking" or "being rational." Those who are intellectually healthy are able to learn and apply new information. An intellectually healthy person can solve problems, adapt to surroundings, and develop effective strategies as they carry out responsibilities.

One key component of intellectual health is cognition. By definition, **cognition** refers to our processes of perception, learning, and reasoning and problem-solving.

© Winthrop University

- **Perception** refers to interpreting data that you sense (hear, see, smell, feel, taste, etc.).
- **Learning** refers to the process of taking the cues that you perceived and applying them to previous ones to store as memory.
- **Reasoning** and **problem-solving** refer to the ability to rationalize a plan to solve a problem.

Cognition is also a link between the intellectual and emotional dimensions of the brain and can often drive our behavior about a situation, or emotional intelligence. Cognition is the pathway in which emotional intelligence works. Here is where you can identify the emotions and use the information to inform the next set of thoughts and behaviors.

Intellectual Health and Learning

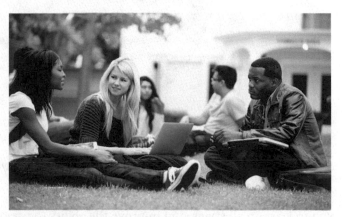

Intellectual capacity, or IQ, refers the ability to think, learn, plan, and execute with discipline. To figure out one's IQ, an individual is tested on how they respond to visual imagery and input, and how they use those skills to solve a problem. When people talk about how intellectual they are, they are talking in particular about their IQ. This is often mistaken with how smart they are, which leads to a society of snobbery and misconception. More recent studies have shown this to be too narrow a focus on the intellect. Howard Gardner (1983) has proposed the idea of multiple intelligences. To put it simply, it is important to understand the difference in the meanings of

© Monkey Business Images/Shutterstock.com

the words "intelligent" and "smart." Once you understand the meaning of learning and how to learn, your knowledge will grow. This will allow your mind to expand and to help others know the differences.

Learning Styles—Are They Real?

Individuals often believe that they have one **learning style** or way in which they can learn. There are four ways that information can be presented, thereby leading to the perceptions that learning best happens during one of the four teaching methods. The four methods, or learning styles, are visual, auditory, reading, and kinesthetic based (as seen in Figure 3.2). Research does not support that individuals only have one style or way of learning, but instead *prefer* to learn new information in the way that suits them best. In fact, most people learn through multiple styles and not just through one particular style.

- Visual learning is a learning style with a preference to imagery, like pictures, diagrams, and body languages. Individuals store what they see, and can remember the visual cues more than written or hearing cues.

- Auditory learning is a learning style with a preference to hearing cues and information. Auditory learners store information by the way it sounds, and have an easier time remembering spoken word than written.

- Reading learners show a preference to reading information. They comprehend and remember what they read, and they often enjoy writing.

- Kinesthetic/tactile learning is a learning style with a preference to touch and interactions. These learners enjoy the "hands-on" component of the information. They are able to refer to the experience for learning.

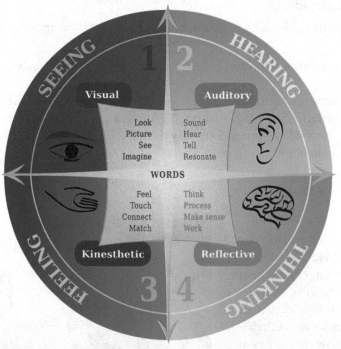

© artellia/Shutterstock.com

Figure 3.2 There Are Four General Ways in Which We Prefer to Learn

Which style do you believe suits you best? While we may prefer one particular style, it is possible for you to learn in all styles, and improve the ability to use other learning methods. In order to get the most out of your learning experience, it is suggested that you focus on your primary learning preference, but incorporate as many of the learning styles as possible in order to get a full learning experience.

Learning, Process, and Application Disciplines

There is discipline when it comes to learning. It is best experienced as an active process, meaning that the learning takes a shared interest in the interchange of information. The ability to identify the different areas of learning can help you assess where you are with each discipline. The three disciplines discussed in this section are categorized as learning, process, and application constructs of intellectual health. Think of these disciplines as your ability to accept, process, and apply new information.

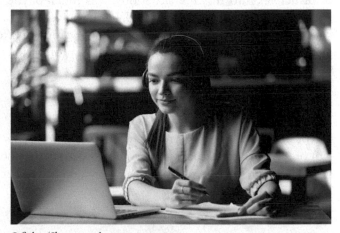

© fizkes/Shutterstock.com

The **learning discipline** refers to the intake of new information. It is your posture of considering new thoughts and ideas, and consists of curiosity, persistence, humility, and a willingness to learn. **Curiosity** is the desire to learn more about something. Curious people have an excitement for knowledge and truth. They will accept and consider new information, thoughts, and ideas. **Persistence** is the continual search for information. Those who are persistent keep on pursuing information despite obstacles, warnings, or setbacks. **Humility** refers to having a modest view of one's own importance. It does not mean that an individual is unimportant, but just one part of a bigger picture, ideal, or movement. Finally, a **willingness to learn** is a discipline that includes a teachable spirit. Those who are willing to learn are open to diverse views and forms of knowledge and information.

The process discipline refers to how you process the information that you receive. It is what you decide to do with the information after you are exposed to it and involves integrity, critical thinking, and patience. **Integrity** refers to the quality of being honest and upholding moral principles. In learning, it refers to a focus on the facts, and the absence of misinformation or twisting what is true. **Critical thinking** is the mental process of reaching an answer or conclusion through conceptualizing, analyzing, synthesizing, and evaluating information. It is an active process of using information, often using multiple steps, to get to a solution. Critical thinkers can consider multiple options, and then make a decision on the **best** option based on the available information. **Patience** is the ability to wait and pause on a final judgment until all facts and information are considered.

The application discipline refers to the process of applying information and knowledge in a practical way. It is the active outcome of the process discipline, and includes courage, systematic thinking, and advancement. **Courage** is the quality of spirit that enables a person to face the unknown or new ideas without fear of implications or repercussions. It is a strength in the face of adversity or persecution of

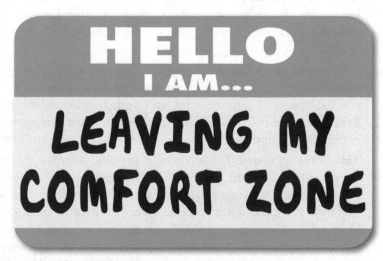

© iQoncept/Shutterstock.com

the truth and knowledge. **Systematic thinking** is the application of an organized set of concepts, ideas, or principles into real life situations. It is much of the "practical" to the term "practical application." New ideas can easily be formulated, but if they cannot be practically applied to real life, they may not be very useful. Advancement refers to the application of information to improve on what is already known or understood to be true. Advancement of information is critical to grow one's thoughts and ideas and to the application of a particular concept.

Steps to Improve Intellectual Health

Devoting time and energy to keep your mind healthy is just as important as improving physical health. Not only does intellectual wellness improve all of the above, but engaging in mentally stimulating activities may also reduce cognitive impairment and put you at a lower risk for dementia and Alzheimer's.

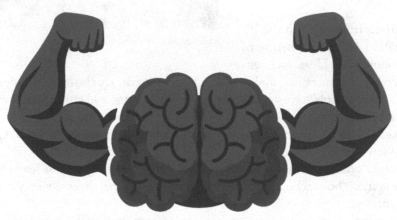

© vectorlab2D/Shutterstock.com

1. **Try Something New.** Research shows that the brain can continue growing and changing throughout one's lifespan. It is up to you to give your brain the chance to change and adapt through new experiences. Is there a new hobby you have been wanting to try? Do you want to learn a new language? These are examples of new experiences that your brain will love, and your intellectual health will grow.

2. **Read, Read, Read.** Read on topics that expand your mindset, your views, your experiences, and your knowledge. It can be on or about anything...fun, interesting, stimulating, or historical....just find something to read. Keeping the neural pathways active through reading influences overall brain health.

3. **Be Curious and Creative.** Curiosity increases brain activity, improves learning, and increases your overall learning and retention capabilities, too. Identify one thing that you wish you understood better and explore it! Creativity stimulates your intellectual wellness and improves your overall health. Research has shown that problem-solving, memory, processing speed, and cognition were enhanced in musicians compared to non-musicians. Get creative through hobbies, jobs, and new experiences!

4. **Take Care of Yourself.** You know, things like exercise, healthy diet, and sleep habits can influence your intellectual health. Research has shown that regular aerobic exercise can increase the size of the brain involved in memory and learning and support the growth of new connections in your brain. The food you eat can influence how your brain feels, from alert and ready to foggy and slow. Staying hydrated and consuming healthy fruits and vegetables can influence brain health, and these are discussed more in the nutrition chapter. Healthy sleep allows the brain to remove stored toxins and takes out the "mental trash," thus, improving its overall function.

5. **Be Social.** Studies have shown that people who socialize often have higher levels of happiness than those who do not have the same social time. Make an effort to grow and nurture your social strengths to increase your intellectual health and wellness.

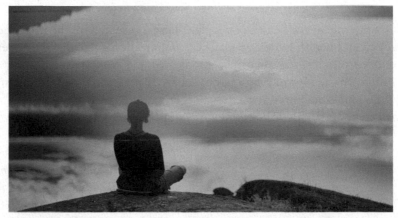

© sun ok/Shutterstock.com

6. **Practice Self-Reflection and Mindfulness. Self-reflection** is serious thought about one's character, actions, motives, life, behavior, and beliefs. Taking time to reflect can increase self-awareness and helps to reframe the perspective of life. Self-reflection can enable learning opportunities and improve self-confidence. Meditation, deep breathing, and mindfulness are steps that you can take during self-reflection. **Meditation** is a practice that allows you to calm your thoughts and achieve greater mental and emotional clarity. Deep breathing increases circulation by bringing oxygen to your muscles and brain.

Intellectual Health on Overall Wellness

Your brain controls your body and your overall health and well-being—it is time to commit to actively increasing intellectual wellness. Intellectual health is deeply connected to your mental, emotional, social, and spiritual health and wellness. Sustainable strategies for stress coping are critical for overall psychological health, including areas within the intellectual dimension.

SPIRITUAL HEALTH

People often confuse religion and spirituality, and even though they are connected, they are different concepts. **Spiritual health** refers to the state of harmony within yourself and with others, focusing on a balance of self needs and world demands (Edlin & Golanty, 2014).

    Religion is defined as a specific system of beliefs, practices, rituals, and symbols for a purpose (Marr & Wilcox, 2015). Religions have similarities, including specific beliefs and worship practices, and a sacred physical space of a church, temple, mosque, synagogue, monastery, or meeting house. The believers of a religion participate in religious ceremonies,

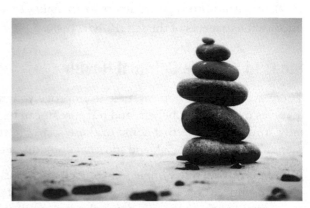

© Michal Bednarek/Shutterstock.com

listen to leaders, and refer to a written word in a book, tablet, or scroll that contains the written word of their God. Religions contain symbolism in practice of customs, readings, and prayers that provides comfort, faith, and support from the group who is practicing the religion's beliefs. Religion is found throughout history, and it is the reason for many wars and conflicts that the world has experienced and continues to reckon with.

Religion can play a big role in the health of people. There is research on the impact of religion, and its effect on daily behaviors and health beliefs. Today, it is important for people of different religions to respect each other and to learn to live together in harmony.

Spirituality is similar to the idea of religion, but is based on personal beliefs and inner balance. It includes the idea that individuals belong to something larger than themselves.

Realistically, one can be spiritual without following a specific religion.

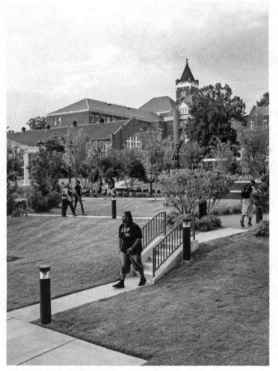

© Winthrop University

When we discuss spirituality, thoughts, and feelings, we all have some concept of what we feel connected to. Usually, many people say that their spiritual makeup occurs when they are within the natural world. Others may find comfort in being surrounded by people on a busy street, and the energy that exists there helps them feel connected and ready to face the day's challenges.[6]

Spirituality is a combination of three integral components: healthy relationships, personal values, and a meaningful purpose in life. Although we cover healthy relationships in much more detail in a different chapter, it is important to see how it relates to spiritual health. Healthy relationships help to foster our own inner wisdom and encourage treatment of respect, honesty, integrity, and love toward ourselves and toward others. Personal values, or principles we hold dear, help to guide our behavior in life situations. Distinguishing personal values is a type of individual spiritual journey, as they will define what we stand for and how we conduct our lives. Spiritually healthy people feel that it is their life goal to live out the purpose they were intended for. They are able to identify a meaningful purpose and work toward fulfilling that mission (Donatelle, 2014). **Spiritual intelligence** refers to an ability to access higher meanings, values, abiding purposes, and unconscious aspects of the self (Zohar, 1998).

Steps to Improve Spiritual Health

There are steps that you can take to improve your spiritual health and wellness. Since spiritual wellness involves one's values, beliefs, and purpose, it can be improved in several ways—both physically and mentally. You will notice that some of these steps are the same or are similar to steps that can improve the mental, emotional, social, and spiritual domains of the psychological dimension of wellness.

1. **Explore yourself.** Simply ask yourself questions about who you are, your purpose, and your meaning. Who am I? What is my purpose? Where do I find the most value? You should consider all possible answers so you can think more in depth about yourself and allow you to fulfill your purpose and meaning.

2. **Find meaning**. Are there patterns that occur in your life? Do you feel like you have control over your destiny? Dig for deeper meaning when you see patterns and events that are significant.

3. **Express yourself.** Allow yourself to feel your emotions, processes, and questions. Find outlets for your negative energy, and direct your positive energy into your thoughts and ideas. Use strategies like writing, creativity, or physical movement to express your deep inner thoughts.

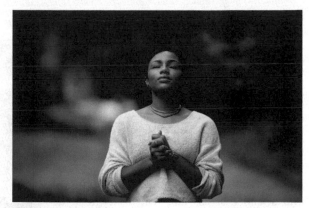

© Kosim Shukurov/Shutterstock.com

4. **Think positively and meditate.** View your life in a positive manner. This will help you to reframe and refocus into a healthy perspective and limit negativity. Try to meditate for 5 to 10 minutes each day to free your mind and increase your spiritual strengths.

MENTAL HEALTH DISORDERS

There are several kinds of mental health disorders such as schizophrenia, depression, general anxiety disorders, bipolar disorders, and panic disorders. These disorders cause mayhem and chaos in the life of the affected individual. People who have these types of disorders usually have frequent feelings that make them feel lost, depressed, or worthless, and can hinder them from living a healthy, enjoyable life. Eliminating the stigma of mental health reduces discrimination and judgment. Several mental health disorders are discussed within this section.

Who Gets Mental Health Disorders?

According to National Alliance on Mental Illness, one out of five Americans currently have a mental illness (Figure 3.3). The different types of mental health disorder affect over 90 million people. Mental illness affects individuals, and their family, friends, and coworkers. There are signs, symptoms, and treatments for many mental health disorders.

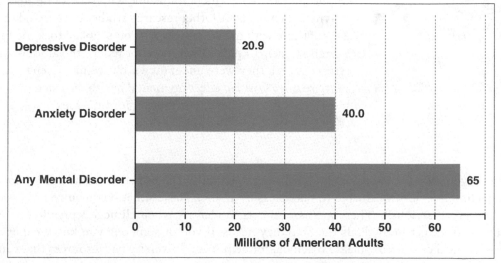

© Kendall Hunt Publishing Company

Figure 3.3 The Number of Americans That Have Mental Health Disorders

Depression

Many people experience occasional bouts of sadness, especially in difficult times. However, clinical depression is a diagnosed mental health disorder that is characterized by persistently depressed mood or loss of interest in activities. Clinical depression is very common, with about 3 million new cases each year, and causes significant impairment of daily life. Biologic, psychological, and social distress can lead to clinical depression, including biologic, psychological, and social distress. These factors cause a change in brain function, specifically altering patterns of neural circuits in the brain. Treatment methods are best when the source is identified, but they usually include medication and/or talk therapy and, in rare cases, medical procedures.

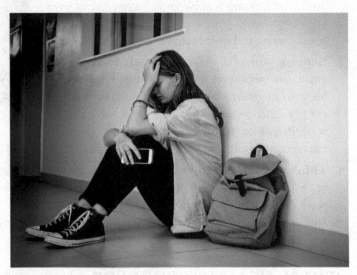
© Rido/Shutterstock.com

Spotlight on . . .

Exercise and Mental Health

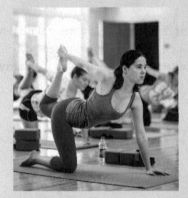
© Winthrop University

There is evidence to support exercise to be effective as a treatment for some types of mental disorders. In a review of over 20 studies, both aerobic exercise and strength training were effective in treating depression. Additionally, exercise can reduce anxiety in patients with panic disorders and can be an important part of treatment for people with schizophrenia (Payne & Hahn, 2000). Other research studies have found that 83% of those with mental health problems looked to some form of exercise to help improve their mood or reduce the amount of stress they felt they were under (news. bbc.co.uk). Even though exercise has a positive effect on mental health disorders, individuals should consult a physician for full care.

While everyone has occasional feelings of being down or sad, depression results in a person crying a great deal, feeling hopeless, or unable to take pleasure in life. These situations require professional help and should be taken seriously. There are assessments to identify when clinical depression is likely, and steps can be taken to get individuals the help they needs. If you or someone you know experiences the symptoms of clinical depression, please reach out for help. Your university has resources that can manage depressive symptoms or clinical depression.

Anxiety Disorder

Similar to occasional sadness, almost everyone has moments of increased nervousness and stress; however, anxiety can be a very serious and debilitating condition. Generalized anxiety disorder (GAD) is a mental health disorder that is much more serious and life changing. Individuals who are diagnosed with GAD often have other anxiety disorders, such as panic attacks, OCD, and post-traumatic stress disorder. There are more than 4 million new cases of GAD each year, and it is characterized by feelings of worry, anxiety, or fear. Individuals with GAD often overthink or think the worst-case scenario of any situations. Those with GAD

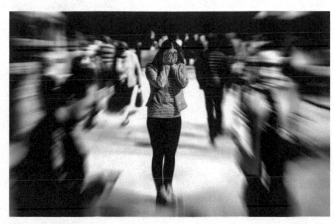

© Tero Vesalainen/Shutterstock.com

struggle with negative thoughts everyday and live in constant fear that their loved ones are in danger or their life will be tossed upside down. GAD most often occurs in children, young adults, and women.

Obsessive-Compulsive Disorder

Those with OCD suffer intensely from recurrent, unwanted thoughts (obsessions) or rituals (compulsions) that they feel they cannot control. People with OCD participate in rituals such as handwashing, counting, checking, or cleaning, hoping to take away any perceived dangers that exist. However, these rituals are often just part of the cycle of anxiety and obsessions that can take over a person's life if left untreated. OCD is often a chronic, relapsing illness that affects over 3 million Americans each year. OCD affects men and women equally. Although it can develop at any age, about one-third of the adult cases of OCD have their be-

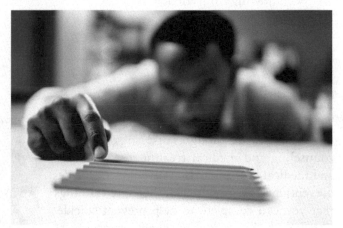

© Andrey_Popov/Shutterstock.com

ginnings in childhood, and many signs and symptoms begin to appear by puberty.

Panic Attacks

Panic attacks are unprovoked and recurring events of tremendous fear that involve chest pains, palpitations, wheezing, and stomach pains. Individuals who experience a panic attack often think they are dying or having a heart attack. In a given year, 1.7% the US population (2.4 million Americans) experiences panic disorder. Although panic attacks usually occur during adolescence, only half of individuals start to experience symptoms by 24 years. Like GAD, women are more common to experience panic attacks than men.

Suicidal Behavior

Each year, approximately one in 10,000 college students commits suicide throughout the United Sates. Many more students report having suicidal thoughts. Many individuals who have attempted suicide note that it was

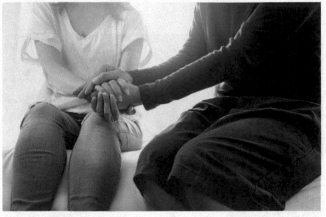

© GBALLGIGGSPHOTO/Shutterstock.com

driven by either one big event or several small events in their life that they wanted to change. Usually, they really do not want to die; they just do not know how to change the situation. Intense pressure or stress, feelings of depression, alcohol misuse, drug abuse, or a personal loss are commonly reported as the cause for suicide/suicidal attempts. Please take anyone who shows signs of suicide seriously, and find ways to help. For students, there are ways to privately report a concerned student to someone who can reach out and help. Each school has a different process, but this can usually be found on the university student resources website or through health services on campus.

Warning signs that a person may be contemplating suicide:

- Skipping classes
- Giving away personal possessions
- Withdrawing from friends
- Withdrawing from "normal" activities
- Engaging in risky behaviors

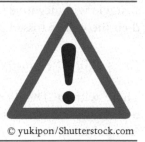

© yukipon/Shutterstock.com

How You Can Help

There are sustainable resources for individuals to get past suicidal thoughts or desires, including counseling and medical treatment. Counselors and medical professionals are trained in suicide-prevention strategies. In fact, there are trainings that you can complete to help prevent suicide. Check with the student engagement services at your school to see when trainings may be offered. There are free online trainings as well those you may be able to complete, such as The Jason Foundation https://jasonfoundation.com/. The key to helping an individual considering suicide is to be aware of warning signs, facts, and possible direction within a difficult moment.

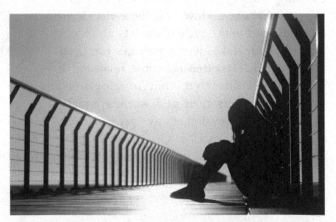

© Antonio Guillem/Shutterstock.com

If you are considering suicide, please take a moment to reach out for help. There are resources to help you, starting with the resources mentioned on campus. If you are not on campus, call the suicide-prevention hotline at 1.800.273.8255 or visit https://suicidepreventionlifeline.org. Please get help.

EATING DISORDERS

Like the other disorders and illnesses mentioned here, eating disorders are psychological conditions that can be medically diagnosed. Those with eating disorders often report struggles with self-esteem and depression. They often have an inner conflict between a desire for perfection and feelings of personal inadequacy. This conflict often leads to distorted views of themselves and their bodies. They believe they see something different than what others see. Eating disorders can be a product of other psychiatric conditions, such as depression, substance abuse, or anxiety disorders. Health concerns are a very serious reality for those with eating disorders and may lead to serious heart conditions, kidney failure, or death. Education on these disorders is critical to reduce their prevalence and incidence, especially among young populations.

Anorexia Nervosa

Anorexia nervosa is a state of starvation and emaciation, resulting from severe dieting and excessive exercise in an effort to control body size. Those with anorexia do not see themselves as they are, even when they have become dangerously thin. They have an extremely distorted body image, where they believe they are overweight.

As seen in Figure 3.5, Symptoms of anorexia includes being very thin, avoiding food or meals, picking out a few "acceptable" foods and eating them in small quantities, or carefully weighing and portioning foods. Other common symptoms of this disease include absent menstruation, dry skin, excessive hair on the skin, and thinning of scalp hair. Additionally, those with anorexia can develop gastrointestinal and orthopedic problems. As a result of starvation, anorexics often experience damage to their bones, organs, and muscles, along with reduced immune system, distorted digestive system, and inefficient nervous system. Often, female anorexics can experience the **female athlete triad** (see Figure 3.4), even if she is not female. The female athlete triad is a viscous cycle that consists of disordered eating that leads to **amenorrhea** (loss of the menstrual cycle) that, in turn, leads to **osteoporosis** (loss of bone mass).

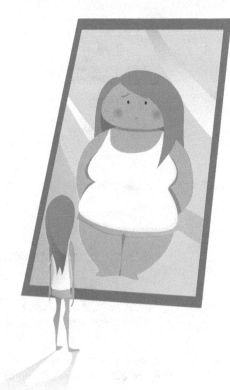

© stefanolunardi/Shutterstock.com

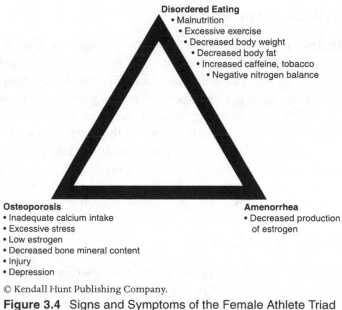

Disordered Eating
- Malnutrition
- Excessive exercise
- Decreased body weight
- Decreased body fat
- Increased caffeine, tobacco
- Negative nitrogen balance

Osteoporosis
- Inadequate calcium intake
- Excessive stress
- Low estrogen
- Decreased bone mineral content
- Injury
- Depression

Amenorrhea
- Decreased production of estrogen

© Kendall Hunt Publishing Company.

Figure 3.4 Signs and Symptoms of the Female Athlete Triad

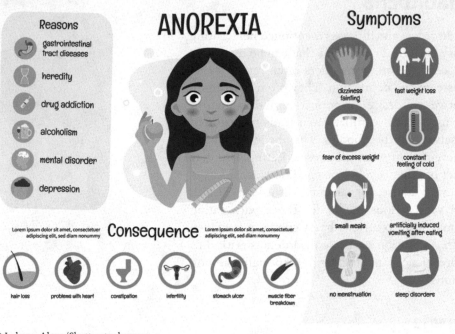

Figure 3.5 Reasons, Symptoms, and Outcomes of Anorexia

Bulimia Nervosa

Bulimia nervosa is an eating disorder that involves bingeing and purging. Bulimia is fairly more common than anorexia. Instead of starving themselves, bulimics will eat copious amounts of food and then almost immediately go to the bathroom to make themselves throw up the food they just ate. Bulimics think that if they throw up the food they just ate, they will not gain any weight. Bulimics are in constant fear of gaining weight and becoming obese, yet they feel like they cannot stop eating or will binge in hiding and then purge, which causes their weight to fluctuate. Bulimics live a vicious cycle of hunger, binge, and then purge because they feel guilty of overeating. Yet, they will become hungry soon after and the cycle will start again. They are obsessed with food. Unless they are caught in the act, it is hard to tell who is bulimic because their weights usually stay the same. A bulimic may have cuts and calluses on their fingers, yellow teeth enamel, or bloodshot eyes from inducing vomiting.

Binge-Eating Disorder

Binge-eating disorder is an eating disorder where individuals will undergo regular periods of binge eating where they continually eat until they cannot anymore. Binge-eating disorder is different from bulimia because individuals who binge eat do not purge the food they just consumed; so, it can be easy to identify these individuals because they are obese. Individuals with binge-eating disorder display at least three of the following symptoms: rapid eating, eating until they are uncomfortable, overeating even when they are not hungry, eating by themselves or in hiding because of the shame of the large amounts of food they are eating. This causes these individuals to feel gross, disgusting, and guilty, which causes them to fall into a deep depression.

PSYCHOLOGICAL HEALTH AND YOU

Are You a Healthy Consumer?

Psychological health is deeply connected to both eustress and distress, so the impact of psychological health can greatly influence your consumer behavior mentioned in chapter 2. Understanding health literacy and consumerism as they relate to psychological health is critical for proactive behaviors. **Health literacy** refers to the ability of an individual to find, understand, and use health-related information, resources, and services that enhance their decisions and actions for improving the individual's health. Can someone find credible information to use in an effective way to promote healthy choices? Individuals with less health literacy are more likely to hesitate to seek credible information regarding their health. So, much of the information on psychological health, like other domains of health, is confounded by miscommunication and misunderstanding of research and can be influenced by family and friends. Where do you turn for answers to questions related to psychological health? If you perceive your feelings to be unhealthy or alarming, or you just have general health questions, you should turn to a physician for answers. While the internet, family, and friends can be informative, they can also provide misleading information. Be a healthy consumer!

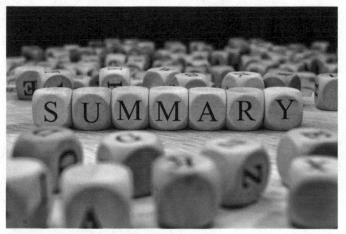

© Fabrick Bilder/Shutterstock.com

In this chapter, we learned about psychological health, and how it affects our lifestyle and overall health. Learning about our psychological health and the different components allow us to take a closer look at our stress-coping behaviors and to better understand them. Additionally, we can learn to value our strengths, and work to improve the areas of psychological health that are not as strong or make us uncomfortable in non-threatening environments. After reading this chapter, you should be able to connect the information from chapters 1 and 2 to this one and visualize how stress, behaviors, and psychological health are related.

PERSONAL REFLECTIONS . . . SO, WHAT HAVE YOU LEARNED?

1. In your own words, describe the difference between self-confidence, self-esteem, self-efficacy, and resilience. Provide an example of each as they relate to you in health-related situations.

2. Reflect on how body image is related to a person's psychological health. Do you think social media plays a positive or negative role in shaping a person's body image?

3. Describe what the term "emotional intelligence" means to you. Provide examples to back up your theory. Do you think teenagers and college students have high emotional intelligence? How can one increase emotional intelligence?

4. In your own words, what is the difference between and introvert and an extrovert? Based on your answer, how do you see yourself? How can this affect your health, both positively and negatively?

5. How are psychological health and stress related? For you, how does your stress impact your social, spiritual, intellectual, and emotional health? How do your stress-coping strategies affect each of those components?

NOTES

RESOURCES ON CAMPUS FOR YOU!

Mission

We believe in the dignity, integrity, growth potential, and innate worth of individuals, and we offer services to foster whole-person health through prevention, education, assessment, treatment, and advocacy.

Counseling

At the initial session, or "Intake," the counselor and the student will explore the presenting problem, contributing factors, and an appropriate plan for intervention. After the Intake, a student and his or her counselor will work together to choose the next best step. The student may continue with individual, couples, or group counseling at Counseling Services; or the counselor may refer the student to a resource in the community for long-term counseling, psychiatric evaluation, or other necessary services. Individual counseling and couples counseling through Counseling Services are short-term (up to 8–12 sessions) and solution-focused, while a student may make unlimited use of group counseling.

REFERENCES

Donatelle, R. J. (2014). *Access to health* (12th ed.). Pearson.

Edlin, G., & Golanty, E. (2014). *Health and wellness* (11th ed.). Jones and Bartlett.

Goleman, D. (1995). *Emotional intelligence: Why it can matter more than IQ.* Bantam Books.

Gardner, H. (1983). *Frames of mind: The theory of multiple intelligences.* New York: Basic Books.

Marr, J., & Wilcox, S. (2015). Self-efficacy and social support mediate the relationship between internal health locus of control and health behaviors in college students. *American Journal of Health Education, 46,* 122–131.

Mayer, J. D., & Salovey, P. (1993). The intelligence of emotional intelligence. *Intelligence, 17,* 433–442.

National Alliance on Mental Illnesses. https://www.nami.org/home.

Payne, W. A., & Hahn, D. B. (2000). *Understanding your health* (6th ed.). Mosby.

Salovey, P., & Mayer, J. D. (1990). Emotional intelligence. *Imagination, Cognition, and Personality, 9,* 185–211.

Zohar, D. (1998). *ReWiring the corporate brain: Using the new science to rethink how we structure and lead organizations.* Bartlett Koehler.

NOTES

Chapter 4

Physical Activity
and Fitness +

OBJECTIVES

Students will be able to:

- Define and explain the benefits of regular physical activity.
- Define key terms related to cardiovascular fitness, muscular fitness, and flexibility.
- Explain the relationship between physical activity and exercise on chronic disease.
- Discuss the benefits of aerobic, muscular, and flexibility fitness on overall health.
- Identify the Centers for Disease Control and Prevention (CDC) and American College of Sports Medicine (ACSM) guidelines for aerobic fitness, muscular fitness, and flexibility using the FITT (frequency, intensity, time, and type) principle.
- Discuss the steps of getting started on a physical activity or exercise program.
- Recognize the risks of injuries with physical activity and exercise.
- Relate healthy consumerism with physical activity and exercise economy.

Physical Activity Readiness Questionnaire and You (ACSM, 2012)

If you are between the ages of 15 and 69 years, the Physical Activity Readiness Questionnaire (PAR-Q) will tell you if you should check with your doctor before you start. If you are over 69 years of age, you should consult a physician before beginning an activity or exercise program. Please read the questions carefully and answer each one honestly.

Check YES or NO:

YES/NO

- ☐ £ 1. Has your doctor ever said that you have a heart condition and that you should only do physical activity recommended by a doctor?
- ☐ £ 2. Do you feel pain in your chest when you do physical activity?
- ☐ £ 3. In the past month, have you had chest pain when you were not doing physical activity?
- ☐ £ 4. Do you lose your balance because of dizziness or do you ever lose consciousness?
- ☐ £ 5. Do you have a bone or joint problem that could be made worse by a change in your physical activity?
- ☐ £ 6. Is your doctor currently prescribing drugs (e.g., water pills) for your blood pressure or heart condition?
- ☐ £ 7. Do you know of any other reason why you should not do physical activity?

Answer Results:

If you answered NO honestly to all PAR-Q questions, the following applies to you:

1. Start increasing your amount of physical activity. Begin slowly and build up gradually.
2. Complete a fitness assessment from a qualified or certified fitness and exercise specialist. This is the best way to identify your strength and weaknesses and to design a practical plan for improvement.

If you answered YES honestly to all PAR-Q questions, then you should:

Talk to your physician before beginning a regular exercise program. Most likely, you will be able to do some activities, but a physician can give you safe guidance.

If you are experiencing an illness, fever, or other unusual symptoms, consult a physician before beginning activity or exercise.

If you are pregnant, you should consult a physician before beginning an activity or exercise program.

If there is any change in your health, consult a physician before beginning or continuing an activity or exercise program.

Critical Thinking . . .

How do your physical activity habits affect your current health status?

Why do you think the majority of people do not engage in regular physical activity or exercise?

What is one physical activity in which you would like to participate?

PHYSICAL ACTIVITY AND EXERCISE

Physical activity is defined as body movement, performed over a period of time. There are many different types of physical activities, and they can range in intensity from easy to very difficult. Examples of physical activity include walking, jogging, dancing, weight training, or practicing a sport.

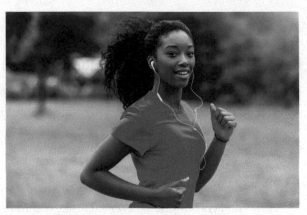

© Samuel BorgesPhotography/Shuttererstock.com

Exercise is considered a structured type of physical activity, meaning that there is a specific purpose or goal to each type of exercise. Whereas physical activity can be unstructured, like walking through an amusement park or playing with a pet, exercise is more focused on a specific component of fitness, such as aerobic endurance, muscular strength, or flexibility.

BENEFITS OF PHYSICAL ACTIVITY AND EXERCISE ON HEALTH

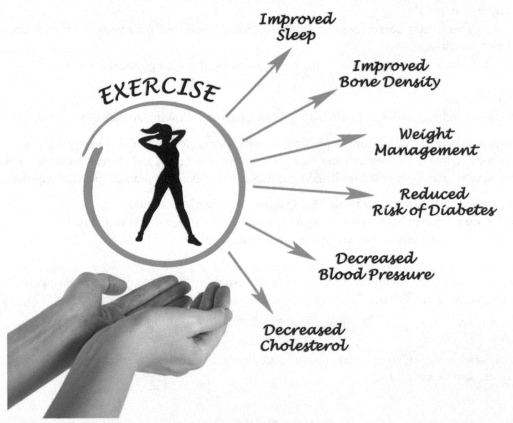

Figure 4.1 The Many Benefits of Physical Activity and Exercise

As seen in Figure 4.1, there is plenty of evidence to support the need for regular physical activity to reduce the risk of disease and early death. Clinical, scientific, and epidemiological studies indicate that physical activity has a positive effect in delaying the development of cardiovascular diseases (ACSM, 2012). A lack of physical activity or exercise can contribute to many cardiovascular diseases and conditions, including heart attack, severe chest pain, and blocked arteries. Additionally, lack of movement can lead to higher risks for diabetes, cancer, joint and bone problems, and even lower mental health. This chapter will discuss several specific benefits on physical activity to overall health, including the impact of physical activity on stress and chronic disease.

Impact on Stress

Physical activity or exercise is a positive strategy for coping with both acute (short-term) and chronic (long-term) stress. Research has shown that regular participation in exercise can decrease overall levels of tension, elevate and stabilize mood, improve sleep, and improve self-esteem. It does not take a long bout of exercise to be effective, as even five minutes of aerobic activity has shown a reduction in anxiety and related symptoms (ADAA, 2016). As you will see throughout this chapter, the benefits of physical activity are incredibly valuable to your overall health, beginning with a sustainable strategy for stress coping.

Impact on Chronic Disease

Physical activity and exercise reduce the risk of many types of chronic diseases, including coronary heart disease, which is the leading cause of death among all populations in the United States. During physical activity, the heart rate becomes elevated owing to the stress of movement. Through regular exercise, the increased heart rate will cause the heart to get stronger. Through healthy habits like regular physical activity, the strength and efficiency of the heart improves, thereby decreasing the **resting heart rate**. Resting heart rate refers to the rate of heartbeat at rest and is an indicator of cardiovascular fitness. Normal resting heart rates are 60 to 100 bpm for the general population, and resting heart rates on the lower end tend to indicate better aerobic fitness. Regular physical activity increases **stroke volume**—or the amount of blood pumped from the heart with each heartbeat—and improves **blood pressure**—or the pressure in the heart to move blood through the body.

Because the heart is stronger, the efficiency of the circulatory system also improves. Blood flow to the skeletal muscles improves owing to an increase in stroke volume, an increase in the number of capillaries, and an increase in the function of existing capillaries. The size of blood vessels increases collateral circulation, providing more efficient circulation both during exercise and during daily activities. The body gets better at delivering oxygen to the working muscles and removing metabolic wastes through improved circulation. Regular physical activity helps lower blood pressure and improve blood cholesterol levels. Additionally, regular exercise can help to maintain a healthy weight, improving the overall performance of the cardiovascular, circulatory, and respiratory systems.

Regular activity and exercise reduce the risk of diabetes, osteoporosis, and even some types of cancer. Physically active individuals show improvements in glucose regulation, which reduces the risk of diabetes or other metabolic conditions. In addition, physical activity increases bone density, making bones stronger and reducing the risk of osteoporosis, or brittle bone disease.

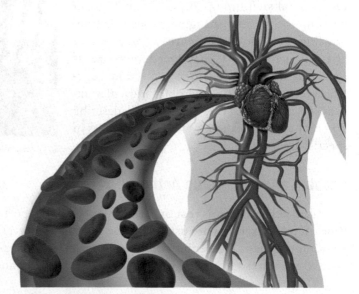

© Lightspring/Shutterstock.com

Impact on Body Composition and Weight Management

Even a small amount of physical activity or exercise can positively influence body composition and is one of the best preventive strategies against undesired weight gain. Regular physical activity can significantly improve body weight and body composition for those who are overweight or obese. One of the leading factors for chronic disease and death is a **sedentary lifestyle**, which includes little to no physical activity. Regular physical activity or exercise prevents premature death through improving the health of the body and reducing the burden of carrying extra body weight.

Impact on Activities of Daily Living

Of course, regular participation in physical activity, and especially exercise, will improve overall health and the ability to perform **activities of daily living (ADLs)**. This is a general term meant to encompass all the different movements that an individual would do each day to support independent living, as shown in Figure 4.2. For example, ADLs could include getting up out of a chair or reaching to get something on a high shelf. Individuals who participate in regular physical activity do not experience as many limitations in ADLs as those who are sedentary. This is critically important as individuals age and hope to maintain physical independence.

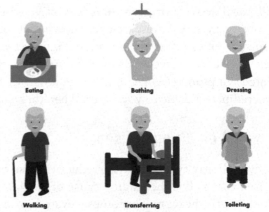
© Namnatt/Shutterstock.com

Figure 4.2 Common Activities of Daily Living or ADLs

TYPES OF PHYSICAL ACTVITY AND EXERCISE

There are different types of physical activity and exercise. Physical activity can be anything, including both unstructured and structured formats. Unstructured physical activity includes playing tag with others, hiking a trail, or recreational swimming. Physical activities can be fun, social, and engaging. Roller skating, bowling, and snow skiing are all examples of physical activity. As mentioned, exercise is more structured and is often focused in a specific area of aerobic, anaerobic, muscular fitness, or flexibility. This section will describe different types of exercise for improvements in specific areas.

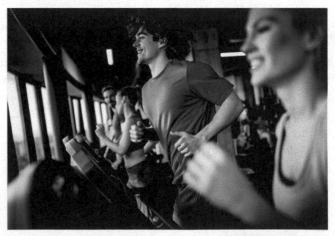
© Gutesa/Shutterstock.com

Aerobic and Anaerobic Activity/Exercise

The term **aerobic** means that oxygen is required to support the completion of the activity over a period of time. Aerobic exercises are usually at a lower intensity level so that they sustain over time. For example, a 30-minute jog is at a lower intensity than a sprint. Aerobic exercise is also synonymous with "cardio" exercise, which refers to exercise that incorporates the heart and lungs in a sustained effort. Aerobic exercise uses large muscle groups in a full-body, rhythmic activity. Examples include walking, jogging, swimming, biking, dancing, or kickboxing. There are examples of cardio exercises shown in Figure 4.3.

As with most exercise, the rate of energy expenditure varies with an individual's skill level and intensity of exercise. Aerobic activities of low intensity are ideal for the beginning or sedentary exerciser because they can be maintained for a longer period of time and have been shown to be effective in promoting weight loss and in enhancing cardiovascular health.

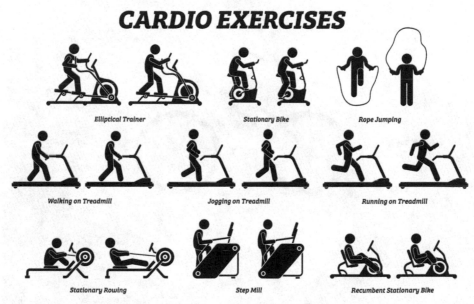

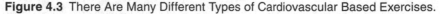

© Leremy/Shutterstock.com

Figure 4.3 There Are Many Different Types of Cardiovascular Based Exercises.

Many activities are too intense to be maintained more than a few minutes; these activities are considered anaerobic. Anaerobic exercises include strength training, sprinting, and interval training. **Anaerobic** refers to exercises performed without the presence of oxygen; so the intensity of these exercises is usually high, but only for a short period. Anaerobic training can improve physical fitness by increasing resistance to fatigue, especially in high-intensity events. Interval training is an example of anaerobic exercise because it uses short bouts of high intensity for exercise. The body does not rely on oxygen during the intense exercise portions, but oxygen is used during the rest breaks. This makes anaerobic exercise beneficial for aerobic fitness.

Benefits of Aerobic and Anaerobic Activity

There are many benefits of aerobic and anaerobic training. **Cardiovascular fitness** or **cardiorespiratory endurance** refers to the ability of the heart and lungs to supply oxygen to the working muscles for optimum levels of exercise for extended periods at moderate to high levels of intensity. Owing to its positive increase in health and optimal performance, cardiovascular fitness is the most important aspect of overall physical fitness. Aerobic exercise and aerobic fitness have shown to have numerous benefits, including better body composition and weight control, improved mental health through reduced anxiety and depression, and better quality of sleep. Additionally, aerobic exercise strengthens connective tissues, which can reduce the risk of injuries and joint pain. Aerobic activity increases cognitive ability and slows down the aging process. There are many health benefits of incorporating aerobic activity into your schedule, as shown in Figure 4.4. What types of aerobic activities do you like best?

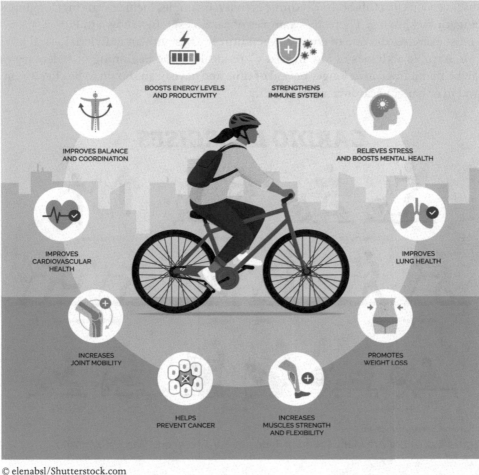

© elenabsl/Shutterstock.com

Figure 4.4 There Are Many Benefits From Regular Aerobic Exercise.

Muscular Strength & Resistance Exercises

Muscular fitness includes exercises that are specific to muscular strength, endurance, or power. **Muscular strength** is the maximum amount of weight a muscle can lift at one time. This is generally not a major goal of exercise for the general population, but it can be a focus for those who are more advanced in strength and resistance training. Exercises that target true muscular strength include big movements with high resistance. Basically, if an individual is interested in improving muscular strength, the individual would incorporate extremely heavy weights while completing the exercises. **Muscular power** refers to the explosive ability of muscles. This is high-intensity movement in a short period of time and includes exercises like box jumps, Olympic lifts, and ball slams. Training for muscular power is generally reserved for more advanced exercisers because the intensity and effort involved are high. **Muscular endurance** is the ability of a muscle to perform sustained contractions over time. This is sometimes referred to as stamina, which much of the general population would greatly benefit from, and should be a primary goal, especially for those starting an exercise program.

Benefits of Strength & Resistance Activity

Through consistent resistance training for endurance, strength, or power, neural and muscular adaptations can take place within the body. Within the first six weeks of training, most changes that occur are

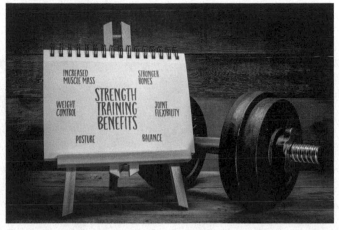

© marekuliasz/Shutterstock.com

neural based. This means that the brain gets better at doing these movements. Think of the first time you performed a push-up versus performing push-ups several nights a week for four weeks. You would get better at push-ups, with little to no changes within the muscle size. As resistance training activities continue, there is an increase in the size of the muscle fibers, known as **muscular hypertrophy**. Benefits of resistance training extend beyond the brain and muscles to also include bone and connective tissue (ligaments and tendons). Bone and connective tissue undergo changes from resistance training as well— such as increase in bone matrix, increases in bone mineral density, and increase in mass and tensile strength of ligaments and tendons. All muscular changes help to prevent injury and decrease the changes of developing osteoporosis later on in life.

Research has shown that improving elements of muscular fitness, like strength and endurance, can improve overall health in many ways (see Figure 4.5). Increased muscular fitness improves overall strength and endurance, reduces risk of injuries, and improves activities of daily living. Muscular fitness includes a component of incorporating functional exercises. **Functional exercise** refers to exercise that mimics everyday movements. For example, a squat mimics getting out of a chair, and a lunge exercise mimics walking up the stairs. Additional benefits are reduced body weight; reduced body fat; and improved **body composition**, which is the ratio of body fat to lean body mass. More muscle mass increases the basal metabolic rate, or how fast we use the calories we consume. This is why increased muscular fitness can help control body weight. Improved muscular fitness can lower the risk of diseases, including heart disease, cancer, diabetes, and osteoporosis. Benefits extend to improved mental health as strength and resistance training has shown increases in body image and self-esteem.

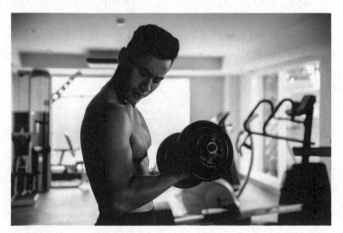

© wear it out/Shutterstock.com

an increase in muscular strength, power and endurance	increased metabolic rate	increased energy & vitality
a higher percent of muscle mass	increased resistance to fatigue	weight loss
increased strength of tendons & ligaments	improved posture	higher self-esteem
increased bone mass	improved movement	improved well-being
	decreased risk of low back pain or other injuries	

Figure 4.5 There Are Many Benefits to Muscular Fitness

Flexibility

Flexibility is defined as the range of motion that exists at a specific joint. As we age, our flexibility begins to decline, mostly owing to inactivity and sedentary lifestyles. The loss of flexibility can greatly affect a person's quality of life because it reduces mobility and increases dependence to complete activities of daily living. There are several factors that can affect flexibility, including gender, age, genetic composition, activity level, muscle core temperature, and previous/current injuries. Women tend to be more flexible than men, and younger individuals tend to be more flexible than older individuals. Those who are active tend to be more flexible owing to their activities. If your parents are active and flexible, then you are more likely to be active and flexible too. Flexibility is specific to individual joints. For example, one could have a full range of motion within their wrist but limited in their shoulder. An individual could also be very flexible on one side of their body, but inflexible on the other side.

For every population, flexibility and balance are a major concern. Including flexibility in exercise and physical activity programs is beneficial for overall health. Benefits of flexibility include improved activities of daily living, reduced risk of injuries, and enhanced physical performance. Flexibility can greatly impact **mobility**, which is the term used to describe how efficient we are with functional and sport-specific movements. Non-impact activities such as tai chi and yoga are popular to incorporate more flexibility within exercise routines. There are several ways to incorporate flexibility into your regular physical activity routine!

There are three categories of stretches that can be used to increase flexibility. Ballistic stretches are more bouncy in nature and are generally not recommended for most of the general population. Static stretches are held stretches that are safe for almost anyone. Dynamic stretches are slow-moving stretches that can increase flexibility and mobility at a joint.

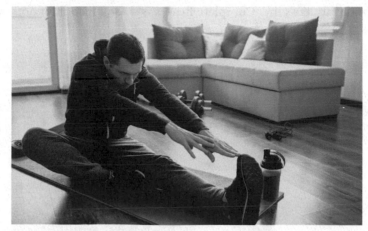

© Dmytrenko Vlad/Shutterstock.com

Types of Stretches

Ballistic stretching involves rapid movements, or "bouncing." Ballistic stretching is not recommended for the general population as a means to improve flexibility. An exception is athletes who have ballistic movement in their sport.

© d13/Shutterstock.com

Static stretching involves a held stretch to the point of mild discomfort and maintaining that angle for 15–60 seconds before allowing the muscle to relax. The entire procedure should be repeated several times for maximum benefit.

© lzf/Shutterstock.com

Dynamic stretches are slow moving stretches that can increase the flexibility and mobility around a joint. For example, big shoulder circles are slow and controlled. They open the shoulder joint and increase the flexibility of the surrounding muscle groups.

© solar22/Shutterstock.com

Health and Skill-Related Fitness

Health-related fitness is the overall ability of the body to function efficiently and effectively. It consists of all types of fitness combined together, including cardiovascular fitness, muscular strength, muscular endurance, flexibility, and optimal body composition. Regular physical activity and exercise can improve health-related fitness. A program that focuses on improvements in specific skills for sport or performance is based on skill-related fitness. **Skill-related fitness** includes agility, balance, coordination, reaction time, speed, and power. These components can increase the athletic performance of an individual but may not necessarily improve overall health. Think of some athletes in sports like football, where the athlete may be quick and powerful but lack aerobic or cardiovascular fitness. This could affect the athlete's overall health at some point in the athlete's life. **Complete fitness** is a combination of both health-related fitness and skill-related fitness as shown in Figure 4.6.

Health-Related Fitness
- Cardiovascular Fitness
- Muscular Strength
- Muscular Endurance
- Flexibility
- Optimal body composition

Skill-Related Fitness
- Agility
- Balance
- Coordination
- Reaction time
- Speed
- Power

Courtesy of Joni Boyd

Figure 4.6 Components of Health-Related and Skill-Related Fitness

GUIDELINES FOR PHYSICAL ACTIVITY AND EXERCISE

You may be wondering how much physical activity and exercise do you need in order to reach health-related fitness? There are evidence-based guidelines for how to improve your health through physical activity and exercise. This section will target each component of physical activity, aerobic fitness, muscular strength and endurance, and flexibility.

Physical Activity Guidelines

Remember, physical activity is any type of full-body movement. It may or may not include structured exercise. The CDC has released Physical Activity Guidelines for Americans. You can read more about those guidelines here: https://health.gov/sites/default/files/2019-10/PAG_ExecutiveSummary.pdf. The following is summary of steps for the Physical Activity Guidelines for healthy adults. The Physical Activity Pyramid provides context of physical activities (Figure 4.7).

- Any physical activity is better than none! The key point is just to get moving. Any increase in physical activity levels will promote health benefits.
- For health-related benefits, adults should accumulate 150 minutes (2 hours and 30 minutes) to 300 minutes (5 hours) a week of moderate-intensity activities; 75 minutes (1 hour and 15 minutes) to 150 minutes (2 hours and 30 minutes) a week of vigorous-intensity aerobic physical activity; or a combination of the two.
- Aerobic activities should be spread throughout the week owing to their heart health benefits.
- Physical activity beyond the equivalent of 300 minutes (5 hours) of moderate-intensity physical activity a week can have additional health benefits.
- Adults should also do muscle-strengthening activities of moderate or greater intensity and those involving all major muscle groups two or more days a week because these activities provide additional health benefits.

Key Point! Adults should average at least 30 minutes a day of accumulated physical activity of at least moderate intensity.

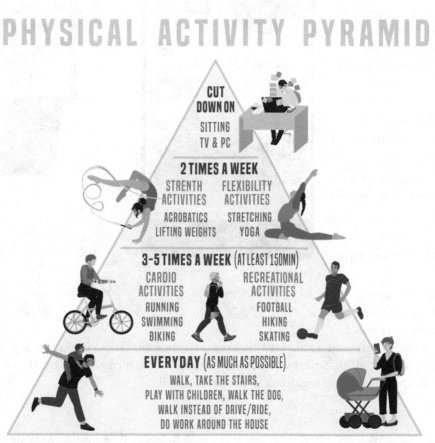

PHYSICAL ACTIVITY PYRAMID

CUT DOWN ON
SITTING
TV & PC

2 TIMES A WEEK
STRENTH ACTIVITIES   FLEXIBILITY ACTIVITIES
ACROBATICS   STRETCHING
LIFTING WEIGHTS   YOGA

3-5 TIMES A WEEK (AT LEAST 150MIN)
CARDIO ACTIVITIES   RECREATIONAL ACTIVITIES
RUNNING   FOOTBALL
SWIMMING   HIKING
BIKING   SKATING

EVERYDAY (AS MUCH AS POSSIBLE)
WALK, TAKE THE STAIRS,
PLAY WITH CHILDREN, WALK THE DOG,
WALK INSTEAD OF DRIVE/RIDE,
DO WORK AROUND THE HOUSE

© Double Brain/Shutterstock.com

Figure 4.7 The Physical Activity Pyramid Describes the Recommended Frequency of Activity

Guidelines to Improve Aerobic Fitness

In order to improve aerobic (or cardiovascular) fitness, the exercise should consist of a right mix of intensity and time and be performed multiple days per week. FITT is the acronym for a method that provides the guidelines for a cardiovascular exercise program. FITT stands for frequency (how many days per week), intensity (how difficulty or easy), time (how long), and type (the kind of exercise), and following the FITT principle is a great way to improve aerobic fitness. The following summarizes the ACSM guidelines for how to improve aerobic fitness using the FITT principle.

- **Frequency = The ACSM recommends performing aerobic activity three to five times during the week.** If you are a beginner or have a low level of fitness, starting a program at two times a week will help you to begin. As you improve, the frequency as well as the intensity should increase to adapt to new challenges.

- **Intensity =** Intensity refers the difficulty of the exercise or activity, and it can be measured by several techniques. **Heart rate, rate of perceived exertion** (**RPE**), and the **talk test** are three ways to measure the intensity level of an exercise or activity.

Target Heart Rate Range

To use heart rate as a measure of intensity, you should first measure your target heart rate range. Target heart rate range is a range where the heart rate should be in order to see positive effects of exercise. **The ACSM recommends working between 50 and 85 % of the heart rate reserve.** You can calculate the heart rate reserve target rate using the following Karvonen formula:

1. 220 − age = maximum heart rate (MHR)

2. MHR − resting heart rate (RHR) = heart rate reserve (HRR)

3. HRR x 50% − 85%

4. %HRR + RHR = heart rate for exercise

For individuals who are very unfit, the recommended range is 40% to 49% of heart rate reserve (Pollock, Gaesser, Butcher, Despres, Dishman, et al., 1998). A heart rate monitor is also useful for monitoring the specific heart rate and intensity. Smart watches are an easy way to measure the heart rate and provide real-time information to you regarding your current level.

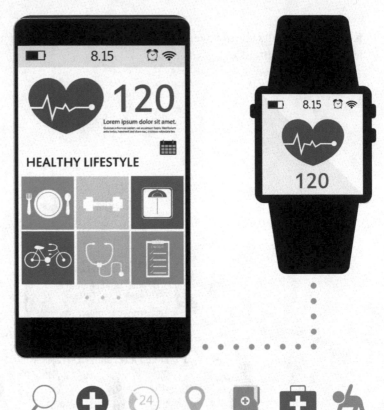

RPE

The **RPE** is a numbered scale from 6 to 20 that you can use to measure how hard or easy the activity is to perform. The modified RPE scale uses a 0 to 10 score. The numbers on the low end represent low intensity or easy effort and numbers on the high end represent very high difficulty involved in performing the activity. Your perception of the intensity is a subjective measure, and each activity could vary from person to person. This scale is a useful tool for estimating the exercise intensity because it is individual and easy to use.

Those that are on medications can use the RPE scale as a better measure of intensity, because some medications could affect heart rate. **The ACSM recommends working between a score of 12 and 16 on the Borg scale, or a score of 3 and 6 on the modified scale.**

Talk Test

The talk test is exactly how it sounds. The test measures your ability to have a conversation while exercising. If it is difficult to participate or maintain a conversation, the exercise intensity is likely too high to sustain. Exercise at this intensity will be difficult to maintain. If you are able to carry a conversation, then you are likely at an intensity that can be maintained.

Table 4.1 chart allows you to compare intensity measures and methods.

TABLE 4.1 A Comparison of the Borg, RPE, Talk Test, and % Max Heart Rate

BORG RPE	Modified RPE	Talk Test	% of Max HR
6	0	No effort/very easy	50–60%
7	·	Very light activity	
8	1		
9			
10	2	Breathing is deeper, but pace can be maintained for long time	60–70%
11			
12	3	You can talk, but holding a conversation is more difficult	70–80%
13			
14	4	Breathing is much deeper and it is uncomfortable to talk	80–90%
15	5		
16	6		
17	7	You do not want to talk at all; focus is on deep, forceful breaths	90–100%
18	8		
19	9	Very difficult to continue for any period of time	
20	10	Total maximum exertion	

- **Time = The ACSM recommends performing aerobic activity between 20 and 60 minutes each bout in order to see improvements in aerobic fitness.** The time bouts can be accumulated in 10 minute sessions throughout the day.
- **Type = The ACSM recommends aerobic exercise incorporating large muscle, full-body, rhythmic movement that increases heart and breathing rates.**

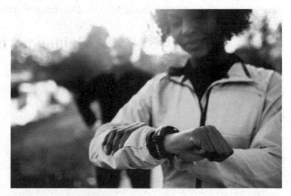

© Uber Images/Shutterstock.com

Key Point! For aerobic fitness, healthy adults should participate in about 30 minutes of aerobic activity at a 60% target heart rate 3 to 5 days per week.

Guidelines to Improve Muscular Fitness

In order to improve muscular fitness for strength and endurance, the exercises should be performed consistently during the week at the right amount of weight, sets, and repetitions. Weight refers to how much weight or resistance is being used. Repetitions (reps) refer to the number of times a move is completed, and sets refers to the block of reps that are performed together. For example, you could perform 3 sets of 10 reps of squats. The ACSM recommends that healthy adults perform 8 to 10 total resistance training exercises 2 to 3 days per week. Each exercise should be performed for 2 to 4 sets, with 8 to 12

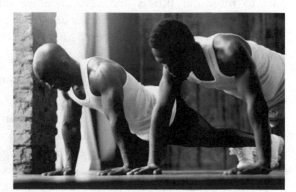

© DmitryStock/Shutterstock.com

repetitions in each set. The weight should be heavy enough to induce volitional fatigue but allow for completion of the set. The following summarizes the ACSM guidelines for how to improve muscular strength and endurance for healthy adults.

- **2 to 3 non-consecutive days per week for major muscle groups**
- **8 to 10 total exercises**
- **2 to 4 sets of each exercise**
- **8 to 12 repetitions of each set to the point of volitional fatigue**

Advanced Muscular Fitness

It should be noted that there are often different goals for muscular fitness based on individual preferences. The ACSM guidelines are to be considered for healthy adults who want improved muscular health overall. If you have more specific goals for muscular fitness, then you may need to adjust your training program accordingly. For example, some people may desire an increase in muscle size or growth. For this to occur, the resistance exercise should include heavier weight, more sets, and less rest in between sets. The following chart compares the differences in goals within muscular fitness. If your goal falls into one of these categories, then you should follow the recommendations in the Table 4.2.

TABLE 4.2 Guidelines for Muscular Fitness Adaptations

Adaptation	Weight	Sets	Reps	Rest Periods
General health	Moderately heavy	2-4	8–12	30 sec–1 min
Endurance	moderate weight	2–3	> 12	< 30 s
Hypertrophy	Mod–heavy weight	3–6	6–12	30 s–1.5 min
Power*	Heavy weight	3–5	1–5	2–5 min
Strength	very heavy weight	2–6	< 6	2–5 min

Muscular Fitness Myths and Half-Truths

We should also discuss some common myths, half-truths, and misconceptions of muscular fitness. Some of these apply to all fitness concepts, but most are specific to muscular fitness and resistance training. A myth is something that is incorrect, a half-truth means that it applies to a specific concept. And a misconception is a basic misunderstanding.

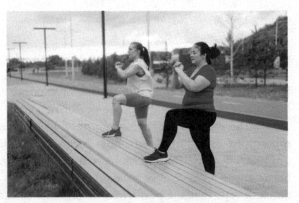

© Dikushin Dmitry/Shutterstock.com

1. *Half-truth: You have to lift hard and heavy in order to see any changes.*

   Truth: Changes can result from programs that are not necessarily "hard and heavy" as long as training is consistent. If the desire is to gain a significant amount of muscle size, then more intense lifts are necessary, but other muscular fitness results can be achieved without heavy weight.

2. *Myth: There is only one way to achieve muscular fitness.*

Truth: There are multiple ways to achieve muscular fitness, and they will produce different positive outcomes. There is no one "perfect" program or routine; they all have benefits and concerns.

3. *Misconception: Women will grow big muscles as quickly as men when undergoing strength training.*

   Truth: Only if they wants to. If muscle hypertrophy is the goal, then a very specific program must be followed in order to see growth in women. Owing to the hormone differences in genders, the average male will increase muscle size at a faster rate than females. Additionally, men generally see a much greater amount of size increase than women.

4. *Myth: If you do not have time to warm-up, then it is not necessary.*

   Truth: Performing a warm-up is the best defense against training-related injuries. Warm-ups prepare the body for activity both physically and mentally. All exercise and training organizations recommend performing a warm-up ANYTIME training will follow.

5. *Misconception: You can "spot-reduce" body fat (i.e., make legs smaller by doing leg exercises).*

   Truth: Resistance training targets the muscle, which will increase strength and toning. However, it does not directly target the fat in the same area. Reducing body fat takes a comprehensive approach of diet and exercise.

6. *Myth: Fat will be converted to muscle with resistance training.*

   Truth: Muscle does not turn into fat, and fat does not turn into muscle. They are separate things and will independently grow or shrink based on diet and exercise.

7. *Half-truth: Dietary supplements will make one bigger and stronger.*

   Truth: Some supplements can be beneficial for some people under very specific circumstances. In most cases, supplements have no effect on the muscular fitness outcome. The overall diet and exercise program is much more impactful. Before using supplements, check with a physician or registered dietician.

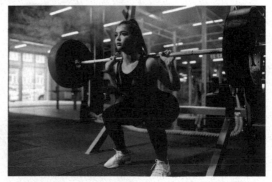

© UfaBizPhoto/Shutterstock.com

8. *Misconception: Stretching is not good for you.*

   Research has shown stretching to be effective in improving flexibility and mobility; reducing injury risk; and reducing tightness, joint, and muscle pain. Stretching should be performed correctly and can be very beneficial. Some athletes should be careful as to what type of stretches they perform; but for the general population, stretching is encouraged.

Spotlight on . . .

Women and Strength/Resistance Training

Women are sometimes concerned that exercises will make them appear less feminine and produce large bulging muscles. Research has disputed this myth. Women have the same muscle properties as men, but they respond to training in different ways. Men develop a greater quantity and gain of muscle mass when they engage in a strength program. In most cases, women will not gain a large amount of muscle mass when training, but they will obtain increased strength and endurance. There is no physiological reason for women not to engage in a strength training program and no need to suggest different training programs on the basis of sex. Both women and men can experience the same general benefits; it is only the degree of gain in muscle tissue that will differ (Allsen, 2009).

Key Point! For muscular fitness, healthy adults should participate in resistance training 2 to 3 days per week, perform 8 to 10 exercises for 2 to 4 sets of 8 to 12 reps to the point of volitional fatigue.

Guidelines to Improve Muscular Flexibility

In order to improve flexibility, stretches should be performed on regular and consistent basis. Once the body is warm and ready to stretch, static stretches are recommended at least 2 days per week, but could be performed every day. Stretches should be held for 15 to 60 seconds at the point of slight discomfort. The following summarizes the ACSM guidelines for how to improve muscular flexibility for healthy adults.

- *Minimum 2 to 3 days per week, could be every day*
- *At least one stretch per muscle group*
- *Hold stretch to the point of slight discomfort*
- *Hold the static stretch for 15 to 60 seconds*

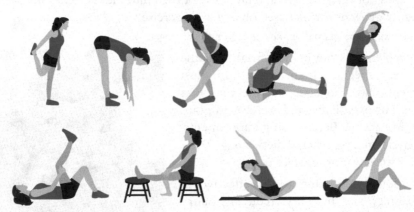

© Lio putra/Shutterstock.com

Figure 4.8 Different Types of Stretches

Flexibility can be improved by simply performing stretches shown in Figure 4.8. For those who want more than just stretching, there are several types of exercise formats for flexibility and mobility, including yoga, Pilates, and stretch/mobility classes. These are optional but great ways to incorporate mindfulness, flexibility, and mobility in an organized way to target major muscle groups.

Spotlight on . . .

Yoga

Yoga is starting to become a favorite pass time within the United States. Yoga is particularly known for its relaxation techniques, but it is also known to increase flexibility and strength. Most forms of yoga increase the core body temperature in order to facilitate movement and increase neural focus. Yoga has been shown in research to reduce anxiety and depression, increase joint mobility, lower injury risk, and improve balance in multiple populations. You can begin Yoga at any time, but it is suggested to begin with beginner or level one yoga practice in order to be at an appropriate intensity.

Pulling It All Together

As you begin or continue your physical activity and exercise routine, work to improve all areas of health and fitness, including aerobic fitness, muscular strength and endurance, and flexibility. Table 4.3 will help you remember the frequency, intensity, time, and type for each adaptation. Just get FITT!

Exercise Prescription Using the FITT Principles

TABLE 4.3 Guidelines for Physical Activity, Aerobic Exercise, Resistance Training, and Flexibility for Americans

Type of Activity	Frequency	Intensity	Time	Type
Physical activity	Most days of the week	Moderate level	At least 30 minutes	Any moderate to vigorous activity
Aerobic exercise	3–5 days per week	30–85% HRR 12–16 RPE scale	20–60 minutes	Any full-body, repetitive activity movement
Resistance training	2–3 nonconsecutive days per week	Point of muscle fatigue	2–4 sets 8–12 reps	8–10 exercises for full body
Flexibility	Minimum 2–3 days per week	Hold stretch until point of discomfort	15–60 seconds Repeat	Static stretches

HRR, heart rate reserve; RPE, rating of perceived exertion scale.
American College of Sports Medicine, 2013
Courtesy of Joni Boyd

GETTING STARTED

Understand that your body type, your experience and fitness levels, as well as your motivation should dictate the type of training that would be best for you. Not every program works at the same rate for every individual. A few rules to remember can ensure that you do not make the typical mistake of doing too much too soon.

Movement Preparation (Warm-Up and Stretch)

Rule number #1 is to always warm-up! A short 5-to10-minute warm-up of light, full-body movement is your best protection against injury and prepares your body for movement. The purpose of a warm-up is to increase core body temperature, increase heart rate, increase blood flow to the working muscles, and include dynamic movements to increase the range of motion. Performing a warm-up before exercise not only decreases the body's risk for injuries, but it also prepares the body mentally to go into high-intensity exercise. You can perform static or dynamic stretches in the warm-up period in order to target the muscle

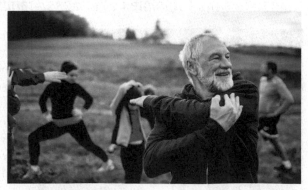
© Halfpoint/Shutterstock.com

specifically. Many athletes choose to perform dynamic, full–range of motion movements that mimic the sport, fitness class, or exercises they will be performing rather than only performing static stretching.

A typical warm-up could look like this:

1. Light aerobic activity (like a jog or walk for 5 to 8 minutes)
2. Light static or dynamic stretching for each muscle group
   Static stretches should be held for 8 to 10 seconds
   Dynamic stretches should be full controlled movement through the joint range of motion
3. A rehearsal of movements you plan to do in the workout; for example, if you will work your lower body, perform body weight exercises to prepare those muscle groups

Listen to Your Body

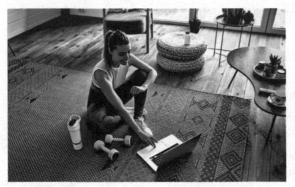

© ORION PRODUCTION/Shutterstock.com

Start light. Do not jump in too quickly. Give your body time to adjust to the demands you place on it. **Stay consistent.** It is going to take time to see changes! You will see changes as long as you stay consistent with SOME type of activity. Trying to do a fitness or exercise program that is not designed for you increases your chance of burnout, injury, and giving up. Be aware of **overtraining**, or lack of enough recovery time, which occurs when someone tries to do too much too fast. These symptoms include increased muscle soreness or pain, increase in resting heart rate, sleep disturbances, eating disturbances, constant fatigue, and loss of interest to exercise. These are symptoms of overtraining that will lead to burnout or to cessation of exercise and activity.

Cooldown and Stretch

After an exercise session, lower the heart rate gradually by reducing the intensity of the exercise. Going into a sudden stop after exercise can lead to muscle cramps, dizziness, and blood pooling in legs. Gradually cooling down, such as walking or light stretching, is highly recommended. Take time to reflect on your physical activity and exercise session. What went well and what would you change? Then, give yourself a big high five!

Remember the Principles of Fitness Training

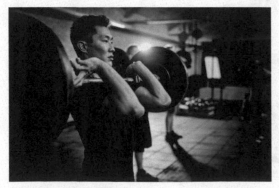

© Ground Picture/Shutterstock.com

The principle of **overload** states that for the body to become more efficient or stronger, it must be stressed beyond its normal working capacity. Therefore, one must overload the body, so that it may adapt. Overloading must occur in order to continue to see results. Being comfortable in the same routine gets the body in a plateau state. The principles of overloading and adaptation can be applied to muscular strength, cardiovascular and muscular endurance, and flexibility training.

Individual differences remind us that individuals will respond differently to the same training programs. Different factors play a role in your response to training, but initial fitness level, age, gender, genetic composition, and previous history will cause different responses to certain activities. Each body type is genetically determined, but body fat distribution and metabolism are individual. With proper training and lifestyle changes, a person's physique changes to a point. However, a large-framed person will never truly be a small-framed person and vice versa.

"If you do not use it, you will lose it" applies to **reversibility**. Cardiovascular benefits can decline with the cessation of aerobic activity. Physiological changes will begin to occur after two weeks of detraining and will continue to decline for several months.

INJURIES AND INJURY PREVENTION

Although injuries are possible, the benefits of regular exercise far outweigh the risk of injury. Injuries usually occur with poor technique, poor exercise prescription, or using equipment incorrectly. If you are injured during exercise, seek medical professionals for advice. Some common injuries resulting from exercise include joint and muscle injuries and soreness. Knowing how to treat an acute, or immediate, injury is important. If an injury causes swelling or pain, then you should do the following until you can see a physician: rest and use ice. Compress (wrap the area), and elevate it to reduce blood flow.

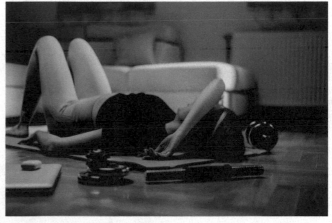

© Zamrznuti tonovi/Shutterstock.com

Making sure the equipment is safe and used properly is a major step for safety. Performing the correct technique of exercises is critical to stay injury-free. Using weight is beneficial for muscular fitness, but make sure it is a weight that you can use safely.

Proper Footwear

The right kind of footwear is critical when being physically active or exercising. This will keep your feet healthy and reduce the chances of injury and pain. Shoes that do not fit well can increase the amount of stress on the feet, ankle, and knee joints. This stress can increase pain throughout the body. You will need to consider the type of activity you will be participating in the most to get the right type of shoe. For example, running shoes are not appropriate for cardio dance, basketball, tennis, or racquetball because they have little lateral support and can increase the chance of ankle or knee injuries. Cross-training shoes are appropriate for most

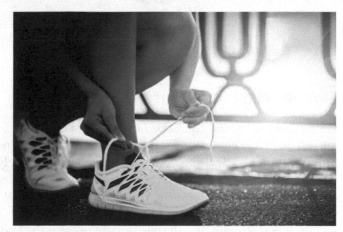

© AlexMaster/Shutterstock.com

activities, except for running and dance. It is also important to identify the surface of exercise and how the shoe will affect movement. Here are a few tips to remember when choosing the right type of shoes for physical activity and exercise.

- Choose shoes based on how they feel on your feet! If they do not feel good, do not use them. Shoes should not be "broken in," they should feel good the first time you wear them!

- Move around in the shoes before you purchase them. Take steps, jog, even hop a bit to see how they feel. Check for laces and tags that may irritate your skin.

- Think about the activities and exercises you will do while you examine the shoe support and sole. Are the shoes sturdy enough to protect you if needed? Are they flexible and provide enough grip?

- Can you wiggle your toes? Does your heel slide inside the shoe? You should be able to wiggle your toes, but you do not want your heel to slide around.

- Try on new shoes after exercise or toward the end of the day because feet tend to swell a bit throughout the day. This will help make sure you get the right size for you.

- Measure your feel everytime you purchase new shoes! Your feet can grow and change over time.

These are a few tips to help you choose a shoe that can provide you support and comfort for physical activities and exercise.

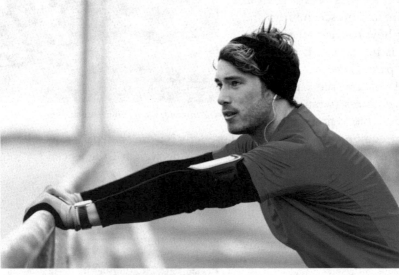
© Maridav/Shutterstock.com

Environmental Conditions

Often, environmental conditions are overlooked when considering exercising outside. When performing outside activity, environmental conditions such as temperature, air pollution, wind-chill, altitude, and humidity can all affect the body's ability to perform safely. There are ways to ensure you are taking precaution when outside. Dressing appropriately for the weather is important when exercising in extreme conditions. In the cold, layering your clothes is advised. Wear clothing that can wick away moisture from the body, unlike wool. Avoiding cotton as the base layer is key in staying warm, for if cotton were to get wet with perspiration, it will stay wet and prevent the body from staying warm.

When exercising in the heat, there are some crucial safety reminders. First, keep in mind your acclamation to the heat. If you have lived in a hot area, you are likely more acclimatized to the heat than someone who has just moved to an area. In the latter, gradually increase the duration and intensity to exercising in the heat. Heat injuries are a real concern for athletes and exercisers, especially during summer months in the southern states.

Heat cramps, heat exhaustion, and heat stroke can all occur with prolonged exposure to heat. **Heat cramps** are painful, brief muscle cramps or spasms. Heat cramps can occur during exercise or work in a hot environment or hours after. Hydration and rest can reduce heat cramps and prevent them from occurring. **Heat exhaustion** is a condition whose symptoms may include heavy sweating and a rapid pulse, as a result of your body overheating. Heat exhaustion is more serious and dangerous than heat cramps, but it is treatable. Some signs and symptoms of heat exhaustion are

- Cool, moist skin with goose bumps when in the heat
- Heavy sweating
- Faintness
- Dizziness
- Fatigue
- Weak, rapid pulse
- Low blood pressure upon standing
- Muscle cramps
- Nausea
- Headache

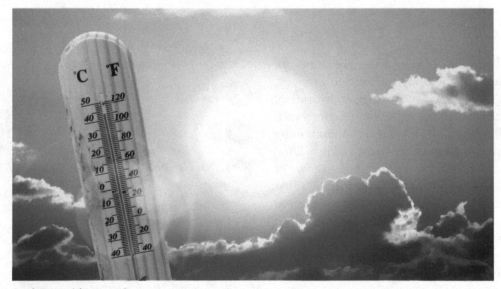
© Ed Connor/Shutterstock.com

If you or someone is experiencing heat exhaustion, stop all activity and rest, move to a cooler place, and drink cool water or sports drinks. Seek medical attention immediately if symptoms worsen or if they do not improve within one hour, if the person becomes confused or agitated and loses consciousness or is unable to drink.

Heatstroke is the most dangerous of heat illnesses. **Heatstroke** is a condition caused by overheating from prolonged exposure to or physical exertion in high temperatures. Heatstroke can occur if your body temperature rises to 104 F (40 C) or higher, and requires emergency treatment. Untreated heatstroke can affect the rest of your body, including the brain, heart, kidneys, and muscles. If treatment is delayed, the risk of serious complications or death greatly increases. Symptoms of a heat stroke are shown in Figure 4.9.

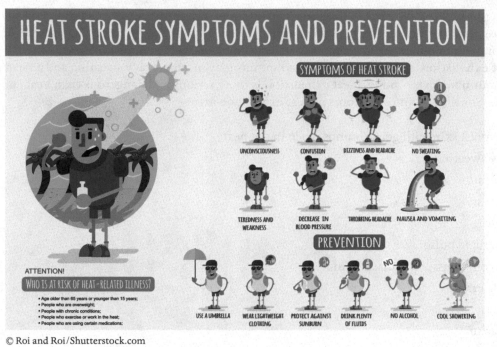

© Roi and Roi/Shutterstock.com

Figure 4.9 Signs & Symptoms of Heat Stroke

Hydration

Adequate hydration is key to the prevention of heat injuries. For the body to function properly, one must take steps toward proper hydration. Water contributes to many bodily functions such as controlling body temperature, maintaining the structure and form of the body, and providing liquid environment for cell processes, as shown in Figure 4.10. Each individual has a specific thirst mechanism relative to the individual's hydration status that informs them that dehydration has already begun. However, to prevent dehydration, pre-hydrating before thirst occurs is important before exercise. The standard recommendation is to drink at least eight 8-ounce glasses of water a day. Exercise increases the body's demand for water owing to an increase in metabolic rate and body temperature. Therefore, if you are consistently exercising, daily recommendations for water intake should be increased to meet the body's demands.

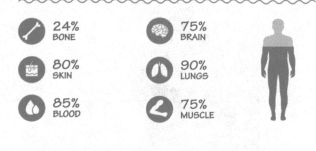

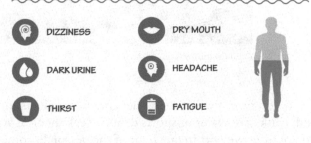

© eveleen/Shutterstock.com

Figure 4.10 Symptoms of Dehydration

PHYSICAL ACTIVITY, EXERCISE, AND YOU
Are You a Healthy Consumer?

Many people would consider themselves a consumer of fitness products . . . but not necessarily of fitness itself. Millions of consumers own fitness memberships, equipment, videos, and apps of exercise, and this does not include the recent popularity of "wellness coaches," also known as personal trainers. Although purchasing these items can be beneficial, efficient, and preferable, they are not always necessary. You do not have to spend money to be physically active, lose or gain weight, or get fit. Make sure you spend wisely when it comes to exercise, and only purchase items in which you see real value. Research products, people, and facilities, and always read the fine print before making big-ticket commitments. The only thing you need to succeed in physical activity is you!

Exercise has shown to increase the quality of life, energy levels, body composition, and self-esteem. Exercise is not limited to a specific group of people. It is for everyone, but exercise might look different for everyone. The first step to a healthy lifestyle is getting started. Choose an exercise routine or activity you enjoy. You are more likely to continue something you enjoy rather than something you do not find interesting. Make a plan of when, where, and how many times you will exercise. Find a workout buddy to help make each other accountable. Lastly, start slowly and listen to your body. If there is pain within the body, something is probably wrong. Do not listen to "no pain, no gain," for it can do more harm than good. Find a balance between activity, leisure time, and rest within each week. Exercise can have a positive impact on numerous health issues and conditions associated with sedentary lifestyles. Exercise helps experience daily benefits such as increased stamina, enthusiasm, enhanced mental state, and more energy. Check out your university's resources on the next page to get you started on your fitness/exercise goals!

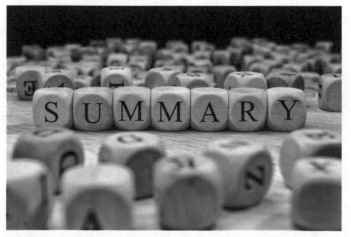

© Fabrick Bilder/Shutterstock.com

In this chapter, we have defined and discussed the elements of physical activity and exercise, including benefits of physical activity and exercise on health and disease risk. We identified guidelines for healthy adults to achieve health improvements with physical activity. We further reviewed ACSM recommendations for increased aerobic and muscular fitness and flexibility. A framework for getting started with physical activity was provided, as well as strategies to reduce injuries and pain. This chapter is a great start to your physical activity and exercise lifestyle! It is up to you to get started!

PERSONAL REFLECTION . . . SO, WHAT HAVE YOU LEARNED?

1. In your own words, summarize (in about five sentences) how participation in a regular physical activity program would affect you specifically. Include information from all sections that describe the impact of physical activity on any health component.

2. What are the ACSM guidelines for physical activity, aerobic exercise, resistance training, and flexibility? Provide one example of each type of activity/exercise.

3. What type of physical activities are available to you at little or no cost?

4. What is one myth about physical activity/exercise from the chapter that surprised you and why?

NOTES

RESOURCES ON CAMPUS FOR YOU!

Recreational services are valuable resources for students, faculty, and staff who wish to pursue a healthy lifestyle. Through participation in various programs, participants can gain a multitude of personal benefits including improved levels of physical fitness and wellness, opportunities for social interaction, time management skills, engagement in a group dynamic setting, a healthy means of stress relief, as well as the creation of a sense of ownership and belonging between students and their college community. Check the services offered on your campus through recreational services.

Examples of services include

- Fitness and wellness
- Group fitness
- Intramural sports
- Club sports
- Personal training
- Aquatics
- Aqua tone water running
- Swimming lessons

REFERENCES

Allsen, P. (2009). *Strength training: beginners, body builders, and athletes* (5th edition). Dubuque, IA: Kendall Hunt Publishing Company.

American College of Sports Medicine [ACSM]. (2012). ACSM's Health/Fitness Facility Standards and Guidelines. Human Kinetics: Champagne, IL.

American College of Sports Medicine. (2013). ACSM information on: Resistance training for health & fitness. Retrieved from www.acsm.org

American College of Sports Medicine, & American Heart Association. (2007). Exercise and acute cardiovascular events: placing risks into perspective." *Medicine and Science in Sports and Exercise*, 39, 5, 886–97.

American Heart Association, & American Stroke Association. (2012). *Heart and Stroke Statistical Update*. Dallas, TX: American Heart Association.

Anxiety and Depression Association of America [ADAA]. (2016). Physical Activity Reduces Stress. Retrieved from: https://adaa.org/understanding-anxiety/related-illnesses/other-related-conditions/stress/physical-activity-reduces-st

Canadian Society for Exercise Physiology. (2002). Physical Activity Readiness Questionnaire. Retrieved from www.csep.ca/forms

Ellingsen, Jan, & The Basics of Barefoot/Minimalist Running Jan. (2012). REI expert advice online. Retrieved from www.physicalactivityplan.org

Pollock, M. L., Gaesser, G. A., Butcher, J. D., Despres, J-P., Dishman, R. K., et al. (1998). ACSM Position Stand on the Recommended Quantity and Quality of Exercise for Developing and Maintaining Cardiorespiratory and Muscular Fitness, and Flexibility in Healthy Adults. *Medicine & Science in Sports & Exercise*, 30, 6, 975–991. 975–991.

Chapter 5

Nutrition +

OBJECTIVES

Students will be able to:

- Review the dietary guidelines for Americans from the USDA
- Identify and describe macronutrients' and micronutrients' sources and nutrition
- Identify essential nutrients and their role in overall health
- Discuss the food nutrition label and the different types of information it present.
- Compare different impacts on diet, such as vegetarianism, food allergies, and Western diet alternatives
- Identify the relationship of nutrition to body composition and weight management
- Describe the role of gut health, probiotics, and prebiotics in overall health

Nutrition Knowledge Assessment. Circle the correct answer.

1. Which of the following is a macronutrient?

   A. carbohydrate   **B.** vitamin D   **C.** water

2. Which of the following food is considered high in fiber?

   A. chicken   **B.** almonds   **C.** eggs

3. Which of the following fats can benefit cholesterol levels?

   A. trans fat   **B.** saturated fat   **C.** unsaturated fat

4. For most adults, how much protein is recommended each day?

   A. 20–25 g   **B.** 45–65 g   **C.** 75–80 g

5. Which of the following nutrients can slow aging by suppressing cell deterioration?

   A. antioxidants   **B.** water   **C.** carbohydrates

6. Superfoods have been shown to reduce the risk of

   A. heart disease   **B.** cancer   **C.** both A and B

7. What type of vegetarian will consume only dairy, fruit, and vegetables?

   A. semivegetarian   **B.** vegan   **C.** lactovegetarian

8. Minerals that the body needs in relatively large quantities are called

   A. microminerals   **B.** macrominerals   **C.** water-soluble vitamins

9. In addition to calcium, milk and dairy products are excellent sources of

   A. vitamin B12   **B.** vitamin C   **C.** zinc

10. Protein amino acids that we must consume in our diet are called

   A. non-essential   **B.** essential   **C.** polyunsaturated

Check your knowledge:

Answers: 1–A; 2–B; 3–C; 4–B; 5–A; 6–C; 7–C; 8–B; 9–A; 10–B

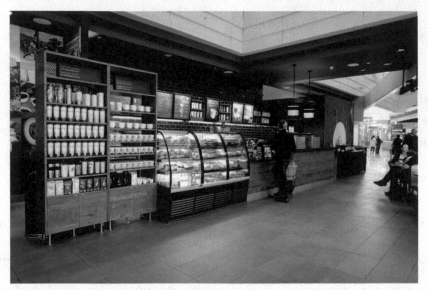

© Sorbis/Shutterstock.com

Introduction to Nutrition

Appropriate, solid nutritional choices are essential for living a healthy lifestyle. Most Americans are not proficient in making the effort to obtain their daily dietary intake. Generally, Americans exceed the recommended intake of salt, sugar, and fat but do not consume the recommended daily allowance (RDA) of vitamins and minerals. Both physical inactivity and poor dietary habits are primary factors that are causing more and more Americans to be overweight or obese. Thus, being overweight or obese is a major risk factor for chronic health problems such as hypertension, cardiovascular disease, diabetes, and certain types of cancers. Keeping this in mind, the importance of building a knowledge base that will allow an individual to develop sound, life-long nutritional habits and practices becomes clear. Once an individual has become proficient enough to make sound nutritional choices, they must then emphasize the necessity to obtain the essential macronutrients and micronutrients through their daily food choices.

In this chapter, we will discuss the different types of nutrients and identify the recommendations and guidelines for healthy diet. Understanding healthy nutrition guidelines can be confusing. The US Department of Agriculture (USDA) and the US Department of Health and Human Services (DHHS) have created guidelines for the general population on healthy dietary practices. We will discuss the guidelines and recommendations in this chapter!

DIETARY GUIDELINES FOR AMERICANS

The Dietary Guidelines for Americans was first published as a scientifically based health promotion in 1980 in an attempt to decrease an individual's risk for chronic diseases through diet and increased levels of exercise. The USDA and the DHHS have since updated and republished these Dietary Guidelines every five years.

The most current version of the Dietary Guidelines was published in late 2015 (http://health.gov/dietaryguidelines/2015/guidelines/executive-summary/). The following is a list of the key recommendations of the Dietary Guidelines.

The Guidelines

1. **Follow a healthy eating pattern across the lifespan.** All food and beverage choices matter. Choose a healthy eating pattern at an appropriate calorie level to help achieve and maintain a healthy body weight, to support nutrient adequacy, and to reduce the risk of chronic disease.

2. **Focus on variety, nutrient density, and amount.** To meet nutrient needs within calorie limits, choose a variety of nutrient-dense foods across and within all food groups in recommended amounts.

3. **Limit calories from added sugars and saturated fats and reduce sodium intake.** Consume an eating pattern low in added sugars, saturated fats, and sodium. Cut back on foods and beverages higher in these components to amounts that fit within healthy eating patterns.

4. **Shift to healthier food and beverage choices.** Choose nutrient-dense foods and beverages across and within all food groups in place of less healthy choices. Consider cultural and personal preferences to make these shifts easier to accomplish and maintain.

5. **Support healthy eating patterns for all.** Everyone has a role in helping to create and support healthy eating patterns in multiple settings nationwide, from home to school to work to communities.

Key Recommendations

Consume a healthy eating pattern that accounts for all foods and beverages within an appropriate calorie level.

A healthy eating pattern includes

- A variety of vegetables from all of the subgroups—dark green, red and orange, legumes (beans and peas), starchy, and others
- Fruits, especially whole fruits
- Grains, at least half of which are whole grains
- Fat-free or low-fat dairy, including milk, yogurt, cheese, and/or fortified soy beverages
- A variety of protein foods, including seafood, lean meats and poultry, eggs, legumes (beans and peas), and nuts, seeds, and soy products
- Oils

A healthy eating pattern limits

- Saturated fats and *trans* fats, added sugars, and sodium
- Consumption of calories to less than 10 percent per day from added sugars
- Consumption of calories to less than 10 percent per day from saturated fats
- Consumption of sodium to less than 2,300 milligrams per day
- Consumption of alcohol (if consumed) in moderation—up to one drink a day for women and up to two drinks per day for men—and only by adults of legal drinking age

Meet the *Physical Activity Guidelines for Americans* (See Chapter 4 Physical Activity & Exercise).

MACRONUTRIENTS

It is important for an individual to ingest more than forty different nutrients in order to maintain good health, including both macro- and micronutrients. It is especially essential to eat a balanced diet because no single food source contains all of these nutrients. **Macronutrients** provide energy in the form of

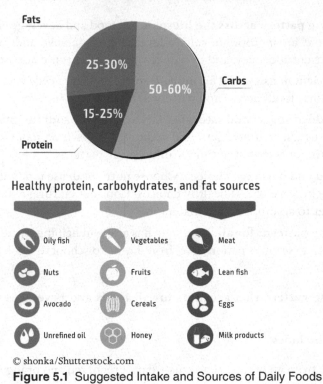

CARB, FAT AND PROTEIN DAILY RATE

Fats

25-30%

15-25%

Protein

50-60%

Carbs

Healthy protein, carbohydrates, and fat sources

Oily fish	Vegetables	Meat
Nuts	Fruits	Lean fish
Avocado	Cereals	Eggs
Unrefined oil	Honey	Milk products

© shonka/Shutterstock.com

Figure 5.1 Suggested Intake and Sources of Daily Foods

calories and include carbohydrates, fats, and proteins within the diet. Eating various food sources will help ensure adequate intake of carbohydrates, fats, and proteins. This section discusses the different types, benefits, and sources of macronutrients.

Carbohydrates

The body's main source of fuel comes from carbohydrates. *Around 55% to 60% of an individual's diet should be composed of carbohydrates. Of this, 45% to 50% of total daily caloric intake should be from complex carbohydrates* (see Figure 5.1). Each carbohydrate provides about 4 calories per gram. **Complex carbohydrates** are carbohydrates that contain a high amount of nutrients, like vitamins, minerals, and fiber. Complex carbohydrates provide the body with a steady source of energy for hours. The best sources of complex carbohydrates are breads, cereals, pastas, and grains. Less than 10% of carbohydrate intake should come from simple carbohydrates. **Simple carbohydrates** are carbohydrates that do not provide a rich source of other nutrients and, therefore, provide empty calories.

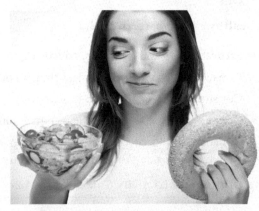

© Juice Team/Shutterstock.com

Dietary fiber, also known as roughage or bulk, is a type of complex carbohydrate that is present mainly in leaves, roots, skins, and seeds and is the part of a plant that is not digested in the small intestine. Dietary fiber helps decrease the risk of certain diseases such as cardiovascular disease and cancer and may lower an individual's risk of coronary heart disease. Dietary fiber can be either soluble or insoluble.

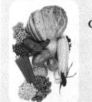

Complex Carbohydrates
- high in micronutrients (minerals & vitamins)
- high in fiber
- more filling
- sustained energy

© Robyn Mackenzie/Shutterstock.com

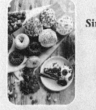

Simple Carbohydrates
- high in sugar (usually processed/refined)
- low in nutrients
- less filling
- can contribute to rapid changes in blood sugar

© Syda Productions/Shutterstock.com

Soluble fiber dissolves in water. It helps the body remove fats and has been shown to lower blood cholesterol levels and blood sugar, as well as helping to control diabetes. Water-soluble fiber travels through the digestive tract in gel-like form, pacing the absorption of cholesterol, which helps prevent dramatic shifts in blood sugar levels. Oats, fruits, barley, and legumes are primary food sources for soluble fiber.

Insoluble fiber is a type of fiber that does not dissolve in water and is not digested by the body, causing softer and bulkier stools and peristalsis (pushing of food through the digestive tract). A diet high in insoluble fiber reduces the risk of cancer within the digestive tract (like colon cancer) by increasing the rate of waste elimination (also known as poops!). Low fiber intake can lead to digestive problems, such as constipation, diverticulitis, hemorrhoids, and obesity. Primary sources of insoluble fiber include wheat, cereals, vegetables, and the skins of fruits. *The recommended daily intake of fiber is 25 to 30 g per day. Although* too much fiber is usually not a problem, in excess, it could lead to diarrhea and nutrient loss. See Figure 5.2 for more healthy sources of fiber.

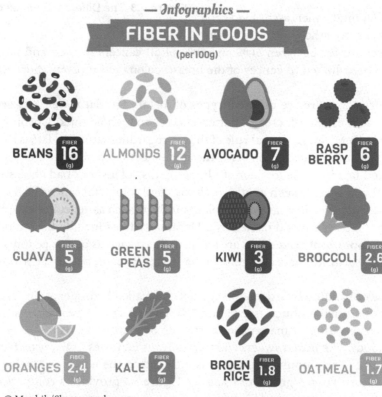

© Monkik/Shutterstock.com

Figure 5.2 These Foods Are Naturally High in Fiber

Fats

Fats are a major source of energy and supply the body with nine calories of energy per gram ingested. Although several Americans get excessive amounts of their daily caloric intake from fats (37% to 40%), dietary fat is not necessarily "bad" for individuals who consume moderate levels in their diet. *In fact, moderate amounts between 25% and 30% of daily calories from fat is necessary for good nutrition.*

Fat has many essential functions: providing the body with stored energy, insulating the body to preserve body heat, contributing to cellular structure, and protecting vital organs by absorbing shock. Fat adds flavor and texture to foods and helps satisfy an individual's hunger owing to gradual digestion; it also supplies the body with essential fatty acids and transports fat-soluble vitamins A, E, D, and K and is necessary for normal growth and healthy skin. Lastly, it is essential in the synthesis of certain hormones.

Fats can have adverse effects on good health when they are consumed in excess. Large amounts of fat in the typical American diet is a major reason why Americans have the highest rates of heart disease globally.

Elevated levels of fat intake increases blood cholesterol levels and leads to atherosclerosis. Diets with too much fat account for between 30% and 40% of all cancers in men and 60% of all cancers in women and have also been linked to cancer of the breast, colon, and prostate more frequently than any other dietary factor.

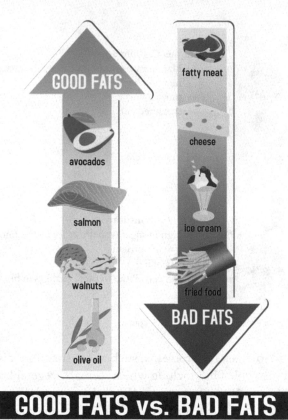

© Elizabeta Lexa/Shutterstock.com

Figure 5.3 The Different Sources of Healthy and Unhealthy Fats

As shown in Figure 5.3, there are different types of dietary fat. **Saturated fats** are found mainly in animal products such as meats, lard, cream, butter, cheese, and whole milk. Coconut and palm oils are two plant sources of saturated fat. A general rule of thumb regarding saturated fats is that they typically do not melt at room temperature (an exception being the abovementioned oils that are "almost solid" at room temperature). Saturated fats increase low-density lipoproteins (LDLs) or "bad cholesterol" levels, which increase one's risk for heart disease such as atherosclerosis and colorectal cancer.

Unsaturated fats are derived primarily from plant products such as vegetable oils, avocados, and most nuts and do not raise the body's blood cholesterol. Unsaturated fats include both monounsaturated and polyunsaturated fats. **Monounsaturated fats** are found in foods such as olives, peanuts, canola oil, peanut oil, and olive oil. **Polyunsaturated fats** are found in margarine, pecans, corn oil, cottonseed oil, sunflower oil, and soybean oil.

Trans fat occurs from adding hydrogen to vegetable oil, called hydrogenation. Trans fat does not occur naturally in plant or animal products (see Figure 5.4). This process increases the shelf life of foods, and include foods such as shortening or margarine shortening or margarine. Trans fat is also found in fried foods and processed foods, like boxed sweets and treats. Trans fat raises LDL (or bad) cholesterol and risk of coronary heart disease. The amount of trans fat is included on the nutrition label and product packaging, unless it contains less than 0.5 grams of trans fat. Figure 5.5 provides a comparison of unsaturated, saturated and trans fat food examples and benefits.

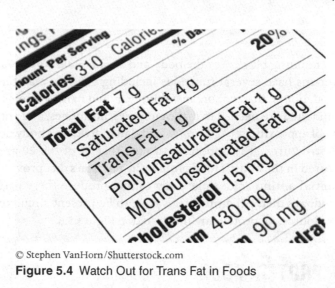

© Stephen VanHorn/Shutterstock.com

Figure 5.4 Watch Out for Trans Fat in Foods

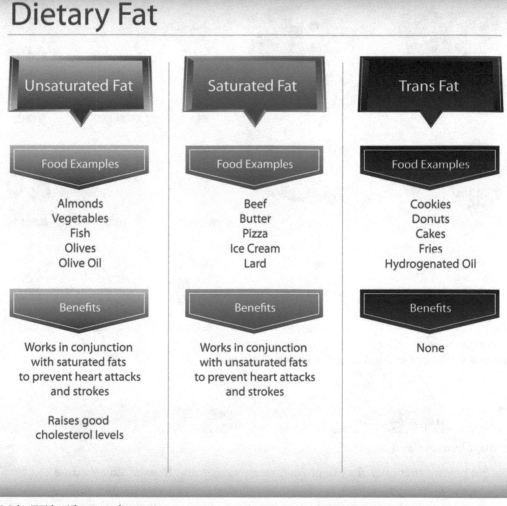

© John T Takai/Shutterstock.com

Figure 5.5 Examples and Benefits of Unsaturated, Saturated, and Trans Fats

Protein

Proteins are the essential "building blocks" of the body and ***should make up approximately 12% to 15% of total calories ingested.*** Proteins have several functions including growth, maintenance, and repair of all body tissues: muscles, blood, bones, internal organs, skin, hair, and nails. Proteins also help maintain the normal balance of body fluids and are needed to make enzymes, hormones, and antibodies that fight infection. Proteins are made up of approximately 20 amino acids; an individual's body needs each amino acid to form the various protein structures. It is important to note that 11 of the 20 are **non-essential amino acids**—they are manufactured in the body if food proteins in a person's diet provide enough nitrogen. The other 9 of the 20 are **essential amino acids**—the body cannot produce these naturally, so they must be supplied through an individual's diet. All amino acids have to be present simultaneously for a particular protein synthesis to occur. Sources of protein are illustrated in Figure 5.6.

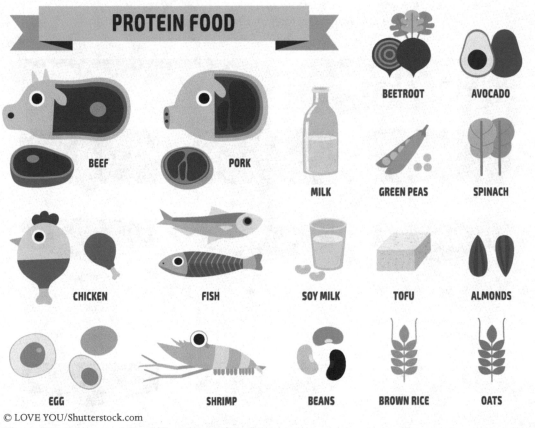

© LOVE YOU/Shutterstock.com

Figure 5.6 Sources of Food That Are High in Protein

Spotlight on . . .

Protein Supplements and Shakes!

Many people believe that once they begin an exercise program, they should consume extra protein through supplements, and most commonly, protein shakes. Although some individuals who train at extremely high levels may need supplementation to address protein needs, this is not the case for most of the general population. "It is inadvisable to consume more protein than the daily recommended dosage (45–65 g/day), particularly in the form of protein supplements. Excessive protein supplementation can damage the kidneys, increase calcium excretion, negatively affect bone health, inhibit muscle growth, and can be detrimental to endurance performance.

Individuals who are trying to maximize muscular strength, endurance, and growth should take in the recommended 1.5 g of protein per kilogram of body weight, as well as an additional 500 calories of complex carbohydrates. The recommended protein and additional complex carbohydrates will work together to provide the extra nutrients and glucose needed for the increased muscular work load."[1]

TABLE 5.1 The Recommended Amount of Each Macronutrient Based on 2000 Calories Per Day

Macronutrient	% of Daily Foods and Calories	Calories per Day
Carbohydrate	45–65	900–1300
Protein	10–35	200–700
Fat	20–35	400–700

MICRONUTRIENTS

Micronutrients do not provide the body with calories but are necessary for regulations and processes within the body. They are also required in smaller amounts than the macronutrients or water. The micronutrients from food are vitamins and minerals.

Vitamins

Vitamins are necessary for normal body metabolism, growth, and development. They are necessary to allow the body to generate energy from the macronutrients of carbohydrates, fats, and proteins. In America, vitamin deficiencies are rare. Vitamins are important because they can reduce the risk of diseases and conditions, and they promote healthy growth, especially in children. Vitamins are especially important during pregnancy and in older populations owing to the increased need for nutrition in this phase. Pregnant women should consume 400 mcg of folic acid per day, and older individuals need to consume more calcium and vitamin D after 70 years than they did when they were younger. Food sources of the different vitamins can be found in Figure 5.7.

There are two types of vitamins—fat-soluble and water-soluble. **Fat-soluble vitamins** are stored and transported by fat and liver cells. Examples of fat-soluble vitamins are A, E, D, and K. Fat-soluble vitamins are stored in the fat cells of body. Over time, fat-soluble vitamins can build up to potentially toxic levels, but this is rare. **Water-soluble vitamins** dissolve in water cells within the body and include the B vitamins and vitamin C. Because they are not stored like fat-soluble vitamins, water-soluble vitamins must be consumed in adequate amounts each day.

Minerals

Minerals are inorganic substances that support many enzyme functions in the body. Approximately 25 minerals have important roles in bodily functions. Minerals are housed in all cells and are concentrated in hard parts of the body—nails, teeth, and bones—they are critical in maintaining water balance and acid–base

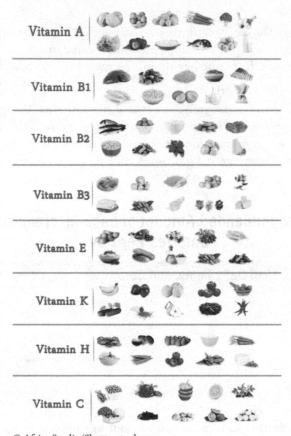

Vitamin A

Vitamin B1

Vitamin B2

Vitamin B3

Vitamin E

Vitamin K

Vitamin H

Vitamin C

© Africa Studio/Shutterstock.com

Figure 5.7 Different Food Sources of Vitamins

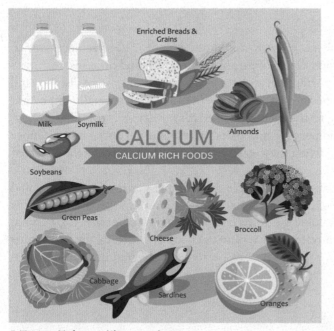

© Tatsiana Tsyhanova/Shutterstock.com

Figure 5.8 Foods That Are High in the Mineral Calcium

balance. Minerals are essential components of respiratory pigments, enzymes, and enzyme systems and also regulate muscular and nervous tissue excitability, blood clotting, and normal heartbeat. Calcium is an example of an important mineral that is critical for bone and muscle health. Foods high in calcium are shown in Figure 5.8.

Macrominerals and microminerals are the two groups of minerals necessary in an individual's diet: **Macrominerals refers to** seven minerals that the body needs to absorb in relatively large quantities (≥100 mg each day). These seven minerals are calcium, chloride, magnesium, phosphorus, potassium, sodium, and sulfur. Usually, these minerals can be acquired by eating a balanced diet. Although **microminerals** are essential to healthy living, they are needed in smaller quantities (<100 mg per day) than macrominerals. Chromium, cobalt, copper, fluoride, iodine, iron, manganese, molybdenum, selenium, and zinc are some examples of microminerals.

Antioxidants

Antioxidants are compounds that assist cells facing an ongoing barrage of damage resulting from daily oxygen exposure, environmental pollution, chemicals and pesticides, additives in processed foods, stress hormones, and sun radiation. Multiple studies suggest that antioxidants possess the ability to suppress cell deterioration and to "slow" the aging process. Americans could realize the potential power of these substances simply by eating a diet with at least five servings of a wide variety of

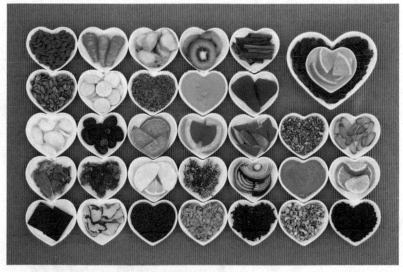

© Marilyn barbone/Shutterstock.com

fruits and vegetables each day. There are numerous proven health benefits of antioxidants. For example, vitamin C speeds the healing process, helps prevent infection, and prevents scurvy. Additionally, vitamin E helps prevent heart disease by stopping the oxidation of low-density lipoprotein (the harmful form of cholesterol); strengthens the immune system; and may play a role in the prevention of Alzheimer disease, cataracts, and some forms of cancer, providing further proof of the benefits of antioxidants. As one can see, sufficient amounts of vitamins, minerals, and antioxidants are crucial to healthy living.

Spotlight on . . .

Organic Foods

Organic foods are foods that are naturally grown without the use of pesticides. These chemical-free foods are much more difficult to grow because they are more vulnerable to disease and pests; thus, they are not "high yield" crops. Because organic foods are less common and harder to grow successfully, they are more expensive. Whether the expense is justified by the improved nutritional quality and overall health benefits is yet to be determined.

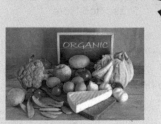

© PIxelbliss/Shutterstock.com

Functional Foods

Functional foods are foods with benefits that go above and beyond basic nutrition. A person's overall health can be greatly affected by the food choices they make. Functional benefits of foods that have been consumed for decades are being discovered and new foods are being developed for their helpful dietary components.

Water

Water is an essential nutrient for life. Although it does not provide calories, we need water in very large amounts. There are many functions of water in the body. Water helps to regulate body temperature, maintains blood volume, and transports fluids throughout the body. Our body is about 70% water, and it

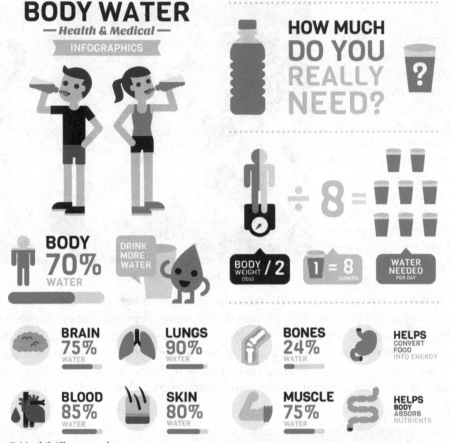

© Monkik/Shutterstock.com

Figure 5.9 Water is Vital to a Healthy Body! Amounts and Benefits Are Presented Here

is a foundational component of physiological functioning. Water should be consumed regularly throughout the day. Any drop in water levels can cause a disruption of the physiological functioning of the body and leads to dehydration. **Dehydration** is a loss of bodily fluid and can be mild to very dangerous. Signs of dehydration can include headaches and confusion. Dehydration that leads to a 10% loss of intracellular water concentration can result in death. People who are overweight; deconditioned or not acclimatized to heat; very old and very young; or do not eat breakfast or drink water are at a higher risk of dehydration.

As shown in Figure 5.9, individuals should aim for at least six to eight 8-ounce glasses of water each day. While exercising, recommendations for water intake are two to three 8-ounce cups of water before exercising, four to six ounces of cool water every 15 minutes during the workout, and rehydrating thoroughly after the activity.

BUILDING A HEALTHY PLATE

MyPlate is an idea that originated from the 2010 Dietary Guidelines for Americans. MyPlate intends to make it easier for consumers to make safer/healthier food choices. MyPlate utilizes the familiar plate setting, using a typical, 9-inch plate in diameter to illustrate the five essential food groups—fruits, vegetables, grains, protein, and dairy—and the relative amounts that should be consumed. Individuals that use MyPlate along with the ChooseMyPlate.gov website have access to practical,

easy-to-understand information that will assist them in building a healthier diet.

ChooseMyPlate uses certain messages to help consumers focus on key behaviors:

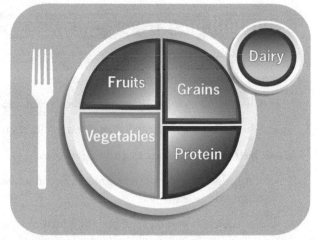

© Basheera Designs/Shutterstock.com

- **Eat the right amount of calories for you.** Everyone has a personal calorie limit. Staying within yours can help you get to or maintain a healthy weight. People who are successful at managing their weight have found ways to keep track of how much they eat in a day, even if they do not count every calorie.

- **Enjoy your food, but eat less.**

- **Cook more often at home, where you are in control of what is in your food. When eating out, choose lower-calorie menu options.**

- **Write down what you eat to keep track of how much you eat. If you drink alcoholic beverages, do so sensibly—limit to one drink a day for women or to two drinks a day for men.**

- **Build a healthy plate.** Before you eat, think about what goes on your plate or in your cup or bowl. Foods like vegetables, fruits, whole grains, low-fat dairy products, and lean protein foods contain the nutrients you need without too many calories. Try some of these options.

- **Keep your food safe to eat—learn more at** www.FoodSafety.gov.

- **Cut back on foods high in solid fats, added sugars, and salt.** Many people eat foods with too much solid fats, added sugars, and salt (sodium). Added sugars and fats load foods with extra calories you do not need. Too much sodium may increase your blood pressure.

- **Choose foods and drinks with little or no added sugars.**

- **Look out for salt (sodium) in foods you buy—it all adds up.**

- **Eat fewer foods that are high in solid fats.**

- Table 5.2 provides details on the amounts of recommendations of food groups for men and women.

TABLE 5.2 Recommendations of Food Groups for Men and Women

Food Group	Examples	Daily Recommendations for Men (Total Calories of 2600–3200)	Daily Recommendations for Women (Total Calories of 1800–2400)
Grains	Breads, cereals, crackers, rice	6–8 oz	9–10 oz
Dairy	Milk, cheese, yogurt	3 cups	3 cups
Fruits	Strawberries, apples, mango	2–2.5 cups	1.5–2 cups
Vegetables	Broccoli, spinach, carrots	2.5–3 cups	3.5–4 cups
Protein-rich	Meats, eggs, legumes, nuts	5–6.5 oz	6.5–7 oz

Spotlight on . . .

MyPlate Food Groups

Make at least half your grains whole.

- Choose 100% whole-grain cereals, breads, crackers, rice, and pasta.

- Check the ingredients list on food packages to find whole-grain foods.

Make half your plate fruits and vegetables.

- Eat red, orange, and dark-green vegetables, such as tomatoes, sweet potatoes, and broccoli, in main and side dishes.

- Eat fruits, vegetables, or unsalted nuts as snacks—they are nature's original fast foods.

Switch to skim or 1% milk.

- They have the same amount of calcium and other essential nutrients as whole milk but less fat and calories.

- Try calcium-fortified soy products as an alternative to dairy foods.

Vary your protein food choices.

- Twice a week, make seafood the protein on your plate.

- Eat beans, which are a natural source of fiber and protein.

Grains

Although it is recommended that grains should make up a good portion of the daily caloric intake, we should recognize that the majority of grains consumed should be whole grains. **Whole grains** are defined as "food made from the entire grain seed, usually called the kernel, which consists of the bran, germ, and endosperm by the American Association of Cereal Chemists (AACC International Board of Directors, 1999). If the kernel has been cracked, crushed, or flaked, it must retain nearly the same relative proportions of bran, germ, and endosperm as the original grain." Some examples of easily accessible whole grains include brown rice, bulgur (cracked wheat), popcorn, whole rye, wild rice, whole oats/oatmeal, whole-grain barley, and whole wheat (see Figure 5.10). These foods also offer a rich supply of dietary fiber and other nutrients. A serving size from the grains group consists of one slice of bread, half a bagel, or one-sixteen-inch tortilla.

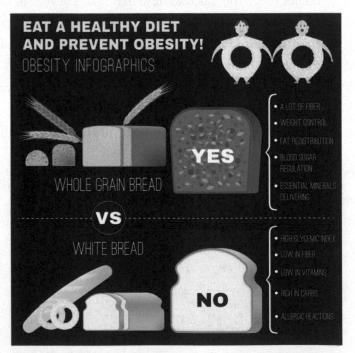

© Double Brain/Shutterstock.com

Figure 5.10 The Differences Between Whole Grain Bread and White Bread

Vegetables

Vegetables are excellent nutritional choices and supply the diet with minerals, vitamins, and fiber. Different colors of vegetables are rich in a variety of vitamins and minerals; therefore, it is important to consume a variety of vegetables. For example, dark green leafy vegetables such as spinach and broccoli are high in calcium, fiber, and vitamin C. Orange vegetables such as carrots provide a high amount of vitamin A. Red vegetables are a great source of lycopene, which is great for heart health. Making vegetables at least one-fourth of your plate for each meal can provide you with healthy, nutrient-rich

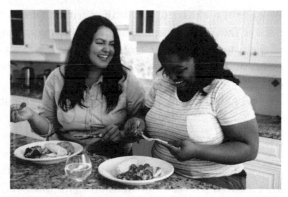
© Monkey Business Images/Shutterstock.com

foods with low calorie intake. One serving from the vegetable group equals one cup of raw, lefty greens; half cup of other chopped vegetables; or three-quarter cup of vegetable juice.

Did you know . . .

What Are Superfoods?

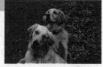
Courtesy of Shelley Hamill

Superfoods are foods that have been shown to reduce the chances of some diseases such as heart disease, cancer, and diabetes. They can also provide valuable nutrients that improve your quality of life, for example by providing immune support and improving memory. Many whole grains, fruits, and vegetables have been shown to have superfood properties! See Figure 5.11.

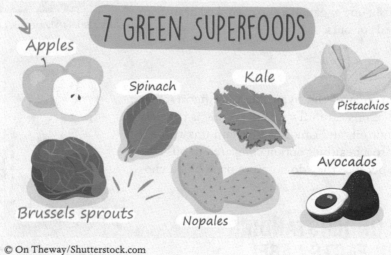
© On Theway/Shutterstock.com
Figure 5.11 Examples of Superfoods

Fruits

Like vegetables, fruits are excellent nutritional choices because they are high in minerals, vitamins, and fiber. Also, like vegetables, the different colors of fruits provide different nutrients to the diet. Aim for a variety of color when choosing fruits. The best source of fruit is fresh fruit, followed by frozen, dried, or canned.

Be careful with dried and canned fruit, as it can be high in sugar, both added and natural. It is also easy to believe that fruit juices are healthy; however, many of them have just as much sugar as a soda with very few of the original nutrition from the fruit. Try to consume the actual fruit as much as possible and reduce fruit juices and canned fruit in syrup. The serving size for fruit is as follows: one serving equals one medium apple, banana, or orange; one melon wedge; half cup of chopped berries; or three-quarter cup of fruit juice.

Milk/Dairy

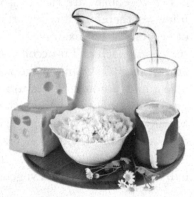

Dairy products are the body's best source of calcium, and they are also an excellent source of protein and vitamin B12. Low-fat and skim alternatives are encouraged to both enhance the benefits of calcium-rich foods and minimize the calories, cholesterol, fat, and saturated fat per selection. One serving from the milk group is equivalent to one cup of milk or yogurt, or one and a half ounces of cheese.

© Madlen/Shutterstock.com

Protein/Meats and Beans

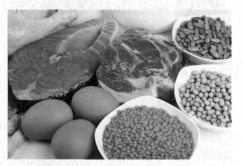

This section of food is very high in protein, iron, zinc, and B vitamins. Aim for foods that are lower in fat from this group because many foods have a high fat content. Because this group contains meat, the foods can be very high in saturated fat, which is the "bad" fat that can lead to other health problems. Lower-fat alternatives within this group that remain a rich source of vitamins and minerals include beans, fish, poultry, and lean cuts of beef. One serving size is about two to three ounces of cooked lean beef, poultry, or fish; one egg; half a cup of cooked beans; or two tablespoons of seeds or nuts.

© Africa Studio/Shutterstock.com

Oils

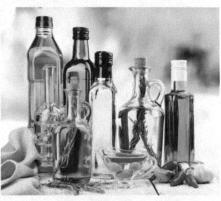

Similar to every other area of the pyramid, it is important to choose your source(s) of oils carefully. A general rule is that oils such as olive oil, peanut oil, and canola oil contain unsaturated fats. Thus, these oils are a healthier option compared to oils that contain saturated fats because they do not raise one's blood cholesterol.

READING AND UNDERSTANDING THE NUTRITION FACTS LABEL

© Africa Studio/Shutterstock.com

Food labels are legally required to include nutrition facts, such as the number of servings per container, serving size, and the number of calories per serving. They must also list the percentage of the daily value of total fat, saturated fat, and trans fat as presented in Table 5.3. Further, food labels must list the percentages of cholesterol, sodium, total carbohydrates (including dietary fiber and sugars), proteins, vitamins, and minerals based on the recommended daily values.[1]

TABLE 5.3 How to Interpret the Information Provided on The Food Label of Nutrition Facts

Food Label: Nutrition Facts

Serving Size

Is your serving the same size as the one on the label? If you eat double the serving size listed, you need to double the nutrient and calorie values. If you eat one-half the serving size shown here, cut the nutrient and calorie values in half.

Calories

Are you overweight? Cut back a little on calories! Look here to see how a serving of the food adds to your daily total. A 5'4", 138-lb. active woman needs about 2,200 calories each day. A 5'10", 174-lb. active man needs about 2,900. How about you?

Total Carbohydrate

When you cut down on fat, you can eat more carbohydrates. Carbohydrates are in foods like bread, potatoes, fruits, and vegetables. Choose these often! They give you more nutrients than sugars like soda pop and candy.

Dietary Fiber

Grandmother called it "roughage," but her advice to eat more is still up-to-date! That goes for both soluble and insoluble kinds of dietary fiber. Fruits, vegetables, whole-grain foods, beans, and peas are all good sources and can help reduce the risk of heart disease and cancer.

Protein

Most Americans get more protein than they need. Where there is animal protein, there is also fat and cholesterol. Eat small servings of lean meat, fish, and poultry. Use skim or low-fat milk, yogurt, and cheese. Try vegetable proteins like beans, grains, and cereals.

Vitamins and Minerals

Your goal here is 100 percent of each for the day. Don't count on one food to do it all. Let a combination of foods add up to a winning score.

Nutrition Facts

Serving Size 1 cup (228g)
Servings Per Container 2

Amount Per Serving

Calories 250   Calories from Fat 110

	% Daily Value*
Total Fat 12g	18%
Saturated Fat 3g	15%
Trans Fat 3g	
Cholesterol 30mg	10%
Sodium 470mg	20%
Total Carbohydrate 31g	10%
Dietary Fiber 0g	0%
Sugars 5g	
Protein 5g	
Vitamin A	4%
Vitamin C	2%
Calcium	20%
Iron	4%

*Percent Daily Values are based on a 2,000 calorie diet. Your Daily Values may be higher or lower depending on your calorie needs:

	Calories	2,000	2,500
Total Fat	Less than	65g	80g
Sat Fat	Less than	20g	25g
Cholesterol	Less than	300mg	300mg
Sodium	Less than	2,400mg	2,400mg
Total Carbohydrate		300g	375g
Fiber		25g	30g

Calories per gram:

Fat 9 • Carbohydrates 4 • Protein 4

More nutrients may be listed on some labels.

Total Fat

Aim low. Most people need to cut back on fat! Too much fat may contribute to heart disease and cancer. Try to limit your calories from fat. For a healthy heart, choose foods with a big difference between the total number of calories and the number of calories from fat.

Saturated Fat

A new kind of fat? No—saturated fat is part of the total fat in food. It is listed separately because it's the key player in raising blood cholesterol and your risk of heart disease. Eat less!

Cholesterol

Too much cholesterol—a second cousin to fat—can lead to heart disease. Challenge yourself to eat less than 300 mg each day.

Sodium

You call it "salt," the label calls it "sodium." Either way, it may add up to high blood pressure in some people. So, keep your sodium intake low—2,400 to 3,000 mg or less each day.*

*The AHA recommends no more than 3,000 mg sodium per day for healthy adults.

Daily Value

Feel like you're drowning in numbers? Let the Daily Value be your guide. Daily Values are listed for people who eat 2,000 or 2,500 calories each day. If you eat more, your personal daily value may be higher than what's listed on the label. If you eat less, your personal daily value may be lower.

For fat, saturated fat, cholesterol, and sodium, choose foods with a low percent Daily Value. For total carbohydrate, dietary fiber, vitamins, and minerals, your daily value goal is to reach 100 percent of each.

g = grams (About 28 g = 1 ounce)
mg = milligrams (1,000 mg = 1 g)

Did you know . . .

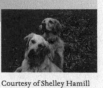

Courtesy of Shelley Hamill

Percent fat of a food refers to the amount of a food that is just fat. You can determine the percent fat of a food by dividing the calories from fat by total calories. For example, for this nutrition label, calories from fat = 100 and total calories = 310.

100/310 = 32% of this food's calories are from fat. Foods that are 35% or higher are considered high-fat food.

Try to limit foods that have higher percentages of fat (Bounds, 2012).

Nutrition Facts

Serving Size 5 oz. (144g)
Servings Per Container 4

Amount Per Serving

Calories 310   **Calories** from Fat 100

	% Daily Value*
Total Fat 15g	**21%**
Saturated Fat 2.6g	**17%**
Trans Fat 1g	
Cholesterol 118mg	**39%**
Sodium 560mg	**28%**
Total Carbohydrate 12g	**4%**
Dietary Fiber 1g	**4%**
Sugars 1g	
Protein 24g	

Vitamin A 1%	•	Vitamin C 2%
Calcium 2%	•	Iron 5%

*Percent Daily Values are based on a 2,000 calorie diet. Your daily values may be higher or lower depending on your calorie needs:

		Calories	2,000	2,500
Total Fat	Less Than		65g	80g
Saturated Fat	Less Than		20g	25g
Cholesterol	Less Than		300mg	300mg
Sodium	Less Than		2,400mg	2,400mg
Total Carbohydrate			300g	375g
Dietary Fiber			25g	30g

Calories per gram:
Fat 9 • Carbohydrate 4 • Protein 4

© Shelby Allison/Shutterstock.com

DIETARY ALTERNATIVES

There are many alternatives to the traditional diet and recommendations based on individuals needs and preferences. In this section, we will discuss vegetarianism, food sensitivities and allergies, and diet styles.

Vegetarianism

Vegetarian diets have become more popular in recent years although different individuals follow these diets for various reasons (religious, ethical, or philosophical). There are four different types of vegetarian diets:

Vegans are considered true vegetarians. Their food selections do not involve animal products, such as meat, chicken, fish, eggs, or dairy products. A vegan's primary sources of protein are vegetables, fruits, and grains (see Figure 5.12). Many vegans choose to supplement their diet with vitamin B12 because it is normally only found in meat products.

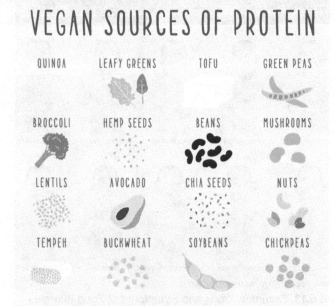

© kondratya/Shutterstock.com

Figure 5.12 Vegan Foods High in Protein

Lactovegetarians eat milk products, fruits, and vegetables but do not consume any other animal products (meat, poultry, fish, or eggs).

Ovolactovegetarians are another type of vegetarian. Although they eat eggs and dairy products and fruits and vegetables, they still do not eat meat, poultry, or fish.

A **semivegetarian** eats fruits, vegetables, dairy products, eggs, and a small selection of poultry, fish, and other seafood but does not consume any beef or pork.

All kinds of vegetarians can meet their recommended nutritional requirements through the foods that are available, but they must be intentional in combining and consuming foods in order to maximize the nutritional value. Without an intentional consumption of food combinations from a wide variety of sources, nutritional deficiencies of proteins, vitamins, and minerals are possible. Without adequate nutrition, proper growth, development, and functionality are affected.

Food Allergies and Sensitivities

Sometimes foods can cause a negative reaction, and this can be a food allergy or food sensitivity, or intolerance. Food allergies and intolerance can cause some of the same symptoms, and one can be confused for the other. A **food allergy** directly affects the immune system, and can cause severe or life-threatening symptoms, including swollen tongue and closed airways. Food allergies involve two parts of the immune system, the immunoglobulin E (IgE) protein that moves through the blood, and mast cells, which you have in all body tissues like your nose, throat, lungs, skin, and digestive tract. When the food allergen is consumed, a process takes place to release chemicals such as histamine, which will cause various symptoms as illustrated in Figure 5.13. Some food allergens can cross into your bloodstream and cause allergic reactions throughout your body. Symptoms of a food allergy include itching in your mouth, vomiting, diarrhea, or belly pain. Food allergens in your blood can cause a drop in blood pressure; in the lungs, they can cause wheezing, and trigger hives or eczema if they reach the skin. This can take place within a few minutes to an hour of consuming the food. Common foods that contain allergens include shellfish, peanuts, tree nuts, milk, and eggs.

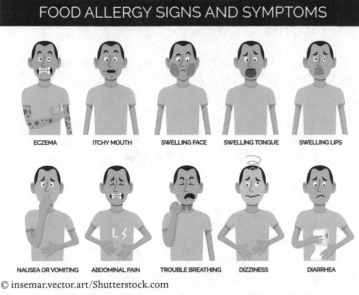
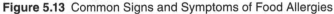

© insemar.vector.art/Shutterstock.com

Figure 5.13 Common Signs and Symptoms of Food Allergies

A **food intolerance** often affects only the digestive system and causes less serious symptoms. Food intolerance is the absence of an enzyme that is necessary to fully digest a food. For example, lactose intolerance is caused by the missing enzyme lactase, which is needed to digest lactose, a milk-derived sugar. Consumption of the foods linked to an intolerance can cause digestive distress, such as cramping, constipation, and diarrhea. People with a food intolerance can sometimes eat small amounts of food without triggering major symptoms or side effects. Sometimes, a food intolerance can be prevented by consuming other foods that may dampen the food-intolerance reaction. For example, those with lactose intolerance may be able to drink lactose-free milk or take lactase enzyme pills to reduce intolerance side effect. Other people can have a sensitivity to food additives. For example, sulfites used to preserve dried fruit, canned goods, and wine can trigger asthma attacks in people who are sensitive to food additives.

Celiac disease is a chronic digestive condition from the protein gluten, found in wheat and other grains. Celiac disease is similar to a food allergy in some ways but is different because anaphylaxis (closed airway) is not a risk. As shown in Figure 5.14, Symptoms often include gastrointestinal issues as well as those unrelated to the digestive system, such as joint pain and headaches. However, people with celiac disease are not at risk of anaphylaxis.

If you have a reaction after eating a particular food, see your doctor to determine whether you have a food intolerance or a food allergy. If you have a food intolerance, your doctor may recommend steps to aid digestion of certain foods or to treat the underlying condition causing your reaction. A registered dietician can also help you find relief with food allergies and sensitivities.

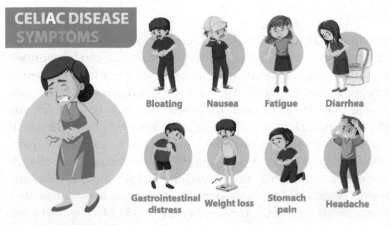

© BlueRingMedia/Shutterstock.com

Figure 5.14 Common Signs and Symptoms of Celiac Disease

Alternatives to the Western Diet

There are alternatives to the typical Western diet, which is high in processed foods, fat, and sugar and low in nutritional value. Some examples of diet alternatives include the Mediterranean diet, Nordic diet, and traditional Okinawa diet. This section provides a brief overview of different alternatives to the typical Western diet.

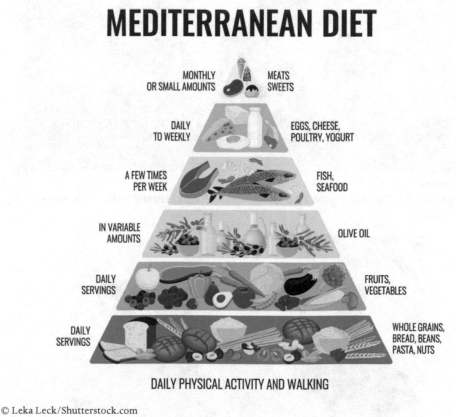

© Leka Leck/Shutterstock.com

Figure 5.15 Foods of the Mediterranean Diet

Mediterranean diet: The Mediterranean diet consists of traditional foods from countries bordering the Mediterranean Sea, including France, Spain, Greece, and Italy. This diet encourages fruits, vegetables, whole grains, legumes, nuts, seeds, and heart-healthy fats, whereas processed foods, added sugar, and refined grains should be restricted. Numerous studies have now shown that the Mediterranean diet can promote weight loss and help prevent heart attacks, strokes, type 2 diabetes, and premature death. This diet is gaining in popularity in other countries owing to its high positive health outcomes. Examples of the Mediterranean Diet are provided in Figure 5.15.

Traditional Okinawa diet: Okinawa is the largest of the Ryukyu Islands located off the coast of Japan between the East China and Philippine Seas and is one of the blue zones of the world. A blue zone is an identified region where people live very long lives compared to the rest of the world (see Figure 5.16). The Okinawa diet reflects the traditional eating patterns of those living on Okinawa and is believed to be a major influence on the lifespan of the Okinawa residents. The traditional Okinawa diet is low in overall calories and fat but high in carbs. It emphasizes vegetables and soy products with limited noodles, rice, pork, and fish. Recently, the diet has shifted to contain more protein and fat, but it is still low-calorie and nutrient-dense. There is a strong emphasis on fruits and vegetables with modest amounts of seafood and lean meat.

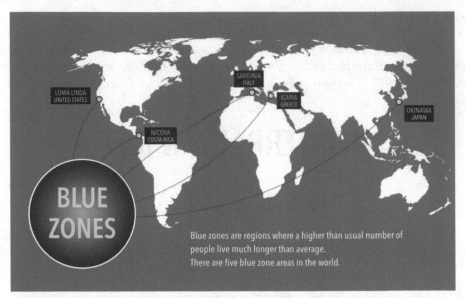

© Dimitrios Karamitros/Shutterstock.com

Figure 5.16 The Blue Zones Represent Areas of Very Healthy Individuals Across the Globe

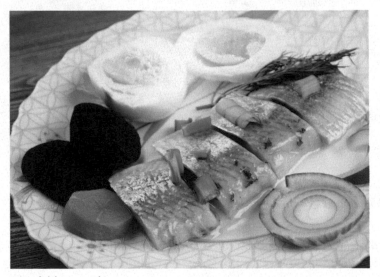

© Fanfo/Shutterstock.com

Nordic diet: The Nordic diet is relatively new, created in 2004 from a group of nutritionists, scientists, and chefs as a way of eating that focuses on locally sourced foods in the Nordic countries—Norway, Denmark, Sweden, Finland, and Iceland. It was created to try to balance the rising obesity rates and sustainable farming. Compared to an average Western diet, it contains less sugar and fat but twice the fiber and seafood. Meat dishes and processed dairy products are limited, but fermented milk and cheese are common ingredients.

French Paradox: The French Paradox diet includes bread, cheese, and wine; the French diet is high in saturated fats but limited in terms of portions. This diet encourages eating smaller amounts of high-quality food rather than overindulging in unhealthy foods.

West African: The West African diet includes lean meat, vegetables, and cereal staples; the West African diet is low in calories and nearly devoid of processed foods. This diet encourages consumption of foods like fruit, vegetables, whole grains, and fish.

GUT HEALTH

Gut health refers to the overall health of the digestive system. Gut microbiota are bacteria that live inside the digestive tract, and they enact a positive influence on the efforts of digestion. The balance of gut microbiota (or good bacteria) is critical for digestive system efficiency and overall health. A diet that includes foods that contain probiotics can help keep the digestive system working effectively, reduce digestive disorders, and improve overall health.

Many of the digestive disorders, including inflammatory bowel disease, Crohn disease, and ulcerative colitis can be identified, prevented, and treated by a qualified nutritional professional, such as a registered dietician. Spend a few extra minutes reviewing the disorders related to nutrition, such as celiac disease, other gluten-related disorders, and irritable bowel syndrome.

Prebiotics and Probiotics

Probiotics are live microorganisms (i.e., bacteria) intended to confer a health benefit on the host. Yogurt and other fermented foods are rich sources of probiotics. Probiotics help to digest food, to destroy disease-causing cells, or to produce vitamins. Probiotics may contain a variety of microorganisms, with the most common bacteria being *Lactobacillus* and *Bifidobacterium*. There are hundreds of different types of microorganisms, but these two are the most commonly researched and have the greatest amount of evidence for positive outcomes. A diet rich in probiotics has shown improvements in gut health, which has been linked to better health outcomes, such as improved mental health, reduced risk for heart disease and diabetes, and improved athletic performance.

Prebiotics are foods that fuel probiotics and provide energy for probiotics. Basically, it is food for the probiotics to eat in order to improve the gut health. Foods rich in prebiotics include vegetables, whole grains, and fruits. Figure 5.17 provides food sources of both prebiotics and probiotics.

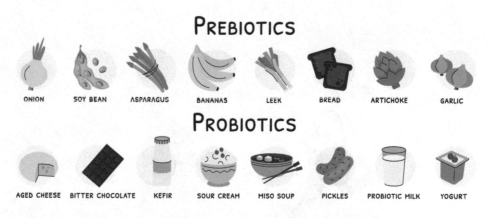

© kanvictory/Shutterstock.com

Figure 5.17 Sources of Probiotics, and the Food that Fuels Them, Prebiotics

BODY COMPOSITION AND WEIGHT MANAGEMENT

Other than physical activity and exercise, nutrition intake plays the biggest role in body composition and weight management. The basis of body weight equals the amount of calories consumed versus the amount of calories burned (or used). If you are participating in higher amounts of physical activity than previously, then you are probably burning more calories than you are consuming, which would lead to weight loss. If you are eating more calories than you are burning through exercise, physical activity, or daily movements, then you have a higher caloric intake, which will lead to weight gain. If you consume the same amount of calories that you burn, then you will stay about the same body weight.

Products that claim to increase the body's metabolism may contain dangerous substances, such as ephedra, or they may just contain increased levels of caffeine, which might have adverse effects. The best weight loss plan is one of balance, as shown in Figure 5.18. Weight is controlled by many factors, including genetics and learned behaviors, but the basics of weight gain or loss is a balance between calories in and calories out. If you burn more calories than you consume, you will lose weight. The rate at which the body burns calories varies and is affected by gender and age, among other factors. The best weight loss plan is one that results in one to two pounds of weight loss a week. Programs that result in drastic weight loss in a short period of time are not easily sustained because most of the weight lost is cause by dehydration (Hamilton, 2010).

If you are trying to lose weight, remember a few important points:

- Body weight and body composition are highly influenced by your genetics.
- Your ability to lose weight is dependent on the types of foods you consume and how much physical activity you perform.
- Never starve yourself. Just consume more healthy foods that are low in calories, fat, and sugar and are higher in nutrients.

If you are trying to gain weight, remember a few important points:

- Body weight and body composition are highly influenced by your genetics.
- Increase your overall caloric intake, but still focus on healthy foods.
- Include resistance training to increase muscle mass.

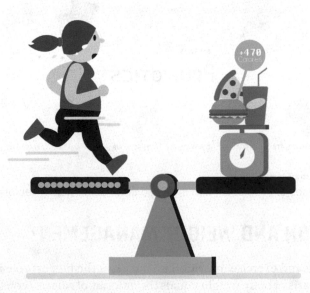

© Mangssab/Shutterstock.com

Figure 5.18 A Balance of Diet and Physical Activity Is the Best Approach to a Healthy Lifestyle

Spotlight on . . .

Diets and Diet Plans

Many Americans have a desire to lose weight. Many diet plans are marketed as quick, easy, and effective, and some of them might live up to this claim. Diets that promote eating only one food for a long period of time are not recommended. Limiting the diet to only one food source is not healthy because this limits vitamin and mineral intake. If a diet asks for the elimination of one energy source, such as carbohydrates, this is also not a healthy choice because it limits the body's source of energy and all sources play a unique role in the maintenance of total wellness.

Diets that severely limit caloric intake or require a period of fasting are never a good idea because this will put the body into starvation mode. If the body perceives that starvation is imminent, it will stop naturally burning calories by shutting down metabolism. It is very difficult to jump start the body's metabolism once it slows.

NUTRITION AND YOU
Are You a Healthy Consumer?

Nutrition and consumerism are strongly related. Most of us do not grow the foods we eat, so we must purchase them from a food market or restaurant. Consumer research within nutrition focuses on various types of behaviors. When do you tend to make your nutrition consumer choices? If you are waiting until you are really hungry or thirsty, you may be more likely to just choose anything, regardless of whether it is healthy or not. Do you use emotions when you purchase your food? If you are sad or anxious or depressed, you may purchase food that you perceive is "comforting." Realistically, most of the "comfort" foods that people gravitate to are not very healthy.

Being a healthy consumer of nutrition products includes a health literacy component. It is easier for those that have some general knowledge or education about nutrition to use tools to make healthy decisions. Understanding how to read and use the information on food labels is critical to becoming a healthy consumer of nutrition products. Beware of "fad" diets or products that make boastful claims about their effectiveness. Be smart about where you are spending your money, even as it relates to your nutrition consumer behaviors!

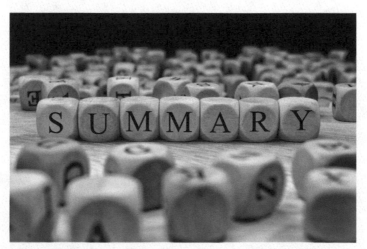

© Fabrick Bilder/Shutterstock.com

In this chapter, we defined and described basic nutrition information regarding macronutrients and micronutrients. We identified sources of both healthy and unhealthy foods and described the current dietary guidelines by the US Department of Health and Human Services. We discussed strategies for individuals to make healthier nutrition choices. This chapter also covered the importance of reading and understanding food nutrition labels, in order to be a more healthy consumer of nutrition products. By understanding one's macronutrient and micronutrient needs and their functions and sources, students can feel in control of their dietary needs, body composition, and weight management.

PERSONAL REFLECTIONS . . . SO, WHAT HAVE YOU LEARNED?

1. Why do you think it is so difficult for most people to eat healthy?

2. In your own words of AT LEAST five sentences, summarize the nutrition guidelines and key recommendations for healthy Americans.

3. List the purpose of the following nutrients: carbohydrates, fats, proteins, and fiber. What is at least one healthy source of each?

4. What impact does your current nutrition choices have on your overall health?

5. Identify at least one change you would like to implement in your nutrition behaviors here. How can you make the change effective?

NOTES

REFERENCES

Bounds, L., Darnell, G., Shea, K.B., & Agnore, D. (2012). *Health and fitness: A guide to a healthy lifestyle* (5th ed.). Dubuque, IA: Kendall Hunt Publishing Company.

Hamilton, A.R. (2010). *Health and the environment: Choices that lead to better health.* Dubuque, IA: Kendall Hunt Publishing Company.

U.S. Department of Agriculture. (2016). *Building a healthy eating style.* Retrieved from http://choosemyplate.gov/MyPlate

U.S. Department of Health and Human Services and U.S. Department of Agriculture. (2015). *2015–2020 dietary guidelines for Americans* (8th ed.). Retrieved from http://health.gov/dietaryguidelines/2015/guidelines/

Chapter 6

Relationships +

OBJECTIVES

Students will be able to:

- Identify the differences in communication patterns.
- Discuss how technology may impact communication
- Identify and describe what makes a healthy relationship.
- Identify and describe the warning signs of an unhealthy relationship.
- Identify the types of abuse
- Discuss the cycle of abuse and why it may be difficult for someone to leave an abusing relationship.

RELATIONSHIP SURVEY

Think about the following questions:

1. What are the top 10 qualities you want in an intimate partner?
2. Which ones are non-negotiable, as in they must have these qualities for you to be with them?
3. Do you think you will have the same requirements in 5 years? Why or why not?
4. What would you say are your own top 10 qualities?

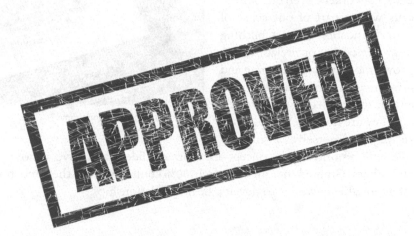

© Mahesh Patil/Shutterstock.com

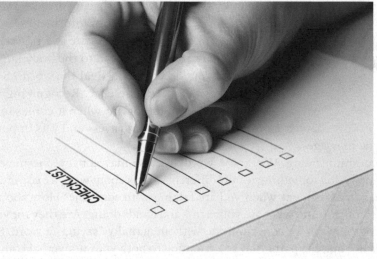

© Di Studio/Shutterstock.com

HEALTHY RELATIONSHIPS

There are many types of relationships. You have those with family, friends, acquaintances, life-long partners, and many in-between. While examining the different types, it is also important to look at how they can grow and change and the different stages they may take.

Positive Self-Esteem

You may have heard along the way that in order to be in a healthy relationship with someone else, you first must value yourself. That is known as positive self-esteem and we develop it over time. Feedback we receive from others is often where we start that process. Family, friends, co-workers, even our accomplishments provide us with a part of our sense of self-worth. While our foundation for establishing positive self-worth may come from our relationships with others, as we grow emotionally, developing and sustaining that positive image from within becomes important. If we continue to rely on others to provide that sense of worth, if they are no longer in our lives for some reason we may find ourselves losing our sense of value.

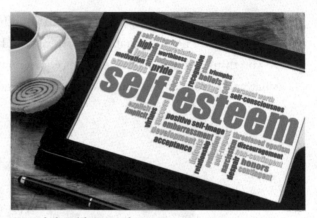

© marekuliasz/Shutterstock.com

People with a positive self-concept are more confident and have a more positive attitude about themselves and others. Granted, not all of us feel 100% confident all of the time, but the better our sense of self-worth the more likely we are to develop healthy relationships.

Communication

According to the Oxford dictionary, communication is the "imparting or exchanging of information by speaking, writing, or using some other medium; the conveying or sharing of ideas and feelings; the means of sending or receiving ideas or information" (Oxford dictionaries).

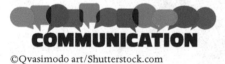

©Qvasimodo art/Shutterstock.com

Tone, pitch, and intonation are additional parts of communication. You are paying attention to the body language, and you hear the words, but do you really **hear** the words? Sometimes the inflection makes all of the difference. Recognizing what someone is really saying is also important when it comes to **consent**, which we will talk about later in this chapter. Communication has many layers and it is important to develop the skill-set to decipher the messages.

We are always communicating. While the words we use may convey one message, our non-verbal communication may be saying something totally different. Think about ways we communicate non-verbally. Do you nod your head in agreement when you are talking with someone? How about your facial expressions? Are you an eye "roller"? And what are your arms and hands doing? Are they moving, open or crossed? These are just some of the ways we communicate without actually "saying" a word. Sometimes it's intentional and sometimes not but, the point is to pay attention to both your nonverbal communication and that of others. It really is true that actions speak louder than words. Make sure your's saying is what you mean.

Another nonverbal to be aware of is the space between two individuals when they are communicating. Some stand close together, while others prefer space in between. This personal space requirement may develop based on culture or experience and may also adjust based on the relationship between the individuals. That said, it is always interesting to watch people with different personal space requirements adjust their postures when they are talking. Be mindful of what your space needs are as well as those you are communicating with.

Communication in the Age of Technology

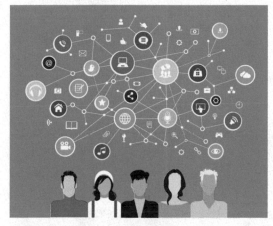
©VLADGRIN/Shutterstock.com

According to the Pew Research Center, 96% of people own a cell phone and 81% own a smart phone. Additionally, ¾ own a laptop and ½ own a tablet (Pew Research Center). And, depending on your source, text messaging is in the hundreds of billions and there is no slowing down! Think about how many text messages you send or receive each day. Of course, that does not include instant messaging, Snapchat, Twitter, Instagram, and the many other electronically-assisted correspondences.

While electronic communication may be fast, it isn't always easy. How do you convey your tone or emotions when you are texting? Do you use emoticons or acronyms? We have a new language where we

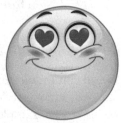
©Yayayoyo/Shutterstock.com

know what "lol" or "btw" means. However, have you ever been misunderstood in a text? There are countless articles citing how electronic communication has impacted our ability to communicate face-to-face. Think about...have you ever seen two people sitting at the table together and instead of talking to one another, they are texting each other? It has become much easier for some people to hide behind the screen rather than engage in an in-person dialog especially if the conversation can be difficult. How you communicate may impact your present and future relationships.

Communicating Effectively

What does it mean to communicate effectively? One key is to actually "be present". Pay attention to the other person(s) with whom you are communicating. Avoid distractions, like looking at your phone or turning your head when someone walks by. Some believe that listening means you are using your eyes to focus on the person, your ears to actually listen, your heart for understanding, and your undivided attention.

Remember to not interrupt or try and complete the other person's sentence. While some people think because they know the other person so well it is "ok" to complete their sentences, it really isn't. Do not formulate your response to something the person is saying until they are finished. Listen to listen, don't listen to respond. Doing so allows you to actually hear everything they are saying rather than blocking it out while you are considering your response. And, don't forget the non-verbals are always "talking".

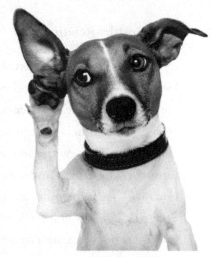
© Javier Brosch/Shutterstock.com

Effective communication entails actually communicating. Some people play "guess what I am thinking" or "if you really cared you would know what I mean," but the reality is we are not mind readers! If you have something to say, say it. If you have an opinion or something is bothering you, let it be known. Making someone guess can create unnecessary stress and misunderstanding in relationships.

Did you know . . .

According to Forbes (2020) there are 12 Concrete Ways to Listen Effectively:

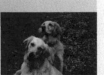

Courtesy of Shelley Hamill

1. Listen with all of the senses.
2. Don't make assumptions.
3. Adopt a posture of deep curiosity.
4. Drop your defensiveness.
5. Ask yourself what matters most.
6. Pay attention to non-verbal communication.
7. Become present physically.
8. Allow yourself 5 seconds of silence.
9. Take one breath.
10. Move around during the conversation (when appropriate).
11. Take notes (when appropriate).
12. Listen from the other person's point of view.

Communication Styles

We all communicate a little differently. Each of us has our own unique style and it can change in any given situation. For example, you probably communicate a bit differently with your friends than with your parents. We typically learn our initial communication styles from our parents, friends, siblings, and others. Combine that with our personality and we have a basic mix of all the above. And, of course, our style may change over time with experience.

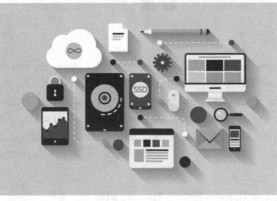

© Bloomua/Shutterstock.com

Spelling a Healthy Relationship
(adapted from Kuriansky, 2002)

Honesty—always tell the truth even if it will initially hurt.

Harmony—enrich one another's differences.

Heart—give your whole heart.

Honor—hold others in high regard.

Happy—be happy with each other.

Empathy—be able to understand what each other feel.

Equality—treat the other as your equal.

Energetic—be spontaneous, relationships take energy.

Enthusiasm—be excited about being together.

Empowerment—support each other.

Acceptance—know that you approve of each other just the way they are.

Accommodation—make adjustments for each other's needs.

Appreciation—be grateful for each other.

Adaptability—be able to make changes when necessary.

Agreements—make an agreement and hold to it.

Love—should be unconditional.

Loyalty—be devoted, never betray each other.

Listening—actively listen, it makes the other person feel important.

Laughter—have fun together.

Lust—sparks the union.

Trust—being able to relax around the other person.

Talking—communication is the key.

Time—spend time together. Nothing is more important than time.

Tenderness—treat each other with kindness.

Thoughtfulness—show consideration in thoughts and actions.

Home—create a safe haven.

Healing—work together to heal new and old wounds.

Humility—admit when you are wrong.

Hope—for a better tomorrow when things are not at their best.

Homework—relationships are not easy, they do require constant work.

YES! Say yes as often as you can.

Recognizing other's communication styles as well as your own can make a difference in relationships, especially in the beginning. Sometimes our differences or misunderstandings are really due to our communication patterns. When we recognize and understand the differences, we can adjust and reduce miscommunication.

Left-Brain vs. Right-Brain . . . there is really no such thing

So, what does this mean? Many people believe they are left brain or right brain thinkers. From books to television programs, you've probably heard the phrase mentioned numerous times or perhaps you've even taken an online test to determine which type best describes you. You've probably spotted at least a few infographics on Pinterest or Facebook claiming to reveal your dominant brain hemisphere (Cherry, 2020).

People who identify as left-brain thinkers might feel that they have strong math and logic skills. Those who profess to be right-brain thinkers, on the other hand, feel that their talents are more on the creative side of things. Given the popularity of the idea of "right brained" and "left brained" thinkers, it might surprise you to learn that this idea is just one of many myths about the brain. Additionally, people are said to prefer one type of thinking over the other. For example, a person who is "left-brained" is often said to be more logical, analytical, and objective. A person who is "right-brained" is said to be more intuitive, thoughtful, and subjective. **The truth is both sides of the brain work together to process whatever is necessary to fulfill the task at hand.**

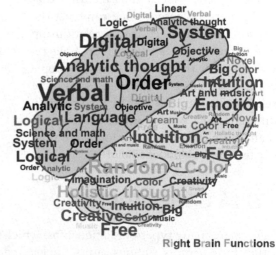

Left Brain Functions

Right Brain Functions

© Photoraidz/Shutterstock.com

That said, some use this concept to note differences in communication patterns. Popular wisdom over the years has stated that men and women communicate differently and listed the specifics of what that looked like. The focus of males being more "logical" and females being more "emotional" continued to be emphasized in communication patterns. The reality is that **gender does not determine a person's communication pattern**. Not only that, a person's pattern of communication may be dependent upon the situation they are in at the time. Perhaps what is more significant is recognizing what that communication pattern is so that the exchange can be more meaningful or less frustrating.

Compromise

Conflict is a part of any relationship at some point. If you and your partner or friend reach an impasse on an issue or situation, it may be necessary to compromise. There are always at least two sides to every issue or situation. If you and your partner cannot reach an agreement, talk about the positives and negatives from your respective positions. Why do you feel something needs to happen and listen to why the other person believes differently? If you still can't reach agreement, then find some middle ground. Of course, sometimes compromise just isn't possible and one person may concede the position. That's fine as long as one person is not always conceding.

Trust

Trust is the foundation for any healthy relationship. It does not matter whether a friend or a partner, establishing trust is key for individuals that are spending time together and sharing their life experiences. Remember, trust takes time to develop and does not happen overnight. Some use the "Onion Theory" of communication when describing building relationships. We share or disclose something about ourselves to another and want them to reciprocate. Nothing too deep or personal until we know we can trust them. As we continue to build trust, those layers of the onion are peeled back. "Be cautious and do not expose deep feelings and internal ideas too early, but at the same time give others a chance to build trust little by little. In a relationship built upon trust one can discuss issues with confidence and know that these ideas will be kept private if necessary. Another element associated with trust is that in this person's absence one can trust the friend's ideas and actions. A relationship built upon trust can have incredible rewards. With this added element, people are comfortable being themselves and the relationship can develop to a completely different level. When complete trust exists many problems such as jealousy are non-existent in the relationship."[1]

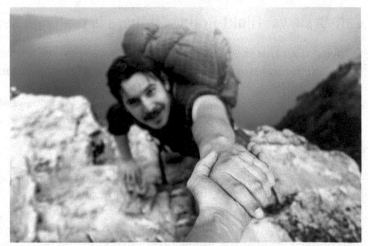

© frankie's/Shutterstock.com

TYPES OF RELATIONSHIPS

"There are many types of relationships, which fulfill many different needs. We begin with our family relationships, parents, siblings, aunts, uncles, and so on. This is the core of our foundation. In today's society we have many different structures that represent 'family.' Some people are raised by both of their biological parents, or maybe just one parent, others by grandparents, and others are adopted, to name a few. These initial relationships have a huge impact upon how we relate with others. What type of relationship do you have with your parents? Is it close? What changes would you make in your relationships with family members if you had the chance? Who has impacted you the most in your family? Was this a positive or negative impact? When there is a good foundation of healthy relationships with family members this typically carries over to friendships and intimate relationships."[1]

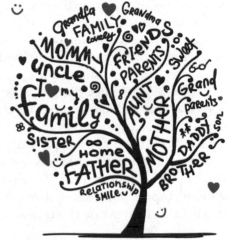

©Kudryashka/Shutterstock.com

Parental Relationship

We have many stages of communication with those who raise us, our parents or guardians. Think about it. We start non-verbal, learn how to talk and, hopefully, progress over time to mutual sharing and engagement as adults. Clearly, there are many different stages along the way. Problems can occur, however, if an adult or child, is ready to transition to the next stage and the other is unwilling or unable. It is very important for adults, and children to be aware of those changing stages and work towards honest open communication to reduce conflicts.

Making the Transition to College

"While there have been many developmental changes along the way, transitioning from high school to college can be a stressful and challenging time for both students and parents. Moving from the position of child or adolescent to young adult in just a few short months after graduation can create uncertainty about roles and responsibilities. The transition from dependence to independence can create difficulties in "deciphering boundaries and expectations. This is especially true if the parents are still paying for living and college expenses. The young adult is experiencing complete independence for the first time in their life. No one is there to tell them when to be home, what and when to eat, who to hang out with, et cetera. This is refreshing and exhilarating to most students, but it can also be a significant unrecognized stressor. It is not uncommon for the new college student to feel anxiety from the new situation, but not immediately recognize its source. Many college freshmen report an internal struggle between their need for complete independence and the relative comfort of the past parent-child bond. This unfamiliar situation can result in a new form of tension when the college student returns home for winter and summer break."[1]

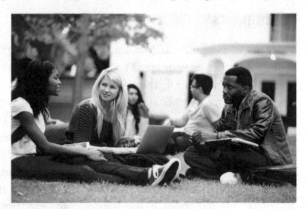

©Monkey Business Images/Shutterstock.com

"It is important to remember that both the college student and the parents have gone through significant transitions in their lives. Confusion and conflict can come from two different realities. Some parents assume the past relationships will be unchanged when the student returns home and hold onto the former expectations. It is still the parent's house and their child is coming back. Many parents believe that if they are under their roof, then the parent's rules apply. The college student, however, has become accustomed to complete freedom and typically does not life the increased control in their life. On the other hand, some parents have moved on to the next stage of their lives. They become accustomed to an empty house with fewer obligations to a dependent child in the home. In this case, tension may arise when the student comes home with the expectation, or even the need, for everything to be as it was when they left. Anxiety can be inadvertently increased when the student realizes that their safety net is no longer the same place they remember. It is likely still there, it just feels or looks different.

"One way to bridge this gap of expectations is to recognize that different perspectives exist and have open dialogue with one another about each other's needs and wants prior to visiting or shortly after arriving. Try to keep emotions calm and allow everyone ample time to speak. It may be helpful for everyone involved to write down and prioritize their expectations and needs before having a discussion. By doing this, it can help identify the areas that are less important and thus can be compromised upon and the areas that cannot be compromised. If at all possible, it is best to try and meet in the middle on the majority of the differing expectations. Recognizing that everyone is in a different stage of life than they were just a year or two before can help ease this transition."[1]

Peer Relationships

College provides the opportunity to meet many new people from diverse backgrounds and experiences. It is the opportunity to expand your circle of friends and to adjust to new relationships with peers. Learning how to navigate through the many opportunities with new peers in various settings can be an important part of the college experience. Take the time to get to know others that are different than you. Campus event, clubs and organizations as well as classes allow you to engage with many people. Expanding your circle of friends and learning different perspectives can be an important part of the college experience.

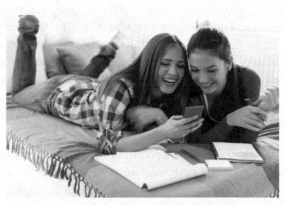
© Stock Rocket/Shutterstock.com

Roommates

"Another important relationship that is typically new to a college student is that of a roommate. Many people think that if they were best friends in high school, they will make perfect college roommates. There are more complicated dynamics that exist with roommates far beyond that of a traditional friendship. Making this assumption can set one up for possible roommate struggles. In some cases, the prior friendship creates barriers to living together harmoniously. Various hygiene habits, different sleep patterns, and different expectations for residence hall or apartment cleanliness can make the best of friends experience difficulty."[1] What about living with a complete stranger, which often happens during the first semester of school? How do you navigate through those expectations while still getting to know the person?

In addition to adjusting to a new living arrangement, one must also learn to balance new-found freedom, and the responsibilities that go along with college education demands. It is helpful to recognize these adjustments and work toward a smooth transition. Any of these changes can cause stress and friction between roommates

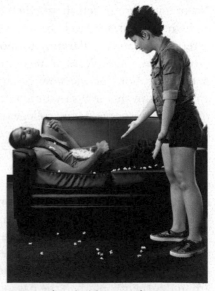
© Rommel Canlas/Shutterstock.com

Spotlight on . . .

Rommate Agreement

It is a great idea for you and your new roommate(s) to agree upon and then document your expectations from each other. In an ideal world, you would be able to do this before you get to campus. If not, make sure to get have the conversation within the first few weeks.

Things you want to agree upon might include:

1. Who does what and when with respect to household cleanup?
2. What is the rule about items in the refrigerator?
3. What about overnight guests?
4. Pet? If yes, what kind and what are the expectations.
5. What are the rules around study time and quiet time?
6. What about borrowing stuff from each other? Does it include clothing or books? What happens if something gets damaged?

These are just a few of the items to think about. Feel free to add more to your agreement. Once you have the answers, make sure to have each person sign and date. Consider revisiting the contract every few months to see what's working or if there needs to be adjustments. Schedules do change from semester to semester and there may well be a need for tweaking.

which can interrupt sleep, study time, and create uncomfortable living arrangements. As previously discussed in the section on communication, people need to talk with one another.

If a problem comes up, or someone isn't holding up their end of the agreement, make sure to address it in a respectful way but do so early. Do not allow a problem to fester as it could hurt your relationship. Sometimes, leaving a note or a reminder may jog someone's memory. If there needs to be a conversation, remember the points discussed earlier in the text on communication.

© Kendall Hunt Publishing Company

When discussions and compromise do not resolve more serious problems, then it is time to consider consulting a third party or a new living arrangement. Most dorms or residence halls have a resident assistant (RA) to help with these types of situations. Be sure that the RA is able to hear all sides of the situation so that they have a good understanding of what is actually happening. Remember, there are always two sides (or more) to every story. If you do not believe that this type of conflict resolution will be helpful to the problem, then it is probably time to consider moving to a different room or find a new roommate.

Types of Friendships

"There different levels of friendship: casual, close, and intimate. Each of these friendships can be very beneficial. The key ingredients to a successful friendship include steadfastness, honesty, reliability, and trust. Casual friendships are good for camaraderie, someone to see a movie with, or eat lunch. In close friendships, there is typically a greater investment of time and emotional energy. Benefits typically seen with close friendships are those that can stand the test of time. There is a connection beyond the surface and a history with this person. Typically close friends know more about you than a casual acquaintance and can be called upon more easily in a time of need."[1]

Consider the many ways people might meet on a college campus: classes, clubs, organizations, sport, events, and residence halls. Each provides different opportunities for interaction. Technology may also play an important role. Now its someone "liking" something you said in a "chat" or "hitting", or "DMing" you back to start a conversation is now the norm. We communicate through our phones through apps that can alter your appearance, your age, even apps that let you know if there is someone

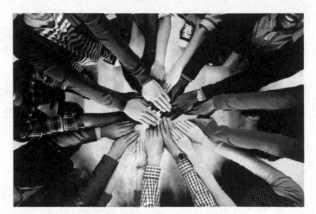
© Rawpixel.com/Shutterstock.com

in your vicinity that you might be a "match" with. But remember, you never know who you might be talking with on the internet. And if you use this method for meeting up with someone, always make sure those initial meetings are in a safe public place. Be cautious when using Facebook, Snapchat, or Tinder type apps. Posting personal information on the Internet can make it easy for those wishing to cause harm to have access to you and your information. It is relatively easy for criminals to piece together random information and figure out where you live or what your usual routine is.

Dating in the Age of Technology

"Dating is the process of getting to know other people as well as yourself while growing with and from each relationship. Typically, a date is stimulated by physical attraction, which can lead to emotional and physical intimacy. One of the outcomes of this process can be finding someone with whom we can happily spend the rest of our life. This process can be incredibly exciting and frustrating all at the same time. Each new relationship exposes one to new and exciting experiences. While dating, your abilities, strengths, and interests can be maxi-

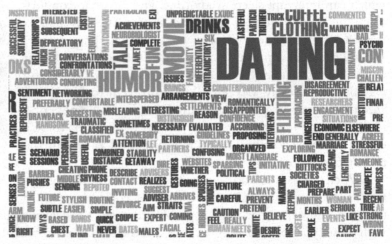
© kentoh/Shutterstock.com

mized. As you are learning who you are and what you like, you should prioritize which characteristics are important and which are not. There is so much to be learned during the dating process. How do you relate to your partner in an intimate setting? What expectations do you have for the person with whom you want to live the rest of your life?"[1]

But how do you find someone you want to date? While many people meet through friends or engaging in activities of mutual interest, in today's world there are many other ways to meet people you may be interested in dating. The internet is full of information on apps you can download to "find your perfect match for dating or hooking up". One study reports that 73% of college students report using Tinder to find a potential date. Other apps like Grindr, Scruff, and Her are designed for the Lesbian, Gay, and Bisexual (LGB) population and a new app has just been released called Thurst for LGBTQ, which includes transsexuals and queer. New apps are springing up regularly like "Friendsy" which offers students matches specific to their own college or university. However, even though there may be many more options to meet people, safety still has to be a consideration when deciding to meet someone from an app.

"As mentioned earlier, after the initial physical attraction, individuals may choose to become emotionally and/or physically intimate. There are many responsibilities that follow when taking this next step. There is more at risk—mentally, physically, and financially. A scenario to contemplate is: How long does it take the average person to decide to buy a car? Or maybe a house? How long will these items be an influence on an individual's life? How long does the average person contemplate sexual intimacy or sexual intercourse? What are some of the repercussions associated with these decisions and how long might they affect an individual's life? It is best to fully consider the consequences before proceeding. Make sure that you and your partner are ready to deal with the consequences."[1] For more information on protection against sexually transmitted infections (STIs) and pregnancy, see Chapter 7.

If you and your partner do decide to become sexually intimate, here is a quick reminder about some sexual activities and their risk for STIs and or pregnancy.

"Rating Safe Sex Activities
Safer sex activities include:

- Dry kissing

- Hugging

- Frottage (rubbing against each other)

- Massage

- Telephone sex

- Tantric sex (extended love-making techniques from the Orient that do not involve penetration)

Riskier activities include:

- Open mouth or deep tongue kissing

- Oral sex (with condoms or dental dams)

- Vaginal intercourse with a condom

Unsafe sex activities include:

- Vaginal intercourse without a condom (even if pulling out before ejaculation)

- Oral sex without a condom (even if pulling out before ejaculation)

- Oral sex or vaginal penetration without a condom during a woman's period

- Anal sex without a condom"[1]

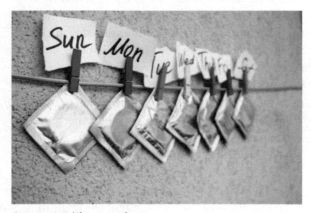

© romantitov/Shutterstock.com

Date Rape

Though this information is discussed in more detail in another chapter, it bears reminding people that sometimes violence can occur in dating situations. Six in ten acquaintance rapes on college campuses occur in dating relationships (New, 2014). Consent means to agree, approve, or permit. If individuals have not mutually consented to a sexual encounter in an unaltered state of mind, then the situation might be considered sexual assault. If a person is intoxicated or unconscious, they would be deemed to be in an altered state and therefore unable to give consent. Remember:

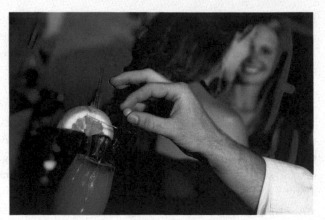

- "Develop clear lines of communication with the person you are dating.
- Communicate and clearly understand what each of you want and expect from the date.
- Do not use psychoactive substances, including alcohol, in dating situations.
- Do not be coerced into unwanted sexual activities.[1]

© Monkey Business Images/Shutterstock.com

If you are a victim of sexual violence, remember that it is not your fault. Please get medical attention as soon as possible as well as counseling support."

What's Love Got to Do with It?

"There are probably as many different definitions of love as there are people in this world. For this reason, it makes answering 'When is it love?' very difficult. One definition of love is a strong affection or liking for someone or something. Some signs it might be love include: verbally expressing affection, such as saying 'I love you'; feeling happier or more secure when this person is present; putting the other person's interests before yours (in a healthy give and-take relationship); respecting the other person for who they are; and not minding the other person's idiosyncrasies (adapted from Yarber et al., 2009).

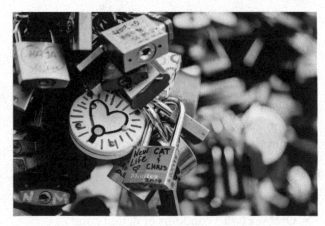

© Grisha Bruev/Shutterstock.com

"Historically, there are several different models of love. Two common ones are described below. The first is Sternberg's (1988) love triangle which includes three components: passion, intimacy, and commitment. Passion tends to occur at the beginning of relationships, peaks relatively quickly, and then reduces to a stable level. Passion generates romance, physical attraction, and sometimes intercourse. Intimacy is the feeling of closeness that exists between two people. Intimacy tends to peak slower than passion and then gradually reduces to a lower level. This level typically changes throughout a relationship. Commitment is the decision to further a loving relationship with another individual. The level of commitment typically rises slowly in the beginning, speeds up, and then gradually levels off. Sternberg describes the various types of love as a composition of different combinations of these three components. These various kinds of love change over time as the relationship matures."[1]

"**John Lee (1973) describes six styles of loving:**

EROS—passionate love

- Become sexually involved quickly
- Intense focus on partner and shares all of him/herself
- Quick to develop, quick to end

LUDUS—game-playing love

- Love and sex are seen only as fun, an activity, a diversion
- Move from partner to partner and often have several at a time
- Passion for the game, not the partner

STORGE—friendship love

- Long-term commitment
- Strong and secure, places less emphasis on passion

MANIA—obsessive love

- Turbulent and ambivalent
- Intense mental preoccupation, but little satisfaction
- Likely to be possessive and jealous

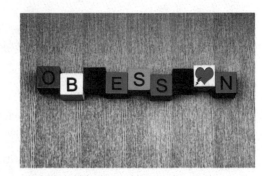

© Ed Samuel/Shutterstock.com

PRAGMA—realistic love

- Rational and practical
- Often for evolutionary and economic purposes
- Intense feelings may develop once a partner is chosen

AGAPE—altruistic love

- Generous, unselfish giving of oneself
- Less emphasis on passion and sexuality"[1]

Taming the Green-Eyed Monster

While some people like to think jealousy is a sign of caring or love, actually jealousy typically comes from a lack of self-esteem and/or lack of confidence. Jealousy will undermine an otherwise healthy relationship and drive potential partners away. Attempting to test your partner to see if they will get jealous may show your own insecurity and can damage the relationship.

If you and your partner find that jealousy is creeping in to your relationship, find a time to talk about what's going on and don't allow it to fester. Make sure you both are on the same page and there are no misunderstandings. Also remember that not only can jealousy come from insecurity, but it can also come from one individual wanting to control another. That may be a sign of an unhealthy relationship developing.

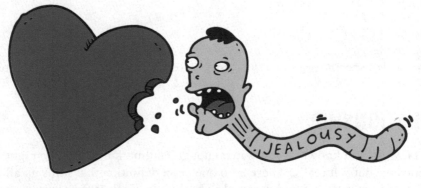

© tetsuu/Shutterstock.com

Every day may not be all sunshine and happiness in most relationships. You will disagree and probably argue from time to time but that is absolutely normal. Problems arise when you find you are disagreeing more than agreeing or when the arguments escalate because you don't actually know how to argue! Some of the most common things couples argue about are listed below. These things, while perhaps changing in order, seem to remain constant over time.

Did you know . . .

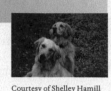

Courtesy of Shelley Hamill

Topics include:

- Lack of communication
- Not paying enough attention to each other
- Jealousy
- Inequity in household responsibilities
- Money
- Frequency of sex
- Religion
- In-laws
- Children
- Goals in life and or future plans (Drevitch, 2019)

When couples do find themselves to have a conflict, the following rules are helpful to go by. Remember, once you say something, you cannot take it back. Though a person may forgive you, it can be very difficult to forget.

Spotlight on . . .

Fighting Fair to Resolve Conflict:

1. Remain Calm
2. Express feelings in words not actions
3. Be specific about what is bothering you
4. Deal with only one issue at a time
5. No "hitting below the belt"
6. Avoid accusations
7. Try not to generalize
8. Avoid "make believe"
9. Don't stockpile
10. Work towards a specific solution (University of Texas, Austin, Counseling Center)

LOVING RELATIONSHIPS

What is "love"? How do you know? If you watch enough Hallmark movies you might think that's the model for romantic love but is it really? There is no one exact definition that sums up all of the meanings of the word love. It is very different and personal to each individual. Different types of love exist with regard to partners, parents, children, and friends. Within a loving relationship there are five important elements:"[1]

1. Honesty
2. Loyalty
3. Thoughtfulness
4. Sharing
5. Sacrifice

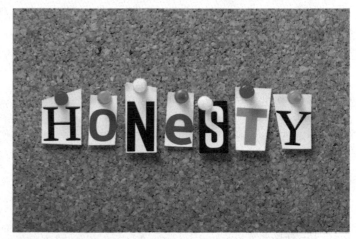
© Thinglass/Shutterstock.com

The foundation for any healthy and long term relationship is honesty and trust. Without it, how do you and your partner share your inner most thoughts or feelings? How do you trust one another with intimacy? As part of that building you are establishing your loyalty to each other and it is important that you are on the same page.

Pair bonded and loving relationships involve doing things together that you both enjoy. They include little things like going to dinner or doing household chores together and they, by nature, include a bit of self-sacrifice and compromise on occasion given freely as a result of the love in the relationship. There are no strings attached.

Lesbian, Gay, Bisexual, Transgender, Queer, Intersex, and Asexual (LGBTQ+)

Students who identify as LGBTQ+ often enter college unsure of how supportive this new environment may be. Adjusting to college is stressful enough for many students, but for some LGBTQ+ students, college may be a time when they first publically acknowledge their sexual identity or sexual orientation. While it may be a liberating experience for some, it can also be a stressful situation filled with fear of rejection from peers and/or family. Some may find their campus community is supportive and accepting, only to find that their family back home is not. While this may create some dissonance, it is important for all students to feel loved and accepted. Having supportive peers, and a welcoming faculty and campus community is important as students are navigating, what for some, may be the first time they have been able to embrace this side of themselves. But remember, any student, no matter their sexual orientation, who is harassed or discriminated against needs to report any incidents to the proper authorities on your campus.

Is Marriage in the Future?

There was a time when this question only pertained to one segment of society. Now that with laws have changed, those of legal age, no matter their sexual orientation, may look at their intimate relationships with the idea of marriage in mind. There are many things to consider when contemplating marriage. Is this the person with whom you really want to spend the rest of your life with? Are you compatible? Do you have similar values? These are just a few of the questions that should be asked.

The question of compatibility is one that takes time to answer. Some characteristics that comprise compatibility include similar interests, ways of doing things, as well as the ability to compromise when you do not see 'eye to eye.' Do you both like to participate in outdoor or indoor activities? Are your activity levels similar? Do you need structure to your life or is spontaneity more your style? Are you both outgoing or do you complement each other with some differences? What are your long-term goals and are they similar to your partner's? Do you have similar views on finances? Are you thrifty or extravagant? Do both of you want children? This is not to say that you and your ideal partner have to be identical. In fact, it is helpful to have some differences (within reason) to help complement the other's weaknesses. For example, if one of you is somewhat over reactive and the other one is more grounded, then you will probably balance one another out. Problems arise when there are so many differences that you cannot relate or the differences simply irritate one another. With this said, it is very helpful to have similar interests and ways of doing things that can carry past the initial infatuation stage.

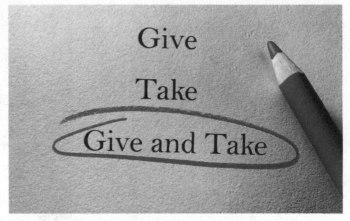

© zimmytws/Shutterstock.com

Another really important part of partner compatibility has to do with values. Do you have similar beliefs or standards? How do you treat others including animals? Is volunteering important to you and giving back to the community? How do you feel about marriage and what does that mean? All of these are things you and you potential life partner need to discuss and find commonality or if there is any room for compromise.

Unhealthy Relationships

"It takes work to have a healthy relationship; they don't just happen. Sometimes there is a process of growing through unhealthy relationships in order to find the right one for you. Some signs of an unhealthy relationship include (Kuriansky, 2002):

- You feel insecure and weak around each other.
- You suffer from low self-esteem because of what happens between you.
- You are dishonest with each other.
- You spend more time feeling hurt than feeling good about how you treat each other.
- You find yourself complaining to others about your relationship.
- You are unable to talk about your feelings or problems with your partner, much less solve them.
- You are unable to resolve your differences together.
- You become unenthusiastic about life because of what goes on between you.
- Your trust is irrevocably broken.
- Seeming small things erode your relationship, like trickling water that wears away at a rock over time.
- Priorities other than each other constantly present themselves.
- What goes on between you interferes with other aspects of your life."[1]

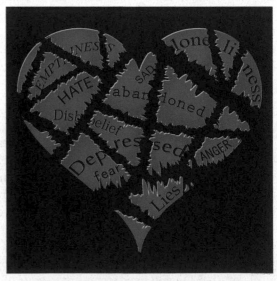

© Athanasia Nomikou/Shutterstock.com

If you or your partner decide that the relationship is not in the best interests of both of you, it may be time to consider ending your time together.

Ending a Relationship

Typically, the first person you date will not be the person you ultimately marry. We continue to learn about ourselves, and each other, and as we grow we often find things about the other person that may not be what we wanted in our lifelong partner. Unfortunately, in many cases, only one partner sees the need for ending the relationship which can make leaving it rather difficult.

If you are the one to end a relationship always, try to be as tactful as possible. Remember that at one point you were interested enough in this person to pursue a relationship. Be open and honest about the reason(s) you wish to end the relationship. Sending a text message or posting on social media that you are no longer in a relationship is NOT the way to let someone know you are no longer interested in being involved. It may be uncomfortable to tell someone face to face but think how you would feel if it happened to you.

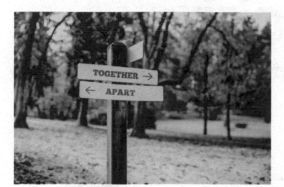
© Gajus/Shutterstock.com

If you are the one being told the relationship is over, listen carefully to what the person is saying and do not respond desperately or defensively. If this truly is the end of this relationship, realize and accept that there will be a better match for you at some point in the future.

Abusive Relationships

To be very clear, **NO ONE** should have to stay in an abusive relationship. Abuse may be subtle at first whether physical or emotional, but these will almost always escalate to dangerous episodes. When signs of abusive behavior appear, it is definitely time to get out of the relationship. Abuse can happen between partners of any sex, sexual orientation, or gender identity and should not be stereotyped as only occurring in certain types of relationships. According to the Center for Disease and Control, about 1 in 4 women and 1 in 10 men have experienced sexual violence, physical violence, and or stalking by an intimate partner during their lifetime. Additionally, over 43 million women and 38 million men have experienced psychological aggression by an intimate partner (CDC, 2021).

Sometimes it is incredibly hard for the abused partner to leave because their self-esteem is so low. They honestly feel the only person that would 'put up' with them is their partner, so they feel trapped. While roughly 70% of young victims may not realize they are being abused by their partners, those that do often resist leaving because of closed social networks on college campuses that can make them feel trapped (Libertin, A., 2017). The abusing partner typically isolates their partner from friends and family over an extended period of time. This evolves into a very controlling and abusive relationship. The abuser may threaten to harm the partner, partner's family, or even the family pet if they try to leave. If this is the case, do not let your partner know you are thinking about leaving. Wait until you know your partner will be gone for an extended period of time and call someone whom your partner does not know for help. It is crucial to reach out for help. Please contact campus police for help. Contact campus police to get assistance and access counseling services for support.

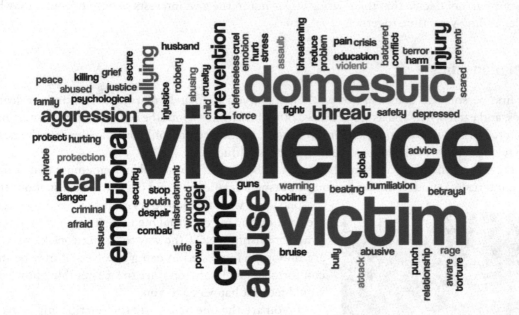

© ibreakstock/Shutterstock.com

If you are being stalked or harassed, you may need to take out a restraining order on the individual. On occasion, these situations have become life threatening. And remember, if you are in a abusive relationship, the abuse is more likely than not to continue until you leave and the relationship is over. And, typically, the abuse will escalate over time. Again, please reach out to campus police! You may need help to leave but support and **resources** are available.

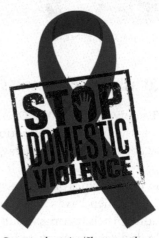

© wow.subtropica/Shutterstock
.com

Are you a wise consumer?

What are you doing to improve your communication skills? Are you really paying attention? Are you participating in your relationships or are you letting others "do all the work"? When you go out with friends in partying situations, do you look out for each other? Are you taking care of you? All of these things matter and you are an active participant.

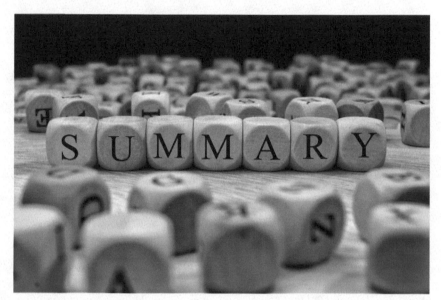

© Fabrik Bilder/Shutterstock.com

Developing and maintaining healthy relationships is a part of developing as well-rounded individuals. Self-confidence and recognizing qualities within ourselves that support our abilities to engage with others in healthy ways is important. Learning the skills necessary for good communication as well as the ability to stand up for ourselves when necessary are all part of our growth. Your campus has many resources to assist students navigate through the challenges of college life. Please make sure to access those services if and when you ever need them.

NOTES

PERSONAL REFLECTIONS . . . SO, WHAT HAVE YOU LEARNED?

1. Answer questions 1–3 under the relationship survey at the beginning of your chapter. Answer these based on what you want not necessarily what you may currently have in a partner.

2. What would you say are your own top 10 qualities? Why do you think these are you best qualities and how will you protect the in a relationship?

3. Of the top 10 steps for being an effective listener, which three do you do well and which three might you need to work on?

4. What advice would you give to incoming freshman regarding their relationships with the following during their transition to college?

   a. Parents and siblings

   b. Living with other students (roommates)

5. What advice would you give to incoming freshman regarding their expectations with dating and intimate relationships in college?

6. Now that you have given such great advice, what do you think someone 5–10 years older than you would give you about your journey once you graduate?

NOTES

RESOURCES ON CAMPUS FOR YOU!

Victims Assistance

Find out if your institution offers any victims assistance services to survivors of sexual assault, domestic violence, dating violence, and stalking on campus. Be sure to take advantage of the educational programs to prevent these crimes from occurring.

In case of an emergency, please call your Campus Police, the local police, or the local rape crisis center in your area.

Health and Counseling Services

Believe in the dignity, integrity, growth potential, and innate worth of the individual, and offer services to foster whole-person health through prevention, education, assessment, treatment, and advocacy.

REFERENCES

Center for Disease Control and Prevention, (2021). Intimate Partner Violence. https://www.cdc.gov/violenceprevention/intimatepartnerviolence/fastfact.html

Cherry K. (2020) about health. *Left brain vs right brain dominance.* Retrieved 2022 from http://www.verywellmind.com/left-brain-vs-right-brain-2795005

Drevitch, G. 2019. 30 Core Disagreements Couples Encounter. Psychology Today. Retrieved 2022 from Psychologytoday.com/us/blog/experimentations/201912/30-core-disagreements-couples-encounter

Floyd, P.A., Mimms, S. E., & Yelding-Howards, C. (2008). *Personal health: Perspectives and lifestyles* (4th ed). Belmont, Calif: Thomson Wadsworth.

Forbes, 2020. 12 Concrete Ways to Listen Effectively. Retrieved 2022 from forbes.com/sites/forbescoaches counesl/2020/08/11/12-concrete-ways-to-listen-effectively/?sh=4d8177863674

Kluger J. (2012) We never talk any more: the problem with text messaging. Retrieved 2016 from http://www.cnn.com/2012/08/31/tech/mobile/problem-text-messaging-oms/index.html

Kuriansky, J. (2002). *The complete idiot's guide to a healthy relationship* (2nd ed). Indianapolis, IN: Alpha

Kuriansky, J. (2003). *The complete idiot's guide to dating* (3rd ed). Indianapolis, IN: Alpha Books.

Lee, J. A. (1973). *Colours of love: an exploration of the ways of loving.* Toronto: New Press.

Libertain, A. (2017) Retrieved 2019. https://hawcdv.org/the-truth-about-domestic-violence-on-college-campuses/

New, J. (2014). *Deadly dating violence.* Retrieved 2016 from https://www.insidehighered.com/news/2014/12/02/domestic-abuse-prevalent-sexual-assault-college-campuses.

Oxford Dictionaries (2016). *Communication.* Retrieved 2016 from http://www.oxforddictionaries.com/definition/english/communication

PEW Institute. Retrieved 2019. https://www.pewinternet.org/fact-sheet/mobile/

Schilling, D. (2012). 10 steps to effective listening. Retrieved 2016 http://www.forbes.com/sites/womensmedia/2012/11/09/10-steps-to-effective-listening/#1d4f230f26fb.

Smith, A. (2015). *U.S. Smartphone use in 2015.* Retrieved 2016 from http://www.pewinternet
.org/2015/04/01/us-smartphone-use-in-2015/

Sternberg, R. J. (1998). *The triangle of love: Intimacy, passion, commitment.* New York: Basic Books.

University of Texas at Austin Counseling and Mental Health Center (n.d.). Fighting Fair to Resolve
Conflict. Retrieved 2022 from cmhc.utexas.edu/fightingfair.html

Yarber, W., Sayad, B., & Strong, B. (2010). *Human sexuality: Diversity in contemporary America* (7th ed).
McGraw-Hill.

CREDITS

1. From *Health and Fitness: A Guide to a Healthy Lifestyle*, 5/e by Laura Bounds, Gayden Darnell, Kristin Brekken Shea, Dottiede Agnore. Copyright ©2012 by Kendall Hunt Publishing Company. Reprinted by permission.

NOTES

Chapter 7

Sexual Health +

OBJECTIVES

Students will be able to:

- Identify female and male anatomical structures
- Explain the stages of the menstrual cycle
- Describe the stages of pregnancy
- List the most common sexually transmitted infections, their pathogens, symptoms, methods of transmission, treatment, and whether or not there is a cure.
- List the methods for the transmission of the HIV virus.
- Explain what makes some sexual behaviors high risk
- Anaylize how the media influences attitudes and beliefs about relationships and sexuality.

The focus of this chapter is on female and male anatomy. We usually know the "main parts" but there are so many more! Additionally, we will examine sexually transmitted infections, their pathogens, and how they are treated. And, we will also analyze various contraceptive methods including the advantages and benefits of each.

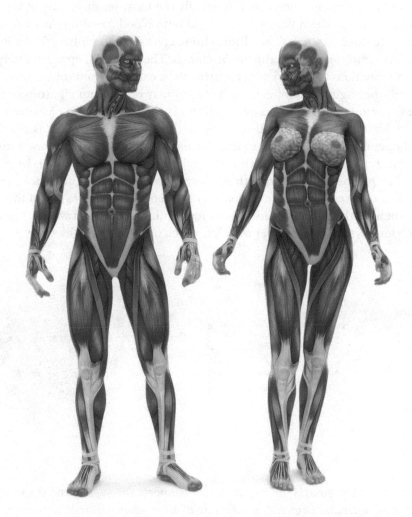

© Digital Storm/Shutterstock.com

ANATOMY

Female Sexual Anatomy

"The female anatomy consists of multiple integral parts both externally and internally (see Figure 7.1 a & b). The **vulva** includes visible external genitalia. The **mons pubis** is the soft fatty tissue covering the pubic symphysis (joint of the pubic bones). This area is covered with pubic hair that begins growing during puberty. The **labia majora** include two longitudinal folds of skin that extend on both sides of the vulva and serve as protection for the inner parts of the vulva. The **labia minora** are the delicate inner folds of skin that enclose the urethral opening and the vagina. These skin flaps, which contain sweat and oil glands, extensive blood vessels, and nerve endings, are hairless and sensitive to touch. When sexually stimulated, the labia minora swell and darken. The **clitoris** is usually the most sensitive part of the female genitalia and consists of erectile tissue, which becomes engorged with blood, resulting in swelling during sexual arousal that enables it to double in size. The **clitoral hood** consists of inner lips, which join to form a soft fold of skin, or hood, covering and connecting to the clitoris. The **urethra** is approximately 2.5 centimeters below the clitoris and functions as the opening for urine to be excreted from the bladder. Because the urethra is located close to the vaginal opening, some irritation may result from vigorous or prolonged sexual activity. The most common problem associated with this is the development of urinary tract infections. The **vagina** is located between the urethral opening and the anus. The **hymen** is the small membrane around the vaginal opening that is believed to tear during initial intercourse, tampon use, while riding a horse, or other various types of athletic activities. The only function of the hymen is to protect the vaginal tissues early in life. The **perineum** is the smooth skin located between the labia minora and the anus. During childbirth this area may tear or be cut (episiotomy) as the newborn passes out of the vagina. The anal canal is located just behind the perineum and allows for elimination of solid waste. The **anal canal** is approximately an inch long with two sphincter muscles, which open and close like valves."[1]

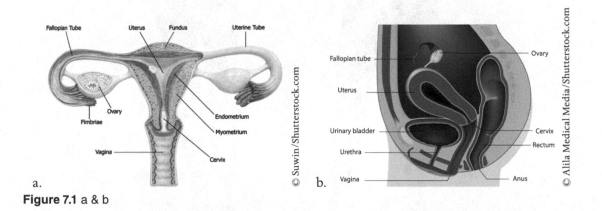

a.   b.

Figure 7.1 a & b

"Internally, just past the vagina, is the cervix, which connects the vagina and the uterus. The uterus is the hollow, pear-shaped muscular organ about the size of a fist when a female is not pregnant. This is the organ in which the fetus develops during pregnancy. The upper expanded portion is referred to as the fundus and the lower constricted part is the cervix. On each side of the uterus are **fallopian tubes**, which are quite narrow and approximately four inches in length. Because of the narrow passageway within these tubes, infection and scarring may cause fertility problems. Most women have a right and a left fallopian tube. These tubes extend from the ovaries to the uterus and transport mature ovum. Fertilization usually takes place within the fallopian tubes. The opening between the fallopian tube and the uterus is only about as wide as a needle. On each end of the fallopian tubes are the **ovaries**, where eggs are produced and released usually once a month. Each ovary is about the size of a large olive. At birth, a female's ovaries contain 40,000 to 400,000 immature ova, of which approximately 450 will mature and be released during the reproductive years. The ovaries also produce the hormones estrogen and progesterone, both of which help regulate the menstrual cycle (Crooks & Baur, 2009)."[1]

"The female *sexual response* consists of four phases:

1. Excitement:

   Vaginal lubrication begins and the vagina, clitoris, labia majora and minora fill with blood. The nipples swell, and there is increased tension in many voluntary muscles.

2. Plateau:

   The vaginal opening usually decreases in diameter due to swelling, the uterus usually increases in size, and the labia majora and minora become more swollen and engorged.

3. Orgasm:

   The muscles of the vaginal wall undergo rhythmic contractions. The number of contractions may range from three to as many as twelve. Involuntary contraction of other muscles may take place as well.

4. Resolution:

   Blood rapidly returns to the rest of the body from the vagina, clitoris, labia majora, and minora, resulting in reduced swelling. At this time the breasts also return to their original size."[1]

Menstrual Cycle

The typical menstrual cycle lasts, on average, about 28 days. Of course, as it is an average, it could be shorter or longer by a few days. The phase at which menstruation begins is the follicular phase and is over when ovulation occurs. Unfortunately, the follicular phase can be unpredictable. While it is typically 14 days, it can be as little as 10 and as long as 25. There are many things that can influence ovulation including stress, illness, and other factors. For those who are trying to control pregnancy, whether to become pregnant or avoid it, this can make things difficult.

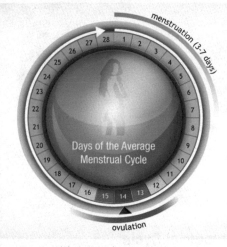

© Janos Levente/Shutterstock.com

Figure 7.2

The length of the luteal phase is more predictable. Typically 13 to 15 days, this phase begins with ovulation and ends when the next menstrual cycle begins. Premenstrual Syndrome (PMS) can begin anywhere from one to ten days before menses (the actual shedding of tissue and fluid, also known as the "period"). During this time, some women experience breast tenderness, bloating, nausea, cramping, diarrhea, backaches, and headaches, among other symptoms. There are psychological symptoms associated with PMS as well. Mood swings, the inability to concentrate, and sleep disturbances may all be a part of the challenges faced by someone dealing with PMS. Additionally, there are often food cravings such as carbohydrates, salty food, and sweets. Think about it. Wouldn't you be a bit cranky if you had these things going on? PMS can also affect sleep. The problem with those cravings is that they may actually make some of those symptoms worse.

So how do you prevent or minimize those challenges? Listed are a few suggestions that may help:

- Modify your diet
- incorporate exercise into your regular routine
- reduce stress

There are also alternative options which include vitamins, herbal remedies, and acupuncture. (Mayo Clinic, 2022)

Ovarian Cycle

"During the ovarian cycle immature eggs (follicles) are maturing and moving toward the surface of the ovary. The follicle and the ovarian surface open and allow the egg to float out. At the time of ovulation some women may feel a twinge or pain in the lower abdomen or back. After ovulation, the egg is swept into a fallopian tube (where fertilization typically occurs) by fimbriae and the cilia (tiny hairs) and travels to the uterus. If the egg is not fertilized, it simply disintegrates or flows out with vaginal secretions, usually before menstruation. If the egg is fertilized, it will attach itself to the endometrium (internal lining of the uterus) in order to develop."[1]

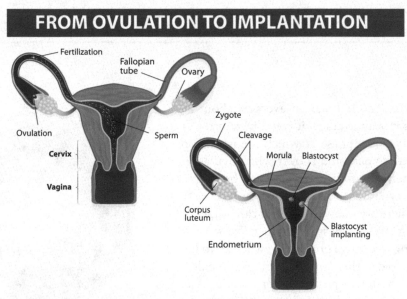

FROM OVULATION TO IMPLANTATION

© Designua/Shutterstock.com

Endometrial Cycle

"The endometrial cycle consists of three phases:

1. Menstrual
2. Proliferative
3. Progestational (secretory).

"The menstrual phase lasts approximately four to seven days, when the lining of the uterus is sloughed off and flows out of the uterus through the vagina, along with blood and other vaginal secretions. The proliferative phase lasts from the completion of the menstrual phase until a day or two after ovulation.

During this time the endometrium is regenerating the layer that was sloughed off with new epithelial cells. During the progestational phase the endometrium becomes twice as thick as it did during the proliferative phase. It develops a cushion-like surface, thereby possessing the ability to nourish an implanted fertilized ovum. During the end of the progestational phase, if fertilization has not occurred, the endometrium begins to deteriorate. These phases repeat throughout the reproductive years until fertilization or menopause occurs."[1]

Male Sexual Anatomy

"The external male sexual structures include the penis and scrotum. The **penis** is an organ through which semen and urine pass, and is structured into three main sections: the root, the shaft, and the glans penis (see Figure 7.3 a & b). The root attaches the penis within the pelvic cavity at the base, while the shaft, or the tube-shaped body of the penis, hangs freely. The **glans penis** is covered by a loose portion of tissue called the **foreskin**, which may be removed during a surgery known as circumcision. A penis without foreskin is circumcised, while one with the foreskin intact is uncircumcised. Uncircumcised men should gently pull the foreskin back when they bathe to wash the foreskin and tip of the penis. At the base of the glans is a rim known as the corona. On the underside is a triangular area of highly sensitive skin called the frenulum, which attaches the glans to the foreskin. The glans penis is the soft, fleshy, enlarged tissue at the end of the shaft, with the urethral opening at the tip. The **scrotum** is the pouch of skin, which hangs from the root of the penis and holds the two testicles. Covered sparsely with hair, the scrotum is divided in the middle by a ridge of skin, showing the separation of the testes. The surface changes of the scrotum help maintain a moderately constant temperature within the testes (93 degrees Fahrenheit), which is important for maintaining good sperm production (Crooks & Baur, 2009).[1]

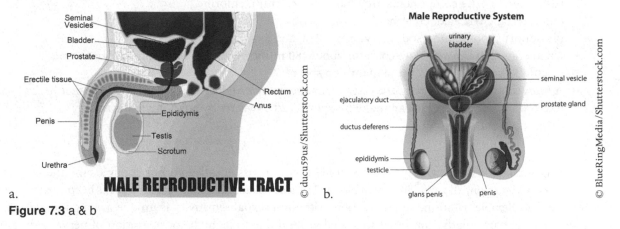

Figure 7.3 a & b

"The male internal sexual structures include the testes, epididymis, vas deferens, seminal vesicles, and prostate and Cowper's glands. The **testes** are the reproductive ball-shaped glands inside the scrotum, which are also referred to as testicles. Sperm and hormone production are the two main functions of the testes (Crooks & Baur, 2007). Sperm are formed constantly, beginning during puberty, inside the highly coiled thin tubes called seminiferous tubules within each testis. Between the seminiferous tubules are cells that produce sex hormones. One such important sex hormone is testosterone, which stimulates the production of sperm. On top of each testis is another tightly coiled tube, the **epididymis**, where nearly mature sperm complete the maturation process (Crooks & Baur, 2009). Mature sperm are stored in the epididymis until they are released during ejaculation. The **vas deferens** is a long tube through which sperm travel during ejaculation. The epididymis is connected to the seminal vesicle via the vas deferens, which is responsible for contracting and pushing the sperm to the seminal vesicle. Located beneath the bladder are the two small seminal vesicles, which secrete a fluid that provides nourishment as well as an environment conducive to sperm mobility. After the sperm have combined with the seminal fluid, they reach the prostate where another substance is added. A thin, milky fluid is produced by the prostate and secreted into the urethra during the time of emission of semen, which enhances the swimming environment for the sperm (Crooks & Baur, 2009). Below the prostate and attached to the urethra are the two pea-sized **Cowper's glands**, responsible for depositing a lubricating fluid for sperm and a coating for the urethra. If there are sperm in the urethra from a previous ejaculation, they will mix with the Cowper's fluid and become a pre-ejaculate lubricant fluid. Ejaculation occurs at peak sexual excitement when the prostate muscle opens and sends the seminal fluid to the urethra where it is then forced out through the urethral opening, forming semen."[1]

"The shaft of the penis can change dramatically during sexual arousal."[1] "The average penis is approximately 3 to 4 inches when flaccid (soft). One study noted that , when erect, the average length among subjects was found to be 6.02 inches, with a variation from 3.4 to 9.44 inches. Average penis girth (circumference) at erection was found to be 4.96 inches with a variation from 2.24 to 7.4 inches (Harding & Golombok, 2002). Most of the variation in penis size occurs during erection. Erection has been called "the great equalizer" because smaller penises seem to grow more during erection than larger ones, so the extremes tend to equalize when erect."[5]

Did you know . . .

According to Dr. Laura Burman:

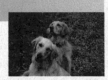

Courtesy of Shelley Hamill

- Sperm can live in a woman's body for up to five days after intercourse!
- There are many ingredients in semen, and its makeup is similar for every man. Some of the components are vitamin C, calcium, chlorine, cholesterol, citric acid, creatine, fructose, lactic acid, magnesium, nitrogen, phosphorus, potassium, sodium, vitamin B12, and zinc.
- An average human ejaculate contains about 180 million sperm (66 million/ml), but some ejaculates contain as many as 400 million sperm
- A man can actually improve the taste of his sperm by avoiding dairy, coffee, and potent herbs like onions and garlic. He can make his sperm taste sweeter by enjoying fruits and by drinking plenty of water.

"During sexual excitement, tiny muscles inside the shaft tissue called corpus spongiosum and corpus cavernosa relax and open, allowing inflow of blood. As these tissues fill with blood, the penis becomes longer, thicker, and less flexible, resulting in an erection. Although sexual sensitivity is unique among individuals, the glans penis is particularly important in sexual arousal due to its high concentration of nerve endings. When a man is either sexually aroused or cold, the testes are pulled close to the body (Crooks & Baur, 2009)."[1]

SEXUAL ORIENTATION

According to the American Psychological Association (APA), sexual orientation refers to an enduring pattern of emotional, romantic and/or sexual attractions to men, women or both sexes. Sexual orientation also refers to a person's sense of identity based on those attractions, related behaviors and membership in a community of others who share those attractions. Research over several decades has demonstrated that sexual orientation ranges along a continuum, from exclusive attraction to the other sex to exclusive attraction to the same sex. However, sexual orientation is usually discussed in terms of three categories: heterosexual (having emotional, romantic or sexual attractions to members of the other sex), gay/lesbian (having emotional, romantic or sexual attractions to members of one's own sex) and bisexual (having emotional, romantic or sexual attractions to both men and women). This range of behaviors and attractions has been described in various cultures and nations throughout the world. Many cultures use identity labels to describe people who express these attractions. In the United States the most frequent labels are lesbians (women attracted to women), gay men (men attracted to men), and bisexual people (men or women attracted to both sexes). However, some people may use different labels or none at all.

"Sexual orientation is distinct from other components of sex and gender, including biological sex (the anatomical, physiological and genetic characteristics associated with being male or female), gender identity (the psychological sense of being male or female)* and social gender role (the cultural norms that define feminine and masculine behavior).

Further, sexual orientation falls along a continuum of possible behaviors and attractions. What was once seen as binary with respect to heterosexual/homosexual, now recognizes a range of possibilities including pan-sexual, asexual, bisexual, just to name a few.

There is no consensus among scientists about the exact reasons that an individual develops their sexual orientation. Although much research has examined the possible genetic, hormonal, developmental, social and cultural influences on sexual orientation, no findings have emerged that permit scientists to conclude that sexual orientation is determined by any particular factor or factors. Many think that nature and nurture both play complex roles; most people experience little or no sense of choice about their sexual orientation (APA).

Lesbian, gay, bisexual, and transgender people in the United States encounter extensive prejudice, discrimination and violence because of their sexual orientation. The CDC notes that in 2015 according to the national Youth Risk Behavior of LGBT students:

- 10% were threatened or injured with a weapon on school property
- 34% were bullied on school property
- 28% were bullied electronically
- 23% of LGBT students who had dated or went out with someone during the 12 months before the survey had experienced sexual dating violence in the prior year
- 18% of LGBT students had experienced physical dating violence
- 18% of LGBT students had been forced to have sexual intercourse at some point in their lives.

Intense prejudice against lesbians, gay men, and bisexual people was widespread throughout much of the 20th century. Public opinion studies over the 1970s, 1980s and 1990s routinely showed that, among large segments of the public, lesbian, gay, and bisexual people were the target of strongly held negative attitudes. More recently, public opinion has increasingly opposed sexual orientation discrimination, but expressions of hostility toward lesbians and gay men remain common in contemporary American society. Prejudice against bisexuals appears to exist at comparable levels. In fact, bisexual individuals may face discrimination from some lesbian and gay people as well as from heterosexual people. Transgender individuals, people whose sense of personal identity does not match their biological sex, have seen a dramatic rise in the number of violent assaults. According to the Human Rights Campaign (HRC), in 2018 at least 26 deaths due to fatal violence of transgender people, the majority of whom were Black transgender women. As of September 2019, at least 18 transgender people had been murdered in the U.S. (HRC).

Sexual orientation discrimination takes many forms. Severe antigay prejudice i019.s reflected in the high rate of harassment and violence directed toward lesbian, gay and bisexual individuals in American society. Numerous surveys indicate that verbal harassment and abuse are nearly universal experiences among lesbian, gay and bisexual people. Also, discrimination against lesbian, gay, and bisexual people in employment and housing appears to remain widespread (APA).

READINESS FOR SEXUAL ACTIVITY

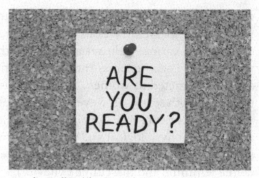

© Ivelin Radkov/Shutterstock.com

How do you know when you are ready for sex? Have you really thought about that question? Being sexually intimate with another person may have a lot of implications across the physical, emotional, and spiritual categories. Typically individuals have very different timelines at which they feel comfortable participating in different types of sexual activity. Different sexual activities may include but are not limited to: vaginal/penal, anal/penal, oral/vaginal, or oral/penal intercourse. Some individuals consider themselves 'virgins' if they have not had vaginal/penal intercourse, but have participated in other sexual activities. It is important to realize there are very real risks associated with some forms of sexual activity, which include but are not limited to sexually transmitted infections (STIs). It is also important that you decide what you would like out of a relationship and when you feel comfortable with beginning a specific sexual activity. Some individuals view sexual activity as a very casual event and others wait until they are married to participate in any sexual activity.

Sexually transmitted infections do not discriminate based on your sexual orientation. If they are present, they can be spread from mucus membrane to mucus membrane based on the sexual activity partners decide to participate in. Gay, straight, bisexual or lesbian, anyone is at risk if you do not know the status of your partner and you do not use a barrier method to prevent transmission.

Communication is one of the most important parts of a good relationship. You must be able to talk with your partner to develop trust and to understand what each individual wants and needs in a relationship. If you cannot talk openly about being physically intimate with your partner, then are you really ready to begin that type of relationship?

If or when you and your partner decide the time is right to begin a sexual relationship you need to discuss some key things. What type of protection should you use? Are you focused on pregnancy prevention, STI protection, or both? If you are a heterosexual couple, have you discussed what might happen if an unplanned pregnancy occurred? After all, nothing is 100% effective except abstinence.

Make sure you have both discussed consent, remembering that "no" means "no: and "stop" means "stop" should either of you hear those words. And remember, avoid using alcohol or drugs prior to sexual encounters as they may alter you decision making ability from either perspective.

Contraception

Many people use the terms birth control, contraception, and family planning interchangeably. Although the terms are similar because they refer to strategies for preventing unintended pregnancy, they are vastly different in terms of their nature and scope.

Family planning implies the desire to have children at some point in time. Planning a family involves postponing childbearing until it is desired, spacing subsequent births and avoiding pregnancy at other times. Family planning may also include all the reproductive technologies available to facilitate a pregnancy as well as adoption. Family planning does not refer to specific methods or techniques to avoid unintended pregnancy.

Contraception refers to all methods designed to prevent conception or fertilization. Contraceptive methods work by preventing the sperm and egg from uniting to cause fertilization. These methods include noninsertive sexual activity, barrier methods, hormonal contraception, withdrawal, fertility awareness, and sterilization. How effective these methods are ranges from 'not very' to 'almost complete' at the other end of the spectrum.

Birth control is a broad term encompassing all methods designed to prevent pregnancy and birth. It includes all contraceptive methods, what may be considered post conceptive methods, and abortion, which is designed to interrupt an established pregnancy.[5]

EFFECTIVENESS: THEORETICAL AND ACTUAL USE

"One of the most important questions regarding any method of fertility control is 'How effective is it?' Effectiveness is measured in two ways: theoretical use and actual use.

The **theoretical effectiveness** (also called perfect use) of any fertility control method estimates how it should work if it is used consistently and correctly. It is the ideal effectiveness of the method, determined through laboratory research and experimental studies. Theoretical effectiveness research designs attempt to control for as many variables as possible that may interfere with correct and consistent use. Failure of the method accounts for most of the ineffectiveness. Theoretical effectiveness is the lowest expected percentage of women who will get pregnant while using the method.

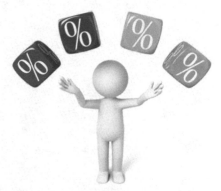

The actual-use effectiveness (also called typical use) of any fertility control method is how it actually works when real people use it under normal circumstances. This is observed effectiveness of the method, determined by following a group of actual users for 1 year to see how many get pregnant (Blonna & Carter, 2013)."[5]

Of course, not everyone engaging in sexual behavior is concerned about pregnancy. Protection from sexually transmitted infections has to also be a part of the consideration.

© Jane0606/Shutterstock.com

Pregnancy

"Pregnancy is usually divided into three trimesters, each of which lasts approximately three months or thirteen weeks. Typically, fertilization occurs twelve to eighteen days after the beginning of the menstrual cycle. There are many variables that can impact the timing of fertilization, including irregular periods, extreme exercise, illness, stress, a missed contraceptive pill, as well as many other factors. As soon as fertilization occurs, the cells begin to divide and multiply. The fertilized egg implants in the uterus after approximately one week after fertilization. For most women the first sign(s) of pregnancy include a missed period, nausea, or excessive fatigue. Home pregnancy kits are 97 to 99 percent accurate if used correctly. These tests can detect human chorionic gonadotropin (HCG) within two to three weeks of fertilization. HCG is the hormone secreted by the placenta to help sustain the pregnancy for the first trimester. During the second and third trimesters the HCG levels decrease and the levels of estrogen and progesterone are sufficient to sustain the pregnancy to term. This is believed to be the reason morning sickness ends for most women after the first trimester. The embryo develops very rapidly during the first trimester. During these three months, all of the major organs are formed. Therefore, it is imperative to see a physician as soon as an individual thinks she may be pregnant to begin and change any habits that could be harmful to the developing embryo. It is also important to remember that no amount of alcohol during pregnancy is safe (CDC). The pregnancy is dated utilizing the first day of the last menstrual period (LMP). The heartbeat can be seen during a sonogram as early as the sixth or seventh week when the embryo is approximately 5 millimeters long. During the second and third trimesters the fetus is growing larger and stronger in preparation for delivery. Typically the mother will begin to feel the movements of the fetus between the sixteenth and twentieth weeks. This is referred to as 'quickening.' After an additional month or so, these movements can be felt externally by friends or family members. Thirty-six weeks is considered a full-term pregnancy, but a typical delivery does not occur until around the fortieth week."[1]

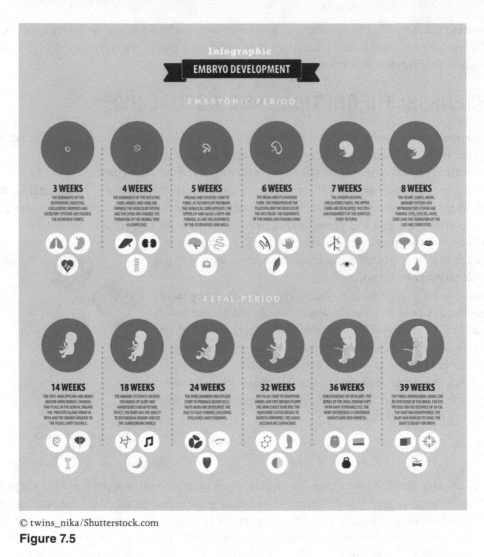

© twins_nika/Shutterstock.com

Figure 7.5

Pregnancy Prevention

Partners select contraceptive methods for a number of reasons. Ease of use, reversibility, knowledge of, disease protection, accessibility are just some of the many factors that are involved in the decision as to which method is right for the people involved. While not all sexual behaviors lead to pregnancy concerns, for those that do, partners need to be informed about which methods offer the most reliability to prevent an unwanted pregnancy.

When looking at advantages and disadvantages, many factors may be involved. Listed below are some of those for each method. Additionally, you will find a fairly wide % effective range. Remember, these ranges are from "typical" use to "perfect use, hence the variance.

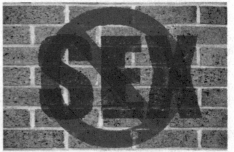

© SergeBertasiusPhotography/Shutterstock.com

"Natural Methods

"Abstinence from Penile/Vaginal Intercourse

Effectiveness:
- in preventing pregnancy: 100 percent
- in preventing STIs—100 percent

Advantages:
- No worries
- No medical or hormonal side effects
- Protects against unwanted pregnancy

Disadvantages:
- Very few people choose lifetime celibacy or abstinence from sexual intercourse.
- People often forget to protect themselves against pregnancy or STIs when they stop abstaining."[1]

"Withdrawal Method

The man will pull his penis out of the vagina before he ejaculates to keep sperm from joining an egg.

Effectiveness:
- in preventing pregnancy: 73–96 percent
- in preventing STIs—NONE

Advantage:
- Can be used when no other method is available

Disadvantages:
- Requires great self-control, experience, and trust
- Not for men who ejaculate prematurely
- Not for men who do not know when to pull out
- Not recommended for teenagers"[1]

"Fertility Awareness-based Methods (FAMs)

- A woman must chart her menstrual cycle and must be able to detect certain physical signs in order to predict 'unsafe' days.
- She must abstain from intercourse or use barrier contraceptives during nine or more 'unsafe' days each menstrual cycle.
- Check temperature daily. Before ovulation waking temperatures remain low, after ovulation temperatures rise until the next menstrual cycle begins.
- Check cervical mucus daily. Before ovulation the mucus is wet and similar to a raw egg white, after ovulation the cervical fluid dries up quickly.
- Record menstrual cycles on calendar to determine if she has regular or irregular cycles. This method is more effective for those with regular menstrual cycles.
- Remember that the sperm can live up to 120 hours after ejaculation. If a female ovulates within 120 hours after unprotected sexual intercourse the possibility of pregnancy exists.

Effectiveness:
- in preventing pregnancy: 75–99 percent
- in preventing STIs—NONE

Advantages:
- No medical or hormonal side effects
- Calendars, thermometers, and charts are easy to obtain

Disadvantages:
- Requires expert training before effective use
- Taking risks during 'unsafe' days
- Poor record keeping
- Illness and lack of sleep affect body temperatures
- Vaginal infections and douches change mucus
- Cannot use with irregular periods or temperature patterns"[1]

"Barrier Methods

"Male Condom

The male condom is a latex sheath, placed over the penis prior to intercourse (see Figure 7.6).

Effectiveness:
- in preventing pregnancy: 83–98 percent
- in preventing STIs—85–98 percent

To increase pregnancy prevention effectiveness also use spermicide or have female utilize another form of contraception. Do not use oil-based lubricants such as Vaseline or lotion, which will cause the condom to break. Use only water-based lubricants such as KY jelly once the condom is on the penis.

Advantages:
- Most effective way to prevent STIs besides abstinence
- Easy to buy (inexpensive)
- Easy to carry
- Only way for male to protect himself from unplanned pregnancy
- Can help relieve premature ejaculation

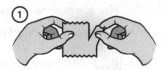
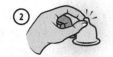
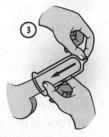

Disadvantages*:
- Possible allergies to latex
- Less sensation
- Condom breakage
- Sometimes interrupts 'the mood'
- Human error: withdrawal without holding the condom in place; using after the expiration date; opening the package with teeth, fingernails, or sharp objects can damage the condom; storage of condoms in a warm place such as a wallet in a back pocket can decrease effectiveness."[1]

© Stanil777/Shutterstock.com

Figure 7.6

"Diaphragm and Femcap

Latex cup (diaphragm) or silicone cup (Femcap) requires fitting by a clinician. The diaphragm or cap is coated with spermicide before placement in the vagina. The diaphragm or cervical cap combined with spermicide act by destroying the sperm and preventing the sperm from reaching the egg. After intercourse, the Femcap should be left in place for eight hours.

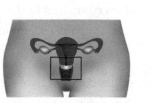
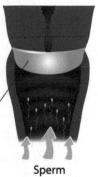

Diaphragm
Barrier method of birth control

Diaphragm blocks sperm

Sperm

© Tefi/Shutterstock.com

Effectiveness:
in preventing pregnancy:
- Diaphragm with spermicide—86–94 percent
- Femcap with spermicide—84–91 percent for women who have never given birth; 68–74 percent for women who have given birth
- in preventing STIs—NONE

Advantages:
- Femcap can be inserted many hours before sexual intercourse
- Diaphragm can be inserted two hours before sexual intercourse
- Does not alter the menstrual cycle; easy to carry with you, comfortable
- No major health concerns
- Can last several years

Disadvantages:
- Can be messy
- Possibility of allergies to latex, silicone, or spermicide
- Cannot use with vaginal bleeding or an infection
- Diaphragm—can only be left in place for up to twenty-four hours
- Diaphragm—increased risk of bladder infection
- Femcap—difficult for some women to use
- Femcap—can only be left in place for up to forty-eight hours"[1]

"Over-the-Counter Contraceptives for Women

- Female condom—insert vaginal pouch deep into vagina prior to intercourse
- Spermicide, foam, jelly, or cream—insert deep into vagina prior to intercourse

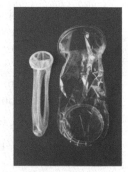

Effectiveness:
in preventing pregnancy:
- Female condom—79–95 percent
- Spermicide, foam, jelly, or cream—71–82 percent in preventing STIs:
- Female condom—similar to the male condom, but not quite as effective, due to possible folding
- Spermicides, foam, jelly, and cream in preventing STIs—NONE

© Image Point Fr /Shutterstock.com

Advantages:

- Easy to purchase in drugstores, supermarkets, etc.
- Increased sensation compared to the male condom
- Erection not necessary to keep female condom in place

Disadvantages:

- Outer ring of female condom may slip into vagina during intercourse
- Possible difficulty inserting the pouch
- More difficult preparation
- Possible allergies to spermicide"[1]

"Hormonal Methods

"The Pill

The pill (oral contraceptive pills) is a prescription medication containing the hormones estrogen and/or progesterone, which usually prevents the release of the egg, thickens the cervical mucus, and reduces the buildup of the endometrial lining within the uterus. The sperm is thus unable to penetrate the egg, and/or the fertilized egg is prevented from implanting in the uterus.

Effectiveness:

- in preventing pregnancy: 92–99.7 percent
- in preventing STIs—NONE

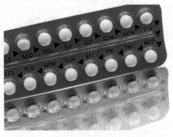

© areeya_ann/Shutterstock.com

Advantages:

- Nothing to put into place before intercourse
- Regular and shorter periods
- Decreases chances of developing ovarian and endometrial cancers, non-cancerous breast tumors, ovarian cysts, pelvic inflammatory disease, and osteoporosis
- Decreased incidence of tubal pregnancies
- Ability to become pregnant returns quickly when use is stopped

Disadvantages:

- Less effective when taken with some drugs
- Must be taken daily (within the same two hour period)
- Rare but serious health risks, including: blood clots, heart attack, and stroke, which are more common for women over 35 and/or who smoke cigarettes (ARHP, 2008). This increased risk is found in most of the hormonal contraceptive methods. This is due to an increased correlation of cardiovascular disease most likely from the formation of atherosclerosis in women who smoke and use hormonal contraceptive methods. This risk also increases as women age, smoke, and use hormonal contraceptive methods.
- Side effects can include temporary irregular bleeding, weight gain, breast tenderness, and nausea.

Women who experience any of the following symptoms while taking the pill should call their physician immediately:

- Abdominal pains (severe)
- Chest pain or shortness of breath
- Headaches (severe)

- Eye problems, such as blurred vision
- Severe leg or arm pain or numbness"[1]

"Mini-pills

Mini-pills (oral contraceptive pills) are a prescription medication containing progesterone only, which usually prevents the release of the egg, thickens the cervical mucus, and reduces the buildup of the endometrial lining within the uterus. The sperm is thus unable to penetrate the egg, and/or the fertilized egg is prevented from implanting in the uterus.

Effectiveness:
- in preventing pregnancy: 87–99.7 percent (slightly less than regular birth control pills)
- in preventing STIs—NONE

Advantages:
- Nothing to put into place before intercourse
- Avoids typical side effects of regular birth control pills
- Has no estrogen
- Ability to become pregnant returns quickly when use is stopped

Disadvantages:
- Less effective when taken with some drugs
- MUST be taken at the same time every day
- Increased risk of ectopic pregnancy
- Increased risk of functional ovarian cysts"[1]

"Vaginal Ring

The female will insert a small, flexible ring deep into the vagina for three weeks and take it out for the fourth week. It releases combined hormones that protect against pregnancy for one month. The ring uses hormones similar to the estrogen and progesterone made by a woman's ovaries to prevent the ovaries from releasing an egg, thickens the cervical mucus, and reduces the buildup of the endometrial lining within the uterus. The sperm is thus unable to penetrate the egg, and/ or the fertilized egg is prevented from implanting in the uterus.

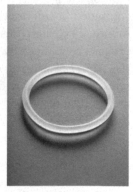

© Image Point Fr /Shutterstock.com

Effectiveness:
- in preventing pregnancy: 92–99.7 percent
- in preventing STIs—NONE

Advantages:
- Protects against pregnancy for one month
- No pill to take daily
- Does not require a "fitting" by a clinician
- Does not require the use of spermicide
- Ability to become pregnant returns quickly when use is stopped
- Nothing to put into place before intercourse
- More regular and shorter periods
- Reduces the risk of ovarian and endometrial cancers, pelvic inflammatory disease, non-cancerous growths of the breasts, ovarian cysts, and osteoporosis
- Fewer occurrences of ectopic pregnancy

Disadvantages:
- Increased vaginal discharge
- Vaginal irritation or infection
- Cannot use a diaphragm or cap for a backup method of birth control
- Rare but serious health risks, including blood clots, heart attack, and stroke—women who are 35 and older and/or smoke are at a greater risk. This increased risk is found in most of the hormonal contraceptive methods. This is due to an increased correlation of cardiovascular disease most likely from the formation of atherosclerosis in women who smoke and use hormonal contraceptive methods. This risk also increases as women age, smoke, and use hormonal contraceptive methods.
- Temporary irregular bleeding, weight gain, breast tenderness, and nausea

Women who experience any of the following symptoms while using the ring should call their physician immediately:
- Abdominal pains (severe)
- Chest pain or shortness of breath
- Headaches (severe)
- Eye problems, such as blurred vision
- Severe leg or arm pain or numbness"[1]

"Contraceptive Patch

The female will place a thin plastic patch on the skin of the buttocks, stomach, upper outer arm, or upper torso once a week for three weeks in a row. Use a new patch each week. Do not use a patch for the fourth week. The patch releases combined hormones that protect against pregnancy for one month. The patch uses hormones similar to the estrogen and progesterone made by a woman's ovaries to prevent the ovaries from releasing an egg, thickens the cervical mucus, and reduces the buildup of the endometrial lining within the uterus. The sperm is thus unable to penetrate the egg, and/or the fertilized egg is prevented from implanting in the uterus.

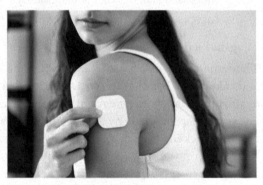

© Image Point Fr/Shutterstock.com

Effectiveness:
- in preventing pregnancy: 99 percent (for women who weigh 197 pounds or less) 92 percent (for women who weigh 198 pounds or more)
- in preventing STIs—NONE

Advantages:
- Protects against pregnancy for one month
- No pill to take daily
- Nothing to put into place before intercourse
- Ability to become pregnant returns quickly when use is stopped
- More regular and shorter periods
- Reduce the risk of ovarian and endometrial cancers, pelvic inflammatory disease, non-cancerous growths of the breasts, ovarian cysts, and osteoporosis
- Fewer occurrences of ectopic pregnancy

Disadvantages:

- Skin reaction at the site of application
- Menstrual cramps
- May not be effective for women who weigh more than 198 pounds
- Rare but serious health risks, including blood clots, heart attack, and stroke— women who are 35 and older and/or smoke are at a greater risk. This increased risk is found in most of the hormonal contraceptive methods. This is due to an increased correlation of cardiovascular disease most likely from the formation of atherosclerosis in women who smoke and use hormonal contraceptive methods. This risk also increases as women age, smoke, and use hormonal contraceptive methods.
- Temporary irregular bleeding, weight gain, breast tenderness, and nausea

Some women may not be able to use contraceptive patches because of the risk of serious health problems. Women over 35 who smoke or have any of the following conditions should not use the patch:

- History of heart attack or stroke
- Chest pain
- Blood clots
- Unexplained vaginal bleeding
- Severe high blood pressure
- Diabetes with kidney, eye, nerve, or blood vessel complications
- Known or suspected cancer
- Known or suspected pregnancy
- Liver tumors or liver disease
- Headaches with neurological symptoms
- Hepatitis or jaundice
- Disease of the heart valves with complications
- Require long bed rest following surgery
- Allergic reaction to the patch

Women who have a family history of breast cancer, diabetes, high blood pressure, high cholesterol, headaches or epilepsy, depression, gallbladder disease, kidney disease, heart disease, irregular periods, or are breast-feeding may not be able to use the patch. Women who experience any of the following symptoms while using the contraceptive patch should call their physician immediately:

- Abdominal pains (severe)
- Chest pain or shortness of breath
- Headaches (severe)
- Eye problems, such as blurred vision
- Severe leg or arm pain or numbness"[1]

"Depo-Provera

Depo-Provera is a hormone shot injected into the arm or buttocks every twelve weeks, which will prevent the release of the egg, less often thickens the cervical mucus and reduces the buildup of the endometrial lining within the uterus thereby preventing conception, and/or the fertilized egg from implanting in the uterus.

Effectiveness:

- in preventing pregnancy: 97–99.7 percent
- in preventing STIs—NONE

Advantages:

- Protects against pregnancy for twelve weeks
- No daily pill
- Nothing to put into place before intercourse
- Can be used by some women who cannot take the pill (oral contraceptive)
- Decreases incidence of endometrial and ovarian cancer, as well as iron deficiency anemia (ARHP, 2008)
- Can be used while breast-feeding

Contraception methods

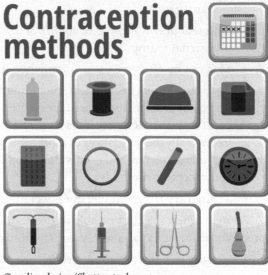

© vadim-design/Shutterstock.com

Figure 7.7

Disadvantages:

- Studies released in 2004 show that Depo-Provera is associated with a loss of bone density resulting in an increased risk of osteoporosis. The bone loss appears not to be reversed when the woman stops the Depo-Provera injections (U.S. Department of Health and Human Services).
- Side effects include irregular bleeding, headaches, depression, nausea, loss of monthly period, weight gain, nervousness, and dizziness
- Side effects cannot be reversed until medication wears off (up to twelve weeks)
- May cause delay in getting pregnant after shots are stopped (up to twelve to eighteen months)
- Should not be used continuously for more than two years."[1]

"IUD

The intrauterine device (IUD) requires a health care professional to insert a small plastic device through the cervix and into the uterus. The IUD contains copper or hormones that impede conception or rarely prevent implantation of a fertilized egg. IUDs can last one to ten years.

Effectiveness:

- in preventing pregnancy: 99.2–99.9 percent
- in preventing STIs—NONE

Advantages:

- Nothing to put into place before intercourse
- Para Gard (copper IUD) may be left in place for up to ten years; Mirena (hormone IUD) may be left in place for up to five years
- No daily pills
- Ability to become pregnant returns quickly when use is stopped

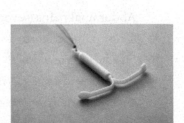

© Image Point Fr/Shutterstock.com

Disadvantages:

- May cause cramping (copper IUD)
- Spotting between periods

- Heavier and longer periods
- Increased risk of tubal infection, which may lead to infertility if inserted when a woman has an STI
- Rarely, the wall of the uterus is punctured"[1]

"Contraceptive Implant

Contraceptive implants are soft capsules, about 1.5 inches long, placed under the skin in a woman's upper inner arm. The capsules release progestin, which usually prevents the release of the egg, thickens the cervical mucus, and reduces the buildup of the endometrial lining within the uterus. The sperm is thus unable to penetrate the egg, and/or the fertilized egg is prevented from implanting in the uterus. Implanon is currently being used in the United States and is a single rod that releases a hormone called etonogestrel which lasts three years. Contraceptive implants can be removed at any time.

Effectiveness:

- in preventing pregnancy: 99 percent
- in preventing STIs—NONE

Advantages:

- Can be worn for three years
- Affects fertility one month at a time
- Has no estrogen

Disadvantages:

- Increased risk of heart attack
- Increased risk of stroke"[1]

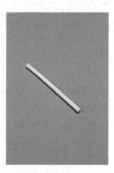

© Michael Kraus /Shutterstock.com

"Sterilization

Sterilization is an operation performed on the female (tubal ligation) or male (vasectomy). The tubal ligation is intended to permanently block a woman's fallopian tubes, where sperm typically unite with the eggs. A vasectomy is performed to permanently block a man's vas deferens tubes, which transport sperm.

Effectiveness:

- in preventing pregnancy: 99.5–99.9 percent
- in preventing STIs—NONE

Advantages:

- Permanent protection against pregnancy
- No lasting side effects
- No effects on sexual pleasure
- Protects woman whose health would be seriously threatened by a pregnancy

Disadvantages:

- Mild bleeding or infection after the surgery
- Some people eventually regret being unable to have children later in life

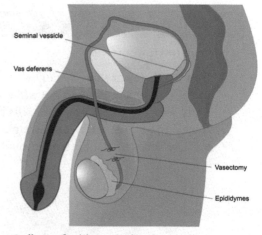

© ellepigrafica/Shutterstock.com

- Reaction to anesthetic
- Not usually reversible if you change your mind
- Rarely, tubes reopen, allowing pregnancy to occur
- Rare complications with tubal ligation include bleeding and injury to the bowel
- Vasectomy—infection or blood clot can occur in or near the testicles; often there is temporary bruising, swelling, or tenderness of the scrotum

Go to www.arhp.org/Method Match and use this interactive program to help you choose the birth control method that is right for you."[1]

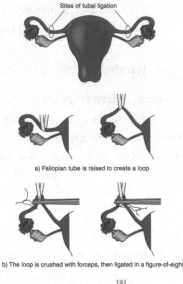

a) Fallopian tube is raised to create a loop

b) The loop is crushed with forceps, then ligated in a figure-of-eight

c) The loop is excised at the crushed zone

© Blamb/Shutterstock.com

EMERGENCY CONTRACEPTION "THE MORNING AFTER PILL"

"Emergency contraception refers to contraceptive methods used to prevent pregnancy in the first few days after unprotected intercourse, sexual assault, or contraceptive failure. Although the U.S. Food and Drug Administration approved the first dedicated product for emergency contraception in 1998, numerous barriers to emergency contraception remain. Emergency contraception is effective in preventing pregnancy within 120 hours after unprotected intercourse, but it is most effective if used as soon as possible, especially within 24 hours. Emergency contraception is sometimes confused with medication-induced abortion. Medication-induced abortion is used to terminate an existing pregnancy. All types of emergency contraception are effective only before a pregnancy is established, and, therefore, are not abortifacients. Another misconception is that making emergency contraception more readily available promotes risky sexual behavior and increases the rates of unintended pregnancy 7. Ready access to emergency contraception is not associated with less hormonal contraceptive use, less condom use, or more unprotected sex" (ACOG, 2019). Other pregnancy prevention methods, this one offers no protection against the contraction of STIs.[1]

Did you know . . .

According to Huffpost:

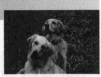

Courtesy of Shelley Hamill

- Every year, fewer than 1 in 100 women will become pregnant if they take the pill every day, but 9 in 100 will if they don't manage to take the pill daily.
- Early versions of birth control pills had higher doses of hormones and caused many women to gain weight, but most modern iterations do not.
- Researchers say that both hormonal and non-hormonal birth control options are on the way!

PREGNANCY PREVENTION CHART

		Effectiveness	Advantages	Disadvantages
Natural Methods:	Abstinence from Penile/Vaginal Intercourse	• In preventing pregnancy: 100% • In preventing STIs: 100%	• No worries • No medical or hormonal side effects • Protects against unwanted pregnancy	• People often forget to protect themselves against pregnancy or STIs when they stop abstaining
	Withdrawal Methods	• In preventing pregnancy: 73-96% • In preventing STIs: NONE	• Can be used when no other method is available	• Requires great self-control, experience, and trust • Not for men who ejaculate prematurely • Not recommended for teenagers
	Fertility Awareness-based Methods (FAMs)	• In preventing pregnancy: 75-99% • In preventing STIs: NONE	• No medical or hormonal side effects • Calendars, thermometers, and charts are easy to obtain	• Taking risks during 'unsafe' days • Illness and lack of sleep affect body temperatures • Cannot use with irregular periods or temperature patterns
Barrier Methods:	Male Condom	• In preventing pregnancy: 83-98% • In preventing STIs: 85-98%	• Most effective way to prevent STIs besides abstinence • Easy to buy (inexpensive); easy to carry • Can help relieve premature ejaculation	• Possible allergies to latex • Condom breakage • Sometimes interrupts 'the mood' • Human error
	Diaphragm	• In preventing pregnancy: 86-94% • In preventing STIs: NONE	• Diaphragm: Can be inserted 2 hours before sexual intercourse • Femcap: Can be inserted many hours before sexual intercourse • No major health concerns • Does not alter the menstrual cycle • Can last several years	• Can only be left in place for up to 24 hrs. • Increased risk of bladder infection
	Femcap	• In preventing pregnancy: 84-91% • In preventing STIs: NONE		• Difficult for some women to use • Can only be left in place for up to 48 hrs.
Over-the-Counter Contraceptives for Women:	• Female Condom • Spermicide, foam, jelly or cream	• In preventing pregnancy: • Female Condom 79-95% • Spermicide 71-82% • In preventing STIs: NONE	• Easy to purchase • Increased sensation compared to male condom • Erection not necessary to keep female condom in place	• Outer ring of female condom may slip into vagina during intercourse • Possible difficulty inserting the pouch • Possible allergies to spermicide

(continued)

		Effectiveness	Advantages	Disadvantages
Hormonal Methods:	The Pill	• In preventing pregnancy: 92-99.7% • In preventing STIs: NONE	• Regular and shorter periods • Nothing to put in place before intercourse	• Less effective when taken with some drugs • Must be taken daily
	Mini-pills	• In preventing pregnancy: 87-99.7% • In preventing STIs: NONE	• Nothing to put into place before intercourse • Has no estrogen • Avoids typical side effects of regular birth control pills	• Less effective when taken with some drugs • MUST be taken at the same time every day • Increased risk of ectopic pregnancy
	Vaginal Ring	• In preventing pregnancy: 92-99.7% • In preventing STIs: NONE	• Protects against pregnancy for one month • No daily pill	• Increased vaginal discharge • Vaginal irritation or infection
	Contraceptive Patch	• In preventing pregnancy: 99% (197 lbs or less) • 92% (198 lbs or more) • In preventing STIs: NONE	• Protects against pregnancy for one month • No daily pill • Nothing to put in place before intercourse	• Skin reaction at the site of application • Menstrual cramps • Temporary irregular bleeding, weight gain, breast tenderness, and nausea
	Depo-Provera	• In preventing pregnancy: 97-99.7% • In preventing STIs: NONE	• Protects pregnancy for 12 weeks • No daily pill • Can be used while breast-feeding	• Increased risk for osteoporosis • Side effects cannot be reversed until medication wears off
	IUD	• In preventing pregnancy: 99.2-99.9% • In preventing STIs: NONE	• Para Gard may be left in up to 10 years, Mirena may be left in up to 5 years	• Increased risk of tubal infection, which can lead to infertility • Rarely, the wall of the uterus is punctured
	Contraceptive Implant	• In preventing pregnancy: 99% • In preventing STIs: NONE	• Can be worn for 3 years • Affects fertility one month at a time • Has no estrogen	• Increased risk of heart attack • Increased risk of stroke
	Sterilization	• In preventing pregnancy: 99.5-99.9% • In preventing STIs: NONE	• Permanent protection against pregnancy • No effects on sexual pleasure	• Some people eventually regret being unable to have children later in life • Mild bleeding or infection after surgery

Courtesy of Caylee King

Male Contraceptives?

While male condoms are certainly popular, easy to find, and provide good protection from STIs, their actual user effectiveness with respect to pregnancy prevention may not be enough for some. There are studies being conducted utilizing injections, a patch, and even a pill to control sperm production. While none of these products are on the market yet, there is progress being made. In the not too distant future, men will have more options for controlling their own fertility.

Unplanned Pregnancy

"This can be a very exciting and/or frightening time in an individual's life. The thought of pregnancy conjures up many emotions, such as the realization of life changes, increased responsibility, happiness, and worry all at the same time. Pregnancy and the responsibilities of parenthood are tremendous. It is important to realize these potential consequences of unprotected intercourse or failed pregnancy prevention. It is a good idea to discuss how you might handle this situation with your potential sexual partner. In the event of an unplanned pregnancy, there are several options, none of which are easy and all can be life altering. These will be discussed in the following sections."[1]

Parenthood

"Parenthood has been described in many words. Many agree it is one of the best things that can happen, while for others parenthood is quite difficult and challenging. For most, this phase of life (given its rewards and demands) is a blend of these two perspectives. These differences of opinion are often influenced by the stage of life during which the individual becomes a parent, combined with factors such as other life circumstances (whether the parent will be a single parent or not), as well as the personality and financial situation of the new parent. Parenthood usually will dramatically alter the lifestyle to which an individual has become accustomed. Initially, it is an end to restful nights, spur-of-the-moment trips, and many social activities. New

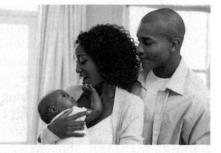

© wavebreakmedia/Shutterstock.com

parents now have an individual who is solely dependent upon them twenty-four hours a day for attention, love, food, clothing, safety, and shelter. This can be overwhelming physically, mentally, and financially even for the most prepared parents. It is also a time of tremendous joy, as well as many special moments, such as your baby's first smile, giggle, word, or step. As the child grows they are less dependent upon you for the basic necessities, but those needs change into dance lessons, soccer practice, and slumber parties, to name a few. The commitment to becoming a parent is large and one that never ends and can be very difficult to face alone."[1]

Adoption

For some, life circumstances may not support becoming a parent at that time. Adoption may be an option for the parent or parents and may be part of the discussion during the pregnancy. There are many factors involved in the decision. While it may be a very difficult one to make, it can be one that is beneficial to both the parent(s) and the child.

"Many adoption agencies exist to help make this option as painless as possible. There are many different types of adoptions. Some allow the biological parents to remain a part of the child's life; others do not, but provide a mechanism whereby the child can eventually obtain information regarding the biological parents. Often this information can be made available only after the adopted child enters adolescence or adulthood."[1]

Abortion

"Some individuals cannot (due to medical reasons) or do not want to carry the embryo to term, and therefore choose abortion. This decision is reached for various reasons. Sometimes this is felt to be the best decision because of the circumstances of conception (such as a rape or incest resulting in pregnancy). Some believe they cannot disclose a pregnancy to their parents or partner and see no other alternative. Others are not ready to become parents and do not want to complete the pregnancy.

"Abortion was made legal throughout the United States in 1973. Today, abortion is about ten times safer than giving birth. There are some potential complications associated with abortion. The complications can include an incomplete abortion, which means the procedure would need to be repeated; an infection, which can usually be treated with antibiotics; or perforation of the uterine wall. There are several types of abortion procedures available, depending on the stage of the pregnancy. Medical abortion (Mifepristone, RU-486, or nonsurgical abortion) is an option up to eight weeks since the last menstrual period (LMP). Surgical vacuum aspiration abortion is the procedure used to empty the uterus and can be performed between six and twelve weeks since the LMP. Last, the dilation and evacuation procedure can be performed between thirteen and twenty-four weeks since the LMP. After and during an abortion there is typically mild to very strong cramping for one to three hours, as well as bleeding and/or spotting for three to six weeks. A normal menstrual period should begin within four to eight weeks. Usually clinics will offer counseling before and after an abortion. Due to the emotional nature of any decision associated with pregnancy, counseling is highly recommended. As mentioned earlier, pregnancy is accompanied by many emotions and lasting effects for both partners. There is no easy route once pregnancy has occurred. It is a good idea to discuss your values and ideas of what you would do in the event of an unplanned pregnancy with your prospective sexual partner. It is best to fully consider all of the options before making a decision."[1]

It should also be noted that abortion laws are being challenged throughout the country. Some states have now enacted laws that prevent termination of a pregnancy after six weeks, no matter the circumstance of conception. Other states are looking to reduce the current window of time for the procedure as well. It is important for partners to be aware of what the laws are in their state with respect to an unplanned pregnancy. And, yes, the United States Supreme Court is now reviewing if they will overturn Roe v Wade which actually affirmed a woman's right to receive an abortion.

SEXUALLY TRANSMITTED INFECTIONS (STIs)

According to the Center for Disease Control, (CDC), the number of sexually transmitted infections, sometimes called sexually transmitted diseases, is on the rise.

STIs are a substantial health challenge facing the United States. On any given day in 2018, the CDC estimates that 1 in 5 sexually active people had an STI. CDC estimates that nearly 26 million new sexually transmitted infections occur every year in this country, half among young people aged 15–24, and account for almost $16 billion in health care costs. Incidence and prevalence estimates suggest that young people aged 15–24 years acquire half of all new STDs and that 1 in 4 sexually active adolescent females have an STD, such as chlamydia or human papillomavirus (HPV). Each of these infections is a potential threat to an individual's immediate and long-term health and well-being. In addition to increasing a person's risk for acquiring and transmitting HIV infection, STIs can lead to severe reproductive health complications, such as infertility and ectopic pregnancy. (CDC, 2021).

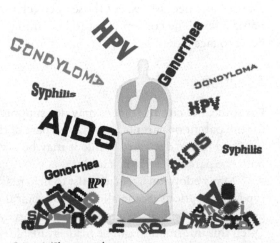

© jcwait/Shutterstock.com

"STIs are transmitted during vaginal, oral, anal sexual activity, or in some cases by simply touching an infected area. STIs can be transferred not only to the genitalia area, but also to the mouth, eyes, nose, and other orifices of the body. You can become infected if someone's blood, semen, vaginal secretions, or pre-cum goes into your body during vaginal, anal, or oral sex. Many individuals who become infected with STIs are asymptomatic (without symptoms) and thus become silent carriers. This is one of the reasons STIs have reached epidemic proportions. There are many health problems that can result if an asymptomatic STI carrier is not treated. Some of these health problems include infertility, ectopic pregnancies, and genital cancers, particularly cervical cancer in women. Therefore, it is very important to know your sexual history and be tested for STIs regularly."[1]

Levels of Risk

"Sexual behaviors have different levels of risk for different STIs. Using condoms lowers the risk of transmitting STIs in association with anal, oral, or vaginal intercourse. The following list depicts risk, assuming no protection is used for the following behaviors.

High Risk
- Anal intercourse
- Vaginal intercourse
- Oral sex on a man with ejaculation
- Oral sex on a man without ejaculation
- Oral sex on a woman
- Oral-anal contact

© Vertes Edmond Mihai/Shutterstock.com

Low Risk
- Intimate kissing
- Casual kissing
- Touching, massage

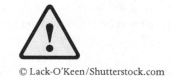

© Lack-O'Keen/Shutterstock.com

No Risk
- Masturbation
- Talking, fantasy"[1]

BACTERIAL STIs

Chlamydia

"Chlamydia is caused by a bacteria-like intracellular parasite called *Chlamydia trachomati*. Chlamydia is typically spread during vaginal, oral, or anal sex and can infect other body parts such as the eyes, nose, or throat where chlamydia can also be contracted. Symptoms in males include a thin, clear-whitish urethral discharge, itching or burning during urination, pain, or swelling in the testes and a low-grade fever. In females, symptoms include moderate vaginal discharge, itching or burning during urination,

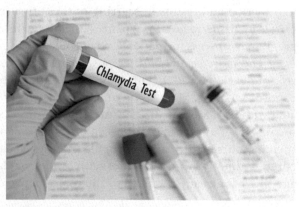

© Jarun Ontakrai/Shutterstock.com

abdominal pain, bleeding between periods, nausea, headaches, and a low-grade fever. If symptoms occur, they will typically begin one to three weeks after infection. 75 percent of infected females and 51 percent of infected males are asymptomatic (without symptoms). The long-term effects of untreated chlamydia can include infertility in both males and females from scarring in the testicles and fallopian tubes. Chlamydia infections are the leading cause of preventable infertility and ectopic pregnancies. In up to 40 percent of women with untreated chlamydia, infection can spread into the uterus and fallopian tubes, causing pelvic inflammatory disease (PID). Most infections respond to tetracycline, doxycycline, or erythromycin, but not penicillin. It is very important that all partners be treated to decrease the spread of infection, as well as prevent reinfection. Chlamydia is estimated to be the most common bacterial STI in the United States, with approximately two million new cases occurring each year (CDC, 2020).

Gonorrhea

"Gonorrhea is caused by the bacterium called *Neisseria gonorrhea*. Infection is found primarily in the linings of the urethra, vagina, mouth, and rectum (Crowley, 2009). Symptoms in males include a foul-smelling thick, creamy white, yellow, or yellow-green discharge from the penis, painful urination, blood or pus in the urine, and enlarged lymph nodes in the groin area. In females, the symptoms include similar discharge from the vagina, pain during urination, pelvic pain, or irregular and painful menstruation. If symptoms are present, they usually appear about one week after exposure. Many individuals are asymptomatic (5 to 20 percent of infected males and 60 to 80 percent

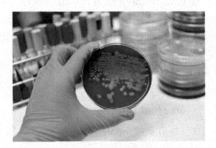

© Jarun Ontakrai/Shutterstock.com

of females). The long-term effects of untreated gonorrhea can cause infertility in both males and females, as a result of infection and scarring in both testicles and in the fallopian tubes. Gonorrhea remains one of the major causes of PID. Most infections respond to penicillin, tetracycline, spectinomycin, cefixime, or ceftriaxone. It is very important that all partners be treated to decrease the spread of the infection, as well as to prevent reinfection."[1]

Pelvic Inflammatory Disease (PID)

"PID is a general term that refers to an infection of the uterus, fallopian tubes, or other reproductive organ. Untreated sexually transmitted infections can cause PID. Chlamydia and gonorrhea are the most common STIs (if left untreated) that lead to PID. Damage to the fallopian tubes and tissues in and near the uterus and ovaries can result from PID. This damage occurs from the inflammation and results in scarring of these tissues. This scarring can lead to serious consequences including infertility, ectopic pregnancy, abscess formation, and chronic pelvic pain."[1]

Pelvic Inflammatory Disease

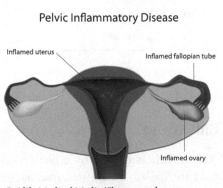

© Alila Medical Media/Shutterstock.com

"The more sexual partners a woman has had, the higher her risk of developing PID. This is because of the potential for more exposure to STIs. Most of the time there are no symptoms associated with PID. Meanwhile, the infection is causing serious long-term damage to the woman's reproductive organs. If symptoms exist, they can include lower abdominal pain, fever, unusual vaginal discharge, painful intercourse or urination, irregular menstrual bleeding, or pain in the right upper abdomen. PID can be cured with Ofloxacin, Levo- floxacin, or Metronidazole. "Antibiotic treatment does not reverse any damage that has already occurred to the reproductive organs. It is critical for any woman who has symptoms

<table>
<tr><td>

Unprotected vaginal or anal intercourse:

Bacterial Vaginosis
Chlamydia
Cytomegalovirus (CMV)
Gonorrhea
Hepatitis B
Herpes Simplex
Human Immunodeficiency Virus (HIV)
Human Papilloma Virus (HPV, Warts)
Pelvic Inflammatory Disease (PID)
Pubic Lice
Scabies
Syphilis
Trichomoniasis
*Safer Sex Tip: Always use condoms.

Unprotected oral sex:
(*"blow job," "giving head," "going down," "rimming"*)

Cytomegalovirus (CMV)
Gonorrhea
Hepatitis B

</td><td>

Herpes (including cold sores)
Human Immunodeficiency Virus (HIV)
Human Papilloma Virus (HPV, Warts)
Syphilis
*Safer Sex Tip: Use dental dams, non-lubricated or flavored condom, or female condoms.

Unprotected manual sex:
(*"hand job" or "fingering"*)

Bacterial Vaginosis
Cytomegalovirus (CMV)
Herpes Simplex
Human Papilloma Virus (HPV, Warts)
Pubic Lice
Scabies
*Safer Sex Tip: Use gloves or condoms.

Source: Adapted from www.scarleteen.com.

</td></tr>
</table>

©Kendall Hunt Publishing Company

Figure 7.8 STI Risk Sheet

of PID to be evaluated by a physician immediately. The longer treatment is delayed for PID the more likely she is to become infertile due to the damage to the reproductive organs."[1]

Syphilis

"Syphilis is a serious bacterial infection caused by the *spirochete Treponema pallidum*. Syphilis can be contracted and spread through vaginal, oral, or anal sex, as well as through blood and blood products. This disease can be debilitating and even fatal if left untreated. A person may be unknowingly infected with syphilis and transmit it to others. It is estimated that for every case of syphilis that is reported, three are not (Crooks & Baur, 2009).

1. "During the first stage, a painless sore (chancre) about the size of a dime may appear at the point where the bacteria first entered the body, usually three weeks after contact. This sore may appear around or in the vagina, on the penis, or inside the mouth or anus. Sores inside the vagina or anus are often unnoticed and may disappear on their own if not treated; however, the bacterial infection remains.

2. "The second stage occurs two to eight weeks after the exposure and includes flu-like symptoms and possible hair loss, a rash on the palms of hands and soles of feet, as well as over the entire body

3. "The tertiary (third stage) syphilis can appear five to twenty-five years after the initial exposure. Symptoms of this stage may include skin lesions, mental deterioration, loss of balance and vision, loss of sensation, shooting pains in the legs, and heart disease (Crooks & Baur, 2009)."[1]

"See a physician immediately if there is any chance you have been exposed to syphilis. A simple blood test can usually determine whether or not you have the disease. However, if you become infected two to three weeks prior to testing, the blood test may not be sensitive enough to detect the antibodies. Syphilis can be treated with the proper antibiotics, most commonly penicillin injections. There have been several

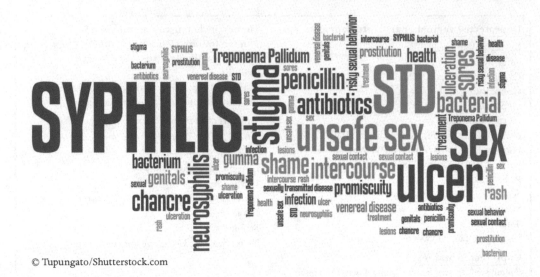

© Tupungato/Shutterstock.com

resistant strains that have developed when individuals did not take the full prescription dose. Always take all of the antibiotics that are prescribed to you; don't save them for later or stop them just because you feel better and NEVER take someone else's medication. Go to www.thebody.com/surveys/sexsurvey.html to take this absolutely anonymous test and discover your risk for HIV or other STIs."[1]

VIRAL STIs

Genital Herpes

"Genital herpes is a chronic, life-long infection caused by the herpes simplex virus (HSV). There are two types of HSV (Type 1 and Type 2), both of which can infect any area of the body, producing lesions (sores) in and around the vaginal area, on the penis, around the anal opening, on the buttocks or thighs, in or around the mouth, and in the eyes possibly causing blindness (Donatelle, 2010). Herpes can be contracted and spread through vaginal, oral, or anal sex, as well as skin-to-skin contact. A newborn may be infected with genital herpes while passing through the birth canal (Crooks & Baur, 2009). Infection in the newborn can cause mental retardation, blindness, or even death. Therefore, it

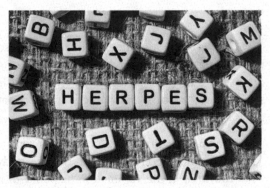

© schatzie/Shutterstock.com

is important that an infected pregnant female inform her physician of the infection so that the physician can watch for an outbreak and perform a cesarean section (C-section) if necessary."[1]

In the United States, about one out of every six people aged 14 to 49 years have genital herpes. Each year there are approximately 750,000 new herpes infections. "There are many more individuals who have genital herpes and are asymptomatic. The symptoms vary, and many people have no noticeable symptoms. Symptoms will most commonly occur within two to twenty days after infection. Early symptoms may include a tingling or burning sensation in the genitals, lower back pain, pain when urinating, and flu-like symptoms. A few days later, small red bump(s) may appear in the genital area. Later, these bumps can develop into painful blisters, which then crust over, form a scab, and heal. Sometimes the diagnosis can be made by physical examination alone. For testing, the physician collects a small amount of fluid from the sores to see if the herpes virus is present. It may take up to two weeks to receive the results. If no sores are present, testing may be difficult. However, a blood test does exist to determine if an individual does have the herpes virus. It is expensive and does not indicate the location of the infection. Although herpes is a chronic, lifelong viral infection, the symptoms can be treated. Treatment of genital herpes outbreaks, especially when begun early, shortens the duration of the outbreak and reduces the symptoms (Marr, 2007)."[1]

HIV/AIDS

"Human Immunodeficiency Virus (HIV)/Acquired Immune Deficiency Syndrome (AIDS) was first identified in the United States in June 1981 by the Centers for Disease Control and Prevention (CDC). HIV is the virus that causes AIDS and is transmitted in one of four ways: 1. vaginal, oral, or anal sex; 2. sharing a needle for piercing, tattoos, or drugs including steroids; 3. blood products infected with HIV; 4. from mother to child during pregnancy, delivery or breast milk. The highest concentrations of HIV are found in bodily fluids such as blood, semen, vaginal secretions, and breast milk (Floyd et al., 2007). Infection can occur when any of these fluids from an infected person comes into direct contact with the bloodstream or mucous membranes of another person. Trace amounts are found in tears, saliva, and other body fluids but have not been found to transmit infection. HIV is not spread by casual contact. It is not known if all individuals infected with this virus will develop AIDS. Women are more likely to become infected with HIV during heterosexual sex than males, because the concentration of virus is higher in semen than it is in vaginal secretions (Floyd et al., 2007). An individual may be asymptomatic or may have some of the symptoms, which include:

- fatigue,
- dry cough,
- fever,
- night sweats,
- diarrhea,
- skin rashes,
- swollen lymph nodes,
- recurrent vaginal yeast infections,
- unexplained weight loss.

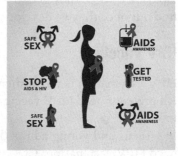

© jennylipets/Shutterstock.com

"Typically six weeks to six months is required after the initial infection to detect the HIV antibodies in a blood test (Floyd et al., 2007). There are numerous drugs/cocktails (mixture of different types of drugs) that exist to boost the immune system and interfere with the replication of the virus, therefore delaying the onset of AIDS. The best way to avoid contracting HIV is to abstain from vaginal, oral, or anal sex or have a mutually monogamous relationship with an uninfected partner. Other ways to protect yourself include HIV testing before becoming sexually active, consistent and correct use of latex condoms with all sexual acts (vaginal, oral, and anal), avoid sharing needles for anything, and do not have sex with anyone known or suspected of using injectable drugs including steroids. There are also new drugs that can prevent the transmission of HIV when taken as directed. PrEP, is a once-a-day pill that prevents HIV and is 99% effective when taken as directed. PEP,(post-exposure prophylaxis) is a medication that can prevent HIV seroconversion after a possible exposure. It should only be used in emergency situations and must be started 72 hours from exposure (CDC, 2022)."[1]

CDC estimates that 1,218,400 persons aged 13 years and older are living with HIV infection, including 156,300 (12.8%) who are unaware of their infection. Over the past decade, the number of people living with HIV has increased, while the annual number of new HIV infections has remained relatively stable. The estimated incidence of HIV has remained stable overall in recent years, at about 50,000 new HIV infections per year.

HPV

HPV is the most common sexually transmitted infection (STI). HPV is a different virus than HIV and HSV (herpes). HPV is so common that nearly all sexually active men and women get it at some point in their lives. There are many different types of HPV. Some types can cause health problems including genital warts and cancers. But there are vaccines that can stop these health problems from happening.

You can get HPV by having vaginal, anal, or oral sex with someone who has the virus. It is most commonly spread during vaginal or anal sex. HPV can be passed even when an infected person has no signs or symptoms. Anyone who is sexually active can get HPV, even if you have had sex with only one person. You also can develop symptoms years after you have sex with someone who is infected making it hard to know when you first became infected.

About 24 million Americans are currently infected with HPV. About 5 million people become newly infected each year. HPV is so common that most sexually-active men and women will get at least one type of HPV at some point in their lives. There is no test to find out a person's "HPV status." Also, there is no approved HPV test to find HPV in the mouth or throat.

There are HPV tests that can be used to screen for cervical cancer. These tests are recommended for screening only in women aged 30 years and older. They are not recommended to screen men, adolescents, or women under the age of 30 years.

Most people with HPV do not know they are infected and never develop symptoms or health problems from it. Some people find out they have HPV when they get genital warts. Women may find out they have HPV when they get an abnormal Pap test result (during cervical cancer screening). Others may only find out once they've developed more serious problems from HPV, such as cancers.

HPV Vaccine

HPV vaccination is recommended at ages 11–12 years. HPV vaccines can be given starting at age 9 years. All preteens need HPV vaccination, so they are protected from HPV infections that can cause cancer later in life.

Teens and young adults through age 26 years who didn't start or finish the HPV vaccine series also need HPV vaccination. CDC recommends that 11- to 12-year-olds receive two doses of HPV vaccine 6 to 12 months apart.

The first dose is routinely recommended at ages 11–12 years old. The vaccination can be started at age 9 years. Only two doses are needed if the first dose was given before 15th birthday. Teens and young adults who start the series later, at ages 15 through 26 years, need three doses of HPV vaccine.

Children aged 9 through 14 years who have received two doses of HPV vaccine less than 5 months apart will need a third dose. Three doses are also recommended for people aged 9 through 26 years who have weakened immune systems. Vaccination is not recommended for everyone older than age 26 years.

Some adults age 27 through 45 years who are not already vaccinated may decide to get HPV vaccine after speaking with their doctor about their risk for new HPV infections and the possible benefits of vaccination for them. HPV vaccination in this age range provides less benefit, because more people in this age range have already been exposed to HPV (CDC, 2021).

Hepatitis B

Hepatitis B is a contagious liver disease that results from infection with the Hepatitis B virus. When first infected, a person can develop an "acute" infection, which can range in severity from a very mild illness with few or no symptoms to a serious condition requiring hospitalization. **Acute** Hepatitis B refers to the first 6 months after someone is exposed to the Hepatitis B virus. Some people are able to fight the infection and clear the virus. For others, the infection remains and leads to a "chronic," or lifelong, illness. **Chronic** Hepatitis B refers to the illness that occurs when the Hepatitis B virus remains in a person's body. Over time, the infection can cause serious health problems.

Unfortunately, many people do not know they are infected.

Hepatitis B is usually spread when blood, semen, or other body fluids from a person infected with the Hepatitis B virus enter the body of someone who is not infected. This can happen through sexual contact with an infected person or sharing needles, syringes, or other injection drug equipment. Hepatitis B can also be passed from an infected mother to her baby at birth.

Hepatitis B is *not* spread through breastfeeding, sharing eating utensils, hugging, kissing, holding hands, coughing, or sneezing. Unlike some forms of hepatitis, Hepatitis B is also not spread by contaminated food or water.

In the United States, Hepatitis B is most commonly spread through sexual contact. The Hepatitis B virus is 50–100 times more infectious than HIV and can be passed through the exchange of body fluids, such as semen, vaginal fluids, and blood.

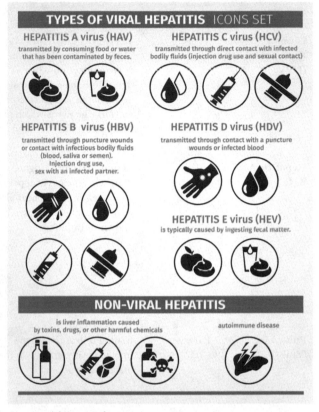

© Leyasw/Shutterstock.com

TABLE 7.1 What Are the Common Sexually Transmitted Infections (STIs)?

STI/D	Pathogen	Symptoms	How Transmitted	Cure?
Herpes	Virus	Fever, headache, blisters at the site of exposure.	Contact with viral shedding at mucus membrane sites.	No, but there are medications to help suppress outbreaks and lesson severity.
Chlamydia	Bacteria	Initially, women in particular may be asymptomatic; painful urination, low back pain; men may experience a discharge.	Vaginal intercourse, oral sex, anal sex and vulva to vulva contact.	Yes, with appropriate antibiotics.
Gonorrhea	Bacteria	Initially for women this is another that may be asymptomatic before eventually leading to PID; men may have discharge, and frequency/ urgency of urination.	Vaginal intercourse, oral sex, anal sex and vulva to vulva contact.	Yes, with appropriate antibiotics.
Syphilis	Bacteria	There are 3 stages for syphilis (see chapter for details). Primary, secondary, and tertiary.	Vaginal intercourse, oral sex, anal sex and vulva to vulva contact.	In the first or second stages, yes, with appropriate antibiotics. However, once the third stage has occurred there may be no repairing the damage already done.

(continued)

STI/D	Pathogen	Symptoms	How Transmitted	Cure?
Human Papillomavirus (HPV)	Virus	There are more than 40 types of HPV. Depending on the type of infection will determine the symptoms. Some of the strains create wart like growths which may be undetectable if located internally.	Vaginal intercourse, oral sex, anal sex and vulva to vulva contact.	There are various treatments available (see text). There is also a vaccine to help prevent infection.
Hepatitis A, B, C	Virus	Abdominal pain, fatigue, diarrhea, and loss of appetite; jaundice can also appear along with headaches, enlarged liver, and vomiting.	Hep A is typically spread by fecal contaminated food, though it can be spread through anal/oral. Hep B is typically through sexual contact. Hep C can be spread through sexual contact but is more commonly spread through blood transfusions.	There are vaccines for both A and B; treatment is available for all three to reduce viral load and assist the body with an immune response.
Pubic Lice "crabs"	Parasite	Itching unless the person infected is not allergic to the insect's saliva.	Contact with person, bedding or clothing infected with lice; they do crawl.	Yes but there are multiple things that must be done to remove the lice and their eggs. There are also creams to help with itching.
Scabies "mites"	Parasite	Rash and intense itching.	Usually spread via skin to skin contact.	Yes but there are multiple things that must be done to remove the lice and their eggs. There are also creams to help with itching.
HIV	Virus	Initial flu like symptoms may appear. However, this virus gradually deteriorates the immune system so additional symptoms will vary (see chapter).	Can be spread through blood, semen, vaginal secretions, breast milk, and perinatal.	There is currently no cure for HIV but there are medications to suppress the viral load.

Courtesy of Shelley Hamill

This chart is designed as a "quick glance" for information on the most common sexually transmitted infections. Further details about each one, along with ways to diagnose, can be found in this chapter.

PARASITIC STIs

Pubic Lice and Scabies

"Pubic lice (often called 'crabs') and scabies (itch mites) are parasitic insects that live on the skin. They are sometimes spread sexually, but are also transmitted by contact with infected bed linens, clothes, or towels. Pubic lice infect hairy parts of the body, especially around the groin area and can be transmitted by fingers to the armpits or scalp

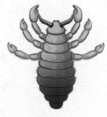

© Matthew Cole /Shutterstock.com

(Crooks & Baur, 2009). With scabies, an itchy rash is the result of a female mite burrowing into a person's skin to lay her eggs. The eggs can be seen on the hair close to the skin, where they hatch in five to ten days.

"Some individuals infected with pubic lice have no symptoms, while others may experience considerable itching in the area infected. Yellowish-gray insects the size of a pinhead moving on the skin or oval eggs attached to body hair may be visible. The primary symptom of scabies is itching, especially at night. A rash may appear in the folds of skin between the fingers or on the wrists, elbows, abdomen, or genitals.

"If you think you may have pubic lice or scabies, see your physician. They can determine whether treatment is necessary or not. The most effective treatments include shampoos and creams that contain lindane or a related compound. Pubic lice can be treated at home with special creams, lotions, and shampoos that are available in drugstores without a prescription. Be certain to follow the instructions carefully and do not exceed the recommended applications. The infestation may be stubborn, requiring an additional treatment.

"Avoid close contact with others if you have pubic lice or scabies until it is treated. Wash clothes, bed linens, and any other materials that may have been infected in hot water and dry on the hottest setting. If you have pubic lice or scabies, be sure to tell your sexual partner(s) or anyone with whom you have had close contact or who has shared your bed linens, clothes, or towels. These individuals should be seen by a physician even if they do not have an itch or rash. The best way to protect yourself is to know your partner's sexual history, don't share towels, swimsuits, or underwear and thoroughly wash any materials that you think may carry pubic lice or scabies in hot water."[1]

Trichomoniasis

"Trichomoniasis is caused by a protozoan parasite, Trichomonas vaginalis. The most common sites of infection are the vagina (in women) and the urethra (in men). The parasite is sexually transmitted through the penis to the vagina during intercourse or vulva to vulva contact with an infected partner. Most men infected with trichomoniasis are asymptomatic, but have the parasites and can infect their sexual partners. Some women will have signs or symptoms from the infection which include a yellowish-green vaginal discharge, a slight burning after urination, or itching in the genital area. These signs or symptoms typically appear five to twenty-eight days after exposure. A health care provider must perform a physical exam and laboratory tests to diagnose trichomoniasis. The treatment for trichomoniasis is a prescription drug (either Metronidazole or Tinidazole) taken by mouth in a single dose. It is important for both partners to be treated at the same time to eliminate the parasite. The best way to avoid contracting trichomoniasis is to abstain from vaginal, oral, or anal intercourse or have a mutually monogamous relationship with an uninfected partner. Utilizing male condoms consistently and correctly can reduce the risk of transmission of trichomoniasis."[1]

STI Prevention

There are several ways to avoid or reduce your risk of sexually transmitted infections:

- **Abstain.** The most effective way to avoid STIs is to abstain from sex.
- **Stay with one uninfected partner.** Another reliable way of avoiding STIs is to stay in a long-term mutually monogamous relationship with a partner who isn't infected.
- **Wait and verify.** Avoid vaginal and anal intercourse with new partners until you have both been tested for STIs. Oral sex is less risky, but use a latex condom or dental dam—a thin, square piece of rubber made with latex or silicone—to prevent direct contact between the oral and genital mucous membranes. Keep in mind that no good screening test exists for genital herpes for either sex, and human papillomavirus (HPV) screening isn't available for men. Different STI's require different screenings (see Table 7.2).

- **Get vaccinated.** Getting vaccinated early, before sexual exposure, is also effective in preventing certain types of STIs. Vaccines are available to prevent human papillomavirus (HPV), hepatitis A and hepatitis B. The Centers for Disease Control and Prevention (CDC) recommends the HPV vaccine for girls and boys ages 11 and 12. If not fully vaccinated at ages 11 and 12, the CDC recommends that girls and women through age 26 and boys and men through age 26 receive the vaccine. The hepatitis B vaccine is usually given to newborns, and the hepatitis A vaccine is recommended for 1-year-olds. Both vaccines are recommended for people who aren't already immune to these diseases and for those who are at increased risk of infection, such as men who have sex with men and IV drug users.

- **Use condoms and dental dams consistently and correctly.** Use a new latex condom or dental dam for each sex act, whether oral, vaginal or anal. Never use an oil-based lubricant, such as petroleum jelly, with a latex condom or dental dam. Condoms made from natural membranes are not recommended because they're not as effective at preventing STIs. Keep in mind that while condoms reduce your risk of exposure to most STIs, they provide a lesser degree of protection for STIs involving exposed genital sores, such as human papillomavirus (HPV) or herpes. Also, nonbarrier forms of contraception, such as oral contraceptives or intrauterine devices, don't protect against STIs.

- **Don't drink alcohol excessively or use drugs.** If you're under the influence, you're more likely to take sexual risks.

- **Communicate.** Before any serious sexual contact, communicate with your partner about practicing safer sex. Reach an explicit agreement about what activities will and won't be OK.

TABLE 7.2 STI Screenings

STI	Type of Test
Chlamydia	Urine test and/or culture
Genital Herpes	Visual inspection, culture and/or blood test
Gonorrhea	Urine test and/or culture
Hepatitis B	Blood test
HIV	Blood test
HPV	Visual inspection
Pubic Lice/Scabies	Visual inspection
Syphilis	Blood test

Are You a Wise Consumer?

If you are or plan on becoming sexually active, are you aware of the different types of contraceptive methods that can prevent pregnancy and or sexually transmitted infections (STI's)? How do you know what works best for you? Are you aware of some of the signs and symptoms of STI's? If you have been sexually active, have you ever been tested to see if you might have been infected, as some may be asymptomatic? We are responsible for our own health, as health literate individuals and wise consumers.

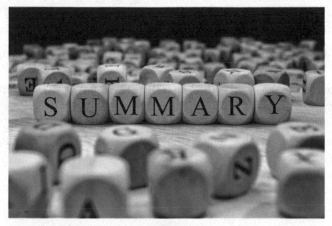

© Fabrik Bilder/Shutterstock.com

Deciding whether you are ready for sexual activity is a very important and personal decision. No one should be pressured in to an action or behavior they are unwilling to engage in nor should they be forced. If you decide the time is right to be sexually active, knowing what forms of protection are available is important. If a pathogen should present itself, knowing where to go and what to do for treatment is equally important.

PERSONAL REFLECTIONS . . . SO, WHAT HAVE YOU LEARNED?

1. In your own words, what is the difference in family planning, contraception and birth control?

2. What is the difference between "theoretical effectiveness" and "actual effectiveness"? Do you think most people actually know the difference? Why or why not?

3. Do you agree with the statement "If you are not mature enough to talk about sex, you are not mature enough to have it?" Why or why not?

NOTES

RESOURCES ON CAMPUS FOR YOU!

Health Services

Health Services is designed to provide confidential, professional, quality, cost-effective, acute, and routine medical care for all enrolled students. The staff of Health Services is committed in obtaining optimum personal health for each student through services and programs provided.

Counseling Services

Counseling Services will provide quality mental health service to enhance the overall mental health of students along cognitive, emotional, personal, and interpersonal dimensions.

Office of Victims Assistance or Campus Police

The Office of Victims Assistance is committed to providing quality services and advocacy to victims and survivors of sexual assault, stalking, and domestic and dating violence through a concentrated community response. Support and provide programming and education directed at eradicating sexual violence both on campus and in the community.

Office of Disability Services

The Office of Disability Services helps to create an accessible campus community where students with disabilities have equal opportunity to fully participate in their educational experience.

REFERENCES

American Cancer Society. (2005.)

American College Health Association (ACHA). (2005). *Sexually Transmitted Infections: What Everyone Should Know.*

American College Health Association (ACHA). (2004).

American College of Obstetricians and Gynecology (ACOG). (2011).

American Phycology Association (APA) Retrieved January, 5, 2016 from http://www.apa.org/topics/lgbt/orientation.aspx.

American Psychology Association. *Sexual orientation and homosexuality.* Retrieved January 5, 2016 from http://www.apa.org/topics/lgbt/orientation.aspx.

American Social Health Association (ASHA). (2009).

American College of Obstetricians and Gynecologists, (2019). https://www.acog.org/clinical/clinical-guidance/committee-opinion/articles/2017/07/access-to-emergency-contraception

Association of Reproductive Health Professionals (ARHP). (2008). Retrieved from www.arhp.org

Berman, L. (2012) Everyday Health. *Facts about male ejaculation.* Retrieved 2016 from http://www.everydayhealth.com/sexual-health-pictures/dr-laura-berman-male-ejaculation-facts.aspx#19

Blonna, R., & Carter, L.C. (2013). *Healthy sexuality.* Dubuque, IA: Kendall Hunt Publishing Company.

Cedar River Clinics Women's Health Specialist. (2016). *Birth control comparison chart.* Retrieved from http://www.birth-control-comparison.info/

Center for Disease Control and Prevention (CDC). (2017). Retrieved from https://www.cdc.gov/lgbthealth/youth.htm

CDC, 2021.https://www.cdc.gov/media/releases/2021/p0125-sexualy-transmitted-infection.html

CDC, 2021. https://www.cdc.gov/vaccines/vpd/hpv/public/index.html

Centers for Disease Control and Prevention (CDC). (2015.) www.cdc.gov/ std/syphilis/STDFact-syphilis.htm www.cdc.gov/std/herpes/STDFact-herpes.htm www.cdc.gov/std/PID/STDFact-PID.htm

Center for Disease Control and Prevention. (2015). *HIV in the United States at a glance.* Retrieved 2016 from http://www.cdc.gov/hiv/statistics/overview/ataglance.html.

Center for Disease Control and Prevention. (2015). *Genital herpes - CDC fact sheet.* Retrieved 2016 from http://www.cdc.gov/std/herpes/stdfact-herpes.htm

Center for Disease Control and Prevention. *Genital HPV infection-fact sheet.* Retrieved 2016 from http://www.cdc.gov/STD/HPV/STDFact-HPV.htm

Centers for Disease Control and Prevention (CDC). (2006). *Guidelines for treatment of sexually transmitted infections.* Retrieved from http://www.cdc.gov/std/treatment/.

Centers for Disease Control and Prevention (CDC). (2016). *Guidelines for treatment of sexually transmitted infections.* Retrieved from http://www.cdc.gov/std/treatment/.

Centers for Disease Control and Prevention. *Hepatitis B.* Retrieved 2016 from http://www.cdc.gov/hepatitis/HBV/PDFs/HepBGeneralFactSheet.pdf

Center for Disease Control and Prevention. (2015). *HIV basics.* Retrieved 2016 from http://www.cdc.gov/hiv/basics

Centers for Disease Control and Prevention (CDC). (2006). *HIV/AIDS surveillance report: Cases of HIV infection and AIDS in the United States and dependent areas.* http://www.cdc.gov/hepatitis/HBV/PDFs/HepBGeneralFactSheet.pdf

Center for Disease Control and Prevention. (2014). *STDs in adolescence and young adults.* Retrieved 2016 from http://www.cdc.gov/std/stats14/adol.htm#foot1.

Centers for Disease Control and Prevention (CDC). (2007). *Youth risk behavior survey.* Retrieved from www.cdc.gov/nchhstp/Newsroom/WADPressrelease-112408.htm

Crooks, R. and Baur, K. (2009). *Our Sexuality* (11th ed). Pacific Grove, CA: Brooks/Cole.

Crowley, L. (2009). *An Introduction to human disease: Pathology and pathophysiology correlations* (8th ed). Boston: Jones and Bartlett Publishers, Inc.

Donatelle, R. (2010). *Access to health* (12th ed). San Francisco: Benjamin Cummings.

Ellertson, C. et al. (2003). Extending the fine limit for starting the Yuzpe regimen of emergency contraception to 120 hours. *Obstetrics and Gynecology,* 101, 1168–1171.

ETR Associates. (2007). *Men's health: What's normal, what's not.*

ETR Associates. (2007). *Not ready for sex: Talking with your partner.*

ETR Associates. (2007). *Women's health: What's normal, what's not.*

ETR Associates. (2008). *Nine sexually responsible behaviors.*

Floyd, P. et al. (2007). *Personal health: perspectives & lifestyles* (4th ed). Englewood, CO: Morton Publishing Co.

Herek, G. et al. (1999). Psychological sequelae of hate-crime victimization among lesbian, gay, and bisexual adults. *Journal of Consulting and Clinical Psychology, 67,* 6.

Huffpost Women. (2013). *Birth control facts: 10 things you should absolutely know.* Retrieved 2016 from http://www.huffingtonpost.com/2013/06/27/birth-control-facts_n_3416638.html

Mayo Clinic, (2022). Mayoclinic.org/diseases-conditions/premenstrual-syndrome/diagnosis-treatment/drc-20376787

Mayo Clinic. (2014). *Sexually transmitted diseases (STDs).* Retrieved 2016 from http://www.mayoclinic.org/diseases-conditions/sexually-transmitted-diseases-stds/basics/prevention/CON-20034128

Marr, L. (2007). *Sexually transmitted siseases: A physician tells you what you need to know.* (2nd ed). Baltimore: Johns Hopkins University Press.

Sexuality Information and Education Council of the United States (SIECUS). (2008.) Retrieved from www. siecus.org/index.cfm?fuseaction=Page.viewPage+pageId=598+ ParentID=477

Trussell, J. and Jordan, B. (2006). Mechanism of action of emergency contraceptive pills. Contraception, 74, 87–89.

U.S. Department of Health and Human Services. (2004). *Bone health and osteoporosis: A report of the surgeon general.* Retrieved from www.cdc.gov/STD/HPV/STDFact-HPV.htm

www.cdc.gov/vaccines/recs/acip/downloads/mtg-slides-feb08/15-4-hpv.pdf

6 modes of HBV transmission in early childhood. Retrieved from www.fwhc.org/birth-control

https://www.hrc.org/resources/violence-against-the-transgender-community-in-2019

CREDITS

NOTES

Chapter 8

Drugs +

Pre-assessment

THINGS TO THINK ABOUT. . .

Tobacco

1. Have you ever tried smoking cigarettes, even one or two puffs?

    A. Yes

    B. No

2. How old were you when you smoked a whole cigarette for the first time?

    A. I have never smoked a whole cigarette

    B. 8 years old or younger

    C. 9 or 10 years old

    D. 11 or 12 years old

    E. 13 or 14 years old

    F. 15 or 16 years old

    G. 17 years old or older

3. During the past 30 days, on how many days did you smoke cigarettes?

    A. 0 days

    B. 1 or 2 days

    C. 3 to 5 days

    D. 6 to 9 days

    E. 10 to 19 days

    F. 20 to 29 days

    G. All 30 days

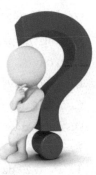

4. During the past 30 days, on the days you smoked, how many cigarettes did you smoke per day?

    A. I did not smoke cigarettes during the past 30 days

    B. Less than 1 cigarette per day

    C. 1 cigarette per day

    D. 2 to 5 cigarettes per day

    E. 6 to 10 cigarettes per day

    F. 11 to 20 cigarettes per day

    G. More than 20 cigarettes per day

5. During the past 30 days, how did you usually get your cigarettes? (Select only one response.)

    A. I did not smoke cigarettes during the past 30 days

    B. I bought them in a store such as a convenience store, supermarket, discount store, or gas station

    C. I got them on the Internet

    D. I gave someone else money to buy them for me

    E. I borrowed (or bummed) them from someone else

    F. A person 18 years old or older gave them to me

    G. I took them from a store or family member

    H. I got them some other way

6. During the past 12 months, did you ever try to quit smoking cigarettes?

    A. I did not smoke during the past 12 months

    B. Yes

    C. No

7. During the past 30 days, on how many days did you use chewing tobacco, snuff, or dip, such as Redman, Levi Garrett, Beechnut, Skoal Bandits, or Copenhagen?

   A. 0 days

   B. 1 or 2 days

   C. 3 to 5 days

   D. 6 to 9 days

   E. 10 to 19 days

   F. 20 to 29 days

   G. All 30 days

8. During the past 30 days, on how many days did you smoke cigars, cigarillos, or little cigars?

   A. 0 days

   B. 1 or 2 days

   C. 3 to 5 days

   D. 6 to 9 days

   E. 10 to 19 days

   F. 20 to 29 days

   G. All 30 days

The next 2 questions ask about electronic vapor products, such as blu, NJOY, or Starbuzz. Electronic vapor products include e-cigarettes, e-cigars, e-pipes, vape pipes, vaping pens, ehookahs, and hookah pens.

9. Have you ever used an electronic vapor product?

   A. Yes

   B. No

10. During the past 30 days, on how many days did you use an electronic vapor product?

   A. 0 days

   B. 1 or 2 days

   C. 3 to 5 days

   D. 6 to 9 days

   E. 10 to 19 days

   F. 20 to 29 days

   G. All 30 days

The next 6 questions ask about drinking alcohol. This includes drinking beer, wine, wine coolers, and liquor such as rum, gin, vodka, or whiskey. For these questions, drinking alcohol does not include drinking a few sips of wine for religious purposes.

11. During your life, on how many days have you had at least one drink of alcohol?

    A. 0 days

    B. 1 or 2 days

    C. 3 to 9 days

    D. 10 to 19 days

    E. 20 to 39 days

    F. 40 to 99 days

    G. 100 or more days

12. How old were you when you had your first drink of alcohol other than a few sips?

    A. I have never had a drink of alcohol other than a few sips

    B. 8 years old or younger

    C. 9 or 10 years old

    D. 11 or 12 years old

    E. 13 or 14 years old

    F. 15 or 16 years old

    G. 17 years old or older

13. During the past 30 days, on how many days did you have at least one drink of alcohol?

    A. 0 days

    B. 1 or 2 days

    C. 3 to 5 days

    D. 6 to 9 days

    E. 10 to 19 days

    F. 20 to 29 days

    G. All 30 days

14. During the past 30 days, on how many days did you have 5 or more drinks of alcohol in a row, that is within a couple of hours?

    A. 0 days

    B. 1 day

    C. 2 days

    D. 3 to 5 days

    E. 6 to 9 days

    F. 10 to 19 days

    G. 20 or more days

15. During the past 30 days, what is the largest number of alcoholic drinks you had in a row, that is, within a couple of hours?

 A. I did not drink alcohol during the past 30 days

 B. 1 or 2 drinks

 C. 3 drinks

 D. 4 drinks

 E. 5 drinks

 F. 6 or 7 drinks

 G. 8 or 9 drinks

 H. 10 or more drinks

16. During the past 30 days, how did you usually get the alcohol you drank?

 A. I did not drink alcohol during the past 30 days

 B. I bought it in a store such as a liquor store, convenience store, supermarket, discount store, or gas station

 C. I bought it at a restaurant, bar, or club

 D. I bought it at a public event such as a concert or sporting event

 E. I gave someone else money to buy it for me

 F. Someone gave it to me

 G. I took it from a store or family member

 H. I got it some other way

The next 3 questions ask about marijuana use. Marijuana also is called grass, weed, or pot.

17. During your life, how many times have you used marijuana?

 A. 0 times

 B. 1 or 2 times

 C. 3 to 9 times

 D. 10 to 19 times

 E. 20 to 39 times

 F. 40 to 99 times

 G. 100 or more times

18. How old were you when you tried marijuana for the first time?

 A. I have never tried marijuana

 B. 8 years old or younger

 C. 9 or 10 years old

 D. 11 or 12 years old

 E. 13 or 14 years old

 F. 15 or 16 years old

 G. 17 years old or older

19. During the past 30 days, how many times did you use marijuana?

    A. 0 times

    B. 1 or 2 times

    C. 3 to 9 times

    D. 10 to 19 times

    E. 20 to 39 times

    F. 40 or more times

The next 10 questions ask about other drugs.

20. During your life, how many times have you used any form of cocaine, including powder, crack, or freebase?

    A. 0 times

    B. 1 or 2 times

    C. 3 to 9 times

    D. 10 to 19 times

    E. 20 to 39 times

    F. 40 or more times

21. During your life, how many times have you sniffed glue, breathed the contents of aerosol spray cans, or inhaled any paints or sprays to get high?

    A. 0 times

    B. 1 or 2 times

    C. 3 to 9 times

    D. 10 to 19 times

    E. 20 to 39 times

    F. 40 or more times

22. During your life, how many times have you used heroin (also called smack, junk, or China White)?

    A. 0 times

    B. 1 or 2 times

    C. 3 to 9 times

    D. 10 to 19 times

    E. 20 to 39 times

    F. 40 or more times

23. During your life, how many times have you used methamphetamines (also called speed, crystal, crank, or ice)?

    A. 0 times

    B. 1 or 2 times

    C. 3 to 9 times

    D. 10 to 19 times

    E. 20 to 39 times

    F. 40 or more times

24. During your life, how many times have you used ecstasy (also called MDMA)?

    A. 0 times

    B. 1 or 2 times

    C. 3 to 9 times

    D. 10 to 19 times

    E. 20 to 39 times

    F. 40 or more times

25. During your life, how many times have you used synthetic marijuana (also called K2, Spice, fake weed, King Kong, Yucatan Fire, Skunk, or Moon Rocks)?

    A. 0 times

    B. 1 or 2 times

    C. 3 to 9 times

    D. 10 to 19 times

    E. 20 to 39 times

    F. 40 or more times

26. During your life, how many times have you taken steroid pills or shots without a doctor's prescription?

    A. 0 times

    B. 1 or 2 times

    C. 3 to 9 times

    D. 10 to 19 times

    E. 20 to 39 times

    F. 40 or more times

27. During your life, how many times have you taken a prescription drug (such as OxyContin, Percocet, Vicodin, codeine, Adderall, Ritalin, or Xanax) without a doctor's prescription?

    A. 0 times

    B. 1 or 2 times

    C. 3 to 9 times

    D. 10 to 19 times

    E. 20 to 39 times

    F. 40 or more times

28. During your life, how many times have you used a needle to inject any illegal drug into your body?

    A. 0 times

    B. 1 time

    C. 2 or more times

29. During the past 12 months, has anyone offered, sold, or given you an illegal drug on school property?

    A. Yes

    B. No

These questions were adapted from the National Youth Risk Behavior Survey (CDC, 2015).

Chapter 8
Tobacco, Alcohol and Other Drugs +

OBJECTIVES

Students will be able to:

- Identify types of tobacco products and the adverse effects associated with each.
- Discuss the concerns with E cigarettes.
- Distinquish between alcoholic beverages and the alcohol content in each
- Describe the risk factors associated with drinking and driving
- Describe the physiological effects of alcohol
- Discuss the societal effects of alcohol
- Analyze factors contributing to binge drinking and alcohol poisoning
- Identify common sources of caffeine
- Discuss varying types of drugs and their potential physiological effects
- Discuss current "club drugs" and their possible effects
- Identify commonly abused prescription drugs

INTRODUCTION

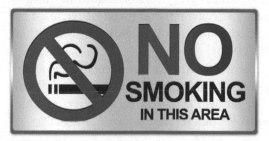

© DeiMosz/Shutterstock.com

Drug use in America has a long history. From hallucinogenic mushrooms and cacti, to alcohol infused enemas and psychoactive dried toad skins, people in the early Americas engaged in many mind altering behaviors.

'Understanding what drugs can do to your children, understanding peer pressure and understanding why they turn to drugs is . . . the first step in solving the problem.' Nancy Reagan

TOBACCO

In 1970, the United States Surgeon General reported that cigarette smoking was dangerous to our health. Yet, people still smoke and some have faced significant health consequences as a result. According to the CDC, smoking leads to disease and disability and harms nearly every organ in the body. It is the leading cause of preventable death and causes the United States billions of dollars each year.

In the U.S., cigarette smoking accounts for more than 480,000 deaths every year or about 1 in 5 deaths (CDC). In 2020, 13 of every 100 U.S. adults aged 18 years or older 12.5% currently* smoked cigarettes. This means an estimated 30.8 million adults in the United States currently smoke cigarettes. More than 16 million Americans live with a smoking-related disease (CDC, 2022).

Tobacco use is started and established primarily during adolescence. Nearly 9 out of 10 cigarette smokers first tried smoking by age 18, and 99% first tried smoking by age 26. If smoking continues at the current rate among youth in this country, 5.6 million of today's Americans younger than 18 will die early from a smoking-related illness. That's about one of every 13 Americans aged 17 years or younger alive today (CDC, 2022).

Tobacco Components

There are approximately 600 ingredients in a cigarette. When those cigarettes are burned, they create over 7,000 chemicals. Of those chemicals, at least 69 are known to cause cancer and many are toxic. Think about that. Why would you knowingly put those substances in your body or around someone you love, including your pets?

So what are some of those chemicals? The picture shows some of them and what they can do, but here are a few more and what they all might be used for:

- **Acetone**—found in nail polish remover
- **Acetic acid**—an ingredient in hair dye
- **Ammonia**—a common household cleaner
- **Arsenic**—used in rat poison
- **Benzene**—found in rubber cement and gasoline
- **Butane**—used in lighter fluid
- **Cadmium**—active component in battery acid
- **Carbon monoxide**—released in car exhaust fumes
- **Formaldehyde**—embalming fluid
- **Hexamine**—found in barbecue lighter fluid
- **Lead**—used in batteries
- **Naphthalene**—an ingredient in mothballs
- **Methanol**—a main component in rocket fuel
- **Nicotine**—used as an insecticide
- **Tar**—material for paving roads
- **Toluene**—used to manufacture paint

Tar, and the many chemicals within it, irritates the lungs and can promote chronic bronchitis and emphysema. Tar is produce from the actual burning of the tobacco. Over time, it can destroy the cilia that line the bronchi and cause "smoker's cough". Longterm use can lead to cancer development (See Figure 8.1).

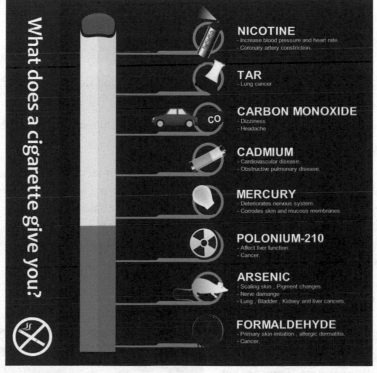

© Wikrom Kitsamritchai/Shutterstock.com

Figure 8.1 Possible Effects From the Various Chemicals Found in Tobacco

Nicotine, the highly addictive and very poisonous when concentrated, is a colorless, oily compound. It's physiological effects include rapid heartbeat, increased blood pressure, and increased blood flow from the heart which can cause narrowing of the arteries. And, nicotine is addictive. While it is debatable if, as some reports state, that nicotine is more addictive than heroin or cocaine, it is has also been reported that nicotine may be harder to quit than other drugs. As such, in 2018, the Food and Drug Administration (FDA), began moving towards regulations on how much nicotine would be allowed in tobacco products.

First, nicotine acts as a stimulant and then it tends to tranquilize the nervous system. The effects depend largely on how one chooses to smoke. Shallow puffs seem to increase alertness because low doses of nicotine facilitate the release of acetylcholine, which creates feelings of alertness. Long, deep drags tend to relax the smoker because high

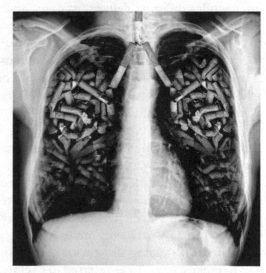

© Protasov AN/Shutterstock.com

doses of nicotine block the flow of acetylcholine. Ninety percent of the nicotine inhaled while smoking is absorbed into the body, while 20 to 30 percent of nicotine is absorbed if the smoke is drawn only into the mouth, not the lungs (Bounds, et al.).

What are some of the other side effects of nicotine? Your sense of taste can be dulled, your throat may become irritated and you skin may appear pale and feel clammy. Nicotine may also reduce your body temperature. And, to underscore it's addictive nature, when you do withdraw from nicotine, irritability, headaches, food cravings, and the inability to concentrate are just a few of the possible side effects.

- According to the CDC, smoking is a major cause of heart disease. One of every three deaths from cardio vascular disease, (CVD), can be attributed to smoking. Smoking can:
- Raise triglycerides (a type of fat in your blood)
- Lower "good" cholesterol (HDL)
- Make blood sticky and more likely to clot, which can block blood flow to the heart and brain
- Damage cells that line the blood vessels
- Increase the buildup of plaque (fat, cholesterol, calcium, and other substances) in blood vessels
- Cause thickening and narrowing of blood vessels (CDC).

Cigar smoking is not a safer alternative to cigarette smoking. In fact, cigar smoking is associated with and increased risk of lung cancer, and cancers of the esophagus, larynx, and lip, tongue, mouth and throat. It has also been linked to gum disease and tooth loss. Those who inhale deeply are more likely to develop CVD and have an increased risk for emphysema (CDC).

Pipe smoking also carries the same inherent risks as cigar smoking though the numbers of people who smoke pipes are far less than those who smoke cigarettes or cigars.

E-CIGARETTES/VAPING

E-cigarettes are known by many names. They have been called "e-cigs", "e-hookahs", "mods", "pens", and "vapes" among others. They are battery powered devices that provide nicotine and others chemicals through and aerosol. Differing brands offer differing delivery systems and flavoring with some of the more popular being fruit, mint, and chocolate. And, their popularity is growing. While some estimates of adult users is over 10 million, use among middle and high school students are growing in spite of FDA regulations on age requirements. In 2021, the CDC reports that nearly 2.8% of middle school students and 11.3% of high school students were using e-cigarettes (CDC, 2021).

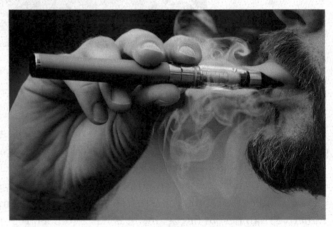

© Marc Bruxelle/Shutterstock.com

Are e-cigarettes less harmful than regular cigarettes? That may be debatable. While they contain fewer toxic chemicals than regular cigarettes, they do contain potentially harmful substances including nicotine (a highly addictive substance), heavy metals like lead, volatile organic compounds, and cancer-causing agents. What's even more troubling is, that in 2019 there were over 805 cases of sever lung disease associated with vaping along with 12 reported deaths.

Kretekes, sometimes referred to as clove cigarettes are "erroneously believed to be safer because they do not contain as much tobacco. In actuality, clove cigarettes are most harmful because they contain **eugenol**, which is an active ingredient of clove. Eugenol deadens sensations in the throat, which allows smokers to inhale more deeply and hold smoke in the lungs longer. Kretekes also contain twice as much tar, nicotine, and carbon monoxide as most moderate brands of American cigarettes."[1]

Bidis are small, thin, hand-rolled cigarettes imported to the United States, primarily from India and other Southeast Asian countries. They comprise tobacco wrapped in a tendu or temburni leaf (plants native to Asia) and may be secured with a colorful string at one or both ends. Bidis can be flavored (e.g., chocolate, cherry, mango) or unflavored (CDC). Though their use is relatively low in the United States, those who do partake are inhaling three to five times the amount of nicotine as regular cigarette users and increasing both the risks of addiction and chronic diseases associated with tobacco use (CDC).

Hookahs are water pipes that are used to smoke specially made tobacco that is usually flavored. They are also called a number of different names, including waterpipe, narghile, argileh, shisha, hubble-bubble, and goza. Hookah smoking is typically practiced in groups, with the same mouthpiece passed from person to person.

Similar to cigarettes, hookah smoking delivers the addictive drug nicotine and it is at least as toxic as cigarette smoking. While many hookah smokers may consider this practice less harmful than smoking cigarettes, hookah smoking carries many of the same health risks as cigarettes.

In recent years, there has been an increase in hookah use around the world, most notably among youth and college students. The Monitoring the Future survey found that in 2018, one in every 13 high school students had used hookah to smoke tobacco in the previous year. About one in every eight young adults 19–30 years had used a hookah to smoke tobacco during the previous year.

Another new addition to the mix **is Kratom.** Kratom is a tropical evergreen tree from Southeast Asia and is native to Thailand. The leaves can be chewed, dried and smoked, put in capsules or tablets or brewed in tea. The effects of can be those of a stimulant at low doses or those of an opiod at higher doses. While this product is not currently regulated, the FDA is examining whether it should be based on possible dangerous side effects. Some states have already banned its sale and distribution.

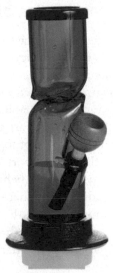

© Yurchyks /Shutterstock.com

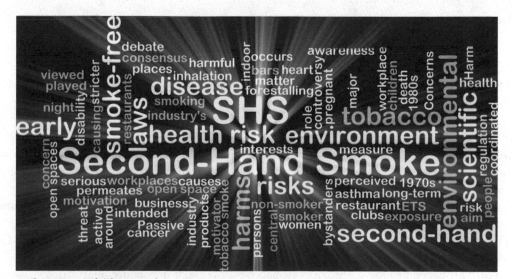

© Kheng Guan Toh/Shutterstock.com

Smoking Cessation

According to the CDC, nearly 7 out of 10 adult cigarette smokers reported they wanted to quit. After all, there are tremendous health benefits to quitting including lowered risk of cancers, reduced risk of heart disease (in as little as 1-2 years after quitting), and reduced risk of stroke to name a few.

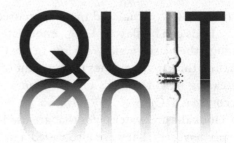

© Jane Rix/Shutterstock.com

And there are many ways to help smokers be successful in their attempt to quit. There are many counseling options including support groups and on-line or telephone connections. There is behavioral therapies and even hypnotherapy. Additionally, there are different products and medications, some are over the counter and some are prescription, that can help people through the withdrawal symptoms that come removing nicotine from your system.

The CDC offers 15 suggested steps for quitting. They are as follows:

- Know Your Reasons for Quitting
- Make a Decision to Quit
- Take Steps to Quit
- Learn About Nicotine Replacement Therapy
- Build Your Quit Plan
- Build Support to Stay Quit
- Manage Your Quit Day
- Prepare for Cravings
- Manage Withdrawal
- Prevent Slips
- Enjoy Benefits of Being Smokefree
- Prepare to Stay Smokefree
- Recognize Signs of Depression
- Reduce Your Stress
- Avoid Secondhand Smoke

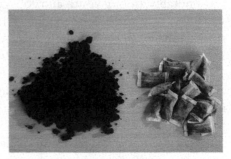

© bildfokus.se/Shutterstock.com

Remember, the best course of action is to not start using any form of tobacco or nicotine product to begin with. Consider your choices.

Smokeless tobacco is tobacco that is chewed, dipped, placed in the cheek of your mouth or sniffed. It come in forms that may involve spitting to remove excess or pouches that lodge in the cheek are absorbed through the lining of the mouth.

There are at least 28 chemicals that have been identified in smokeless tobacco that cause cancer. The most harmful of these are nitrosamines which are formed during the growing and maturing process for tobacco. There are other agents, including polonium, which is a radioactive particle and even formaldehyde, which is found in embalming fluid.

As with other tobacco products, smokeless tobacco is not safe. It may cause heart disease, oral cancers, gum disease, esophageal cancer, and has even been linked to pancreatic cancer. Leukoplakia, precancerous white patches, may also appear in the mouth. In men, smokeless tobacco reduces sperm count and increases the likelihood of abnormal sperm cell.

ALCOHOL

Approximately 52.7% of Americans age twelve and over (139.7 million people) reported being current drinkers in the 2019 National Survey on Drug Use and Health (SAMHSA, 2020). "**Ethyl alcohol**, or ethanol, has been prevalent in our society for centuries. Except for the Prohibition Era in the United States from 1917 to 1932 when alcohol was considered an illegal substance, it has become the legal and accepted drug of choice. There are three major types of alcoholic beverages: distilled spirits (hard liquor), wine or wine coolers, and beer."[1]

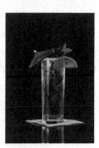

© Wollertz/
Shutterstock.com

When we think distilled spirits, we are talking about gin, rum, scotch, tequila, vodka, and whiskey and all of the variation of each. And, let's not forget about all of the liquors. Alcohol content varies depending on the type and the proof of the beverage is twice the percent of alcohol. So, if scotch is 60 proof, then it is 30 percent alcohol by volume. Of course, some mixed drinks have multiple shots of hard liquor. A "Long Island Ice Tea" for example may have 4–5 shots of different liquors making one drink the equivalent of 4–5 drinks!

For a better look at alcohol content by type, consider the following:

- 12 ounces of beer, or one bottle at 5% ABV.
- 8 ounces of malt liquor at 7% ABV.
- 5 ounces of wine at 12% ABV.
- 1.5 ounces of hard liquor, or one shot, at 40% ABV.
- 8-9 ounces of malt liquor at 7% ABV.

One of the challenges when talking about a "standard" drink is that people don't understand serving size as well as alcohol amount in those servings. The average glass of wine, with a fair pour, is 4-5 ounces. Beer is typically 12 and hard liquor is 1.5 ounces. "Beer is usually served in twelve-ounce cans or bottles, although some pubs sell pints, which are 16 ounces. The average alcohol content of beer is 4.5 percent by volume. To be considered a beer, the alcohol content must not exceed 5 percent by weight and volume. If the amount of alcohol is greater, it is considered ale. **Craft beer** has become a booming industry. According to Fortune.com (2015), 1 out of every 10 beers sold is a craft beer. The average alcohol content of craft beer is 5.9 percent. However, that number is increasing. According consumer research group Mintel, the amount of beers released with more than 6.5 percent alcohol by volume increased by 319 percent in North America from 2011 to 2014, with 46 percent of new beer releases falling into this category (CNN, 2015). Overall U.S. beer volume sales were up 1% in 2021, while craft brewer volume sales grew 8%, raising small and independent brewers' share of the U.S. beer market by volume to 13.1%.

Physiological Effects

Alcohol can have many damaging effects on the body. It can raise blood pressure, increase the risk for many different types of cancer, including liver and brain. It can also have an impact on vision affecting fine muscle control in eyes impacting focus, night vision and color distinction. Another factor with alcohol is, as a depressant, it slows down the nervous system which impacts the respiratory and cardiovascular systems.

Blood Alcohol Concentration (BAC)

BAC is a measure of the concentration of alcohol in blood, expressed in grams per 100 milliliter. An example would be 100 milligrams of alcohol in 10 milliliter of blood would be reported as .10 percent. The higher the alcohol content of the drink, the higher BAC it will produce.

There are many factors that influence how alcohol will effect a person drinking. Obvious things like alcohol content and the size of the drink certainly, but there are also factors like body weight, how quickly the drinks are consumed, did the person eat before or while drinking, all have an influence. Additionally, gender plays a role in BAC. Males tend to have more water weight and therefore dilute alcohol more readily than women who tend t have more body fat. Men also have more of an enzyme called alcohol dehydrogenase than women which also helps them metabolize alcohol slightly faster. The liver can metabolize one standard drink an hour.

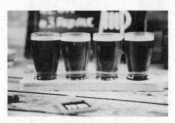
© MaxyM/Shutterstock.com

- And while the above mention factors have an influence, it still takes time for it to leave your system. No amount of sleep, food, exercise or medication can speed up the process. Depending on how it is being measured, alcohol can be detected in a person's system:
- **Blood**: Up to 6 hours
- **Breath**: 12-24 hours
- **Saliva**: 12-24 hours
- **Urine**: 12-24 hours
- **Hair**: 90 Days (See Figure 8.2)

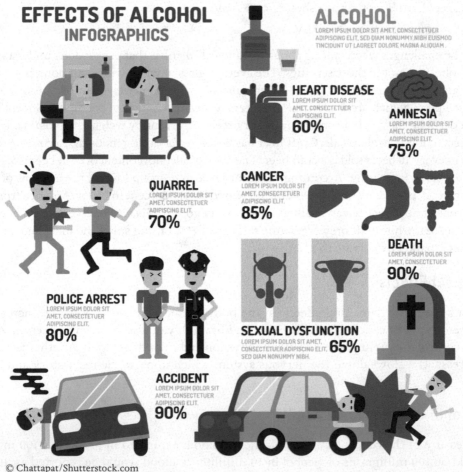
© Chattapat/Shutterstock.com

Figure 8.2 Possible Effects of Alcohol on the Body and the Brain

SIGNS OF INTOXICATION

Once alcohol enters the bloodstream, physical, metal and behavioral changes begin to occur. Signs and symptoms range from:

- Lowered inhibitions.
- Euphoria, excitability.
- Slurred speech.
- Impaired coordination.
- Confusion.
- Trouble remembering things.
- Difficulty concentrating.
- Loss of motor functions.
- Breathing problems (e.g., decreased respiratory effort, respiratory depression).
- Vomiting.
- Unconsciousness.
- Possible death[1]

Societal Problems

While we noted earlier how many people drink alcohol, the National Survey on Drug Use and Health report estimates that 14.8 million people over the age of 12 had an alcohol use disorder in 2018. In addition to health problems, drinking may contribute to motor vehicle accidents, violence, family and school or work problems.

Drinking and Driving

The National Highway Traffic Safety Administration (NHTSA) reported the almost 28 people died every day in the U.S. in 2019 as a result of drink driving crashes. That equates to one person every 52 minutes and more than 10,142 lives per year.

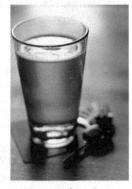
© Arjuna Kodisinghe /Shutterstock.com

"Drunk driving is no accident; it is a crime. The greatest tragedy is that these crashes are preventable, predictable, and 100 percent avoidable. Although most drivers involved in fatal crashes have no prior convictions for DUI, about one-third of all drivers arrested for driving under the influence are repeat offenders, which greatly increases their risk of causing a drunk driving accident. As a nation, we have seen a downward trend in alcohol-related fatalities. Today, all states have lowered their legal level of intoxication to .08 BAC. All states have some form of the zero tolerance law, as well as an open container law. These laws, in addition to stricter enforcement of existing laws, have helped in changing behavior. High school and university education programs, such as non-alcoholic activities for prom nights and designated driver organizations, have also contributed in raising awareness to combat such a serious problem."[1]

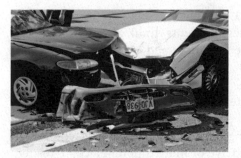
© TFoxFoto/Shutterstock.com

Before letting someone you know drink and drive, consider this:

- There are many ride-sharing companies. Call one! Better yet, call one before heading out for a night of partying.
- If you find you need to take someone's keys, avoid being confrontational. Make a joke and make seem easy.
- When they are distracted by something else, hide the keys so they will have to make another choice.

If it is someone you know well, insist that they give you their keys.

Alcohol Use in College

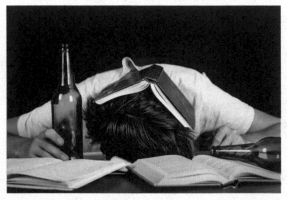

© Sabphoto/Shutterstock.com

In all states, the legal drinking age is 21. Yet, how many people do you know that have been drinking long before they reached that mark? Drinking on colleges campuses is not a new phenomenon and school administrators have struggled over time in dealing with problems associated with alcohol use and abuse. In addition to strict policies, some campuses require students to complete an on-line course on the dangers of alcohol use and others make sure sessions in freshman orientation address the issues. Still, the bottom line responsibility is on students making the best choices when it comes to alcohol use.

The National Institute on Alcohol Abuse and Alcoholism (NIAAA) reports that 1,519 college students die annually from alcohol-related unintentional injuries, including motor vehicle crashes, with 3.36 million students driving under the influence of alcohol. Another 599,000 between the ages of 18 and 24 are injured, and approximately 696,000 students per year are assaulted by a drinking student. Also, approximately 400,000 students between 18 and 24 years old reported having unprotected sex as a result of drinking. One in five college women experience sexual assault on college campuses. A majority of sexual assaults on those campuses involve alcohol or other substances, NIAAA, 2021).

About 23% of college students report academic consequences of their drinking including missing class, falling behind, doing poorly on exams or papers, and receiving lower grades overall. Other consequences include suicide attempts, health problems, injury, unsafe sexual behavior, and driving under the influence of alcohol, as well as vandalism, damage, and involvement with the police (NIAAA, 2021).

Binge Drinking

According to the 2019 National Survey on Drug Use and Health, 33 percent of college students reported binge drinking in the past month. Further 52.5% of full-time college students drank alcohol in the past month (NIAAA, 2021). Binge drinking occurs when men consume 5 or more and women consume 4 or more drinks in a two hour period. It is also most common in people aged 18–34.

"Binge drinkers usually experience more alcohol-related problems than their non-drinking counterparts. These problems affect their health, education, safety, and interpersonal relationships. According to the Harvard School of Public Health College Alcohol Study, these problems include driving after drinking, damaging property, getting injured, missing classes, and getting behind in school work. According to the same Harvard study, one in five students surveyed experienced five or more different alcohol-related problems and more than one-third of the students reported driving after drinking.

"The study also found that the vast majority of non-binge drinking students are negatively affected by the behavior of binge drinkers. It was reported that four out of five students who were non-binge drinkers and who lived on campus experienced secondary effects of binge drinking such as being the victim of a sexual assault or an unwanted sexual advance, having property vandalized, and having sleep or study interrupted."[1]

Did you know . . .

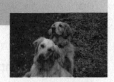

Courtesy of Shelley Hamill

Binge Drinking

According to the National Institute on Alcohol Abuse and Alcoholism:

- **Death:** 1,825 college students between the ages of 18 and 24 die each year from alcohol-related unintentional injuries.
- **Assault:** More than 696,000 students between the ages of 18 and 24 are assaulted by another student who has been drinking.
- **Sexual Abuse:** More than 97,000 students between the ages of 18 and 24 are victims of alcohol-related sexual assault or date rape.
- **Injury:** 599,000 students between the ages of 18 and 24 receive unintentional injuries while under the influence of alcohol.
- **Academic Problems:** About 25 percent of college students report academic consequences of their drinking including missing class, falling behind, doing poorly on exams or papers, and receiving lower grades overall.
- **Health Problems/Suicide Attempts:** More than 150,000 students develop an alcohol-related health problem and between 1.2 and 1.5 percent of students indicate that they tried to commit suicide within the past year due to drinking or drug use.

Alcohol Poisoning

Alcohol poisoning is certainly the most serious consequence of binge drinking. It can lead to unconsciousness and death. As a depressant, when too much alcohol is consumed, it can slow down breathing and heart functions as a result of oxygen depletion to the brain.

Alcohol poisoning signs and symptoms may include:

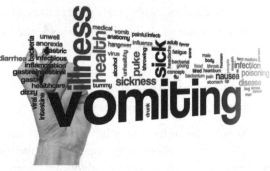

© ibreakstock/Shutterstock.com

- Confusion
- Vomiting
- Seizures
- Irregular breathing
- Blue tinged or pale skin
- Low body temperatures

If you think someone is experiencing alcohol poisoning, call 911 immediately. Do not leave the person alone. If they are unconscious, turn them on their side so that, should they become sick, they will not choke. Some students fear they will get in trouble if they call the police if they are involved in underage drinking. However, Good Samaritan laws protect individuals who offer assistance to someone in need.

Drinking Problems

In 2019, 85.6 percent of people ages 18 or older reported they drank alcohol at some point in their lifetime; 69.5 percent of those reported that they drank in the past year; 54.9% reported that they drank in the past month (NIAAA, 2022). "The National Institute on Alcohol Abuse and Alcoholism (NIAAA) found that the earlier young people begin to drink alcohol, the more likely they are to become an alcohol abuser or alcoholic. According to the report:

- Young people who start drinking before age 15 are four times more likely to become an alcoholic than if they start after age 21.
- Forty percent who drink before age 15 become alcohol dependent; 10 percent if they wait until 21.
- Fourteen percent decreased risk of alcoholism for each year drinking is delayed until age 21.

Alcoholism/Alcohol Use Disorder

When a person can no longer control their use of alcohol, when they compulsively abuse alcohol in spite of its negative health consequences and or if they experience emotional distress when they are not drinking, they may be suffering from Alcohol Use Disorder (AUD) or Alcoholism.

According to the *Diagnostic and Statistical Manual of Mental Disorders (DSM-5)*. To be diagnosed with AUD, individuals must meet any two of the below criteria within the same 12-month period:[2]

- Using alcohol in higher amounts or for a longer time than originally intended.
- Being unable to cut down on alcohol use despite a desire to do so.
- Spending a lot of time obtaining, using, and recovering from the effects of alcohol.
- Cravings, or a strong desire to use alcohol.
- Being unable to fulfill major obligations at home, work, or school because of alcohol use.
- Continuing to abuse alcohol despite negative interpersonal or social problems that are likely due to alcohol use.
- Giving up previously enjoyed social, occupational, or recreational activities because of alcohol use.
- Using alcohol in physically dangerous situations (such as driving or operating machinery).
- Continuing to abuse alcohol despite the presence of a psychological or physical problem that is probably due to alcohol use.
- Having a tolerance (i.e. needing to drink increasingly large or more frequent amounts of alcohol to achieve desired effect).
- Developing symptoms of withdrawal when efforts are made to stop using alcohol.

While alcoholism may have a genetic predisposition, there are a variety of psychological, social and environmental factors that may play a role. A child of an alcoholic parent is not destined to become an alcoholic. It does, mean, however, that they should be mindful of their use, if they decide to drink. Additionally, people with no genetic predisposition may become alcohol dependent.

Alcohol and Pregnancy

There is no known safe amount of alcohol use during pregnancy or while trying to get pregnant (CDC). There is also no safe time during pregnancy to drink. All types of alcohol are equally harmful, including all wines and beer. When a pregnant woman drinks alcohol, so does her baby.

© Stephen Finn/Shutterstock.com

Women also should not drink alcohol if they are sexually active and do not use effective contraception (birth control). This is because a woman might get pregnant and expose her baby to alcohol before she knows she is pregnant. Nearly half of all pregnancies in the United States are unplanned. Most women will not know they are pregnant for up to 4 to 6 weeks.

Chronic Effects

Drinking too much alcohol can cause a wide range of chronic health problems including liver disease, cancer, heart disease, brain, pancreas, nervous system problems, as well as alcoholism. Although moderate amounts of alcohol may not be harmful, there are some major health issues associated with chronic alcohol use and abuse.

Laws Relating to Alcohol

"In every state in the United States, it is illegal for a person under the age of 21 to attempt to purchase, possess, or consume alcohol.

"By operating a motor vehicle in a public place, the driver has given consent to take a breath/blood test to determine alcohol in their system. Refusing or failing the test is considered a violation, and penalties will result in loss of license, regardless of the outcome of the violation. In many states, the legal definition of **driving while intoxicated** (DWI) is not having normal use of your mental or physical faculties because of alcohol or other drugs; or a blood alcohol concentration of .08 or more. It is, however, illegal in all states to drink and drive. In addition, in most states, it is also illegal for anyone in the vehicle to possess an **open container** of alcohol regardless of age."[1]

Cannabinoids

Marijuana refers to the dried leaves, stems, flowers and seeds from the Cannabis Sativa or Cannabis indica plant. This plant contains a mind-altering substance known as THC. Depending on the potency of the THS, differing hallucinogenic effects can occur. THC is fat-soluble, and while its effects may wear off in a fairly short time, it can be detected for up to three weeks after consumption.

Marijuana activates the parts of the brain that contain the highest number of brain receptors. The effects from the 'high" that people feel include:

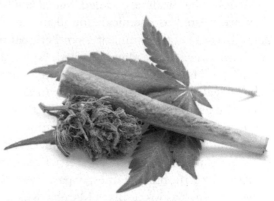

© Luis Carlos Jimenez del rio/Shutterstock.com

- altered senses (for example, seeing brighter colors)
- altered sense of time
- changes in mood
- impaired body movement
- difficulty with thinking and problem-solving
- impaired memory
- hallucinations (when taken in high doses)
- delusions (when taken in high doses)
- psychosis (risk is highest with regular use of high potency marijuana)

Prior to 2015, marijuana was the most commonly used illicit drug in the United States (SAMHSA, 2014). However, laws are changing quickly across the country. As of 2019, there were 11 states plus D.C. plus two US territories states where cannabis is now legal for adults 21 years and older as well as 33 states that allow medical use.

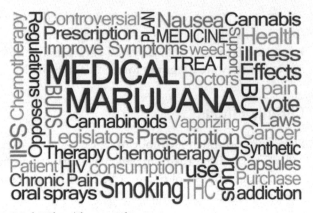

© Rob Wilson/Shutterstock.com

"The long-term effects are still being studied; however, chronic abuse may lead to a motivational syndrome in some. Marijuana smoke is irritating to the lung tissues and may be more damaging than cigarette smoke. There are four hundred chemicals in marijuana linked to lung cancer development. In addition, the immune system and reproductive systems are damaged. There is an increase in birth defects among children whose mothers smoke marijuana during pregnancy. The biggest concern related to marijuana use is the perception that there is no risk or harm associated with occasional use. Other health risks include possible mental health decline and addiction."[1]

Synthetic Cannabinoids

Synthetic cannabinoids refer to a growing number of man-made mind-altering chemicals that are either sprayed on dried, shredded plant material so they can be smoked (herbal incense) or sold as liquids to be vaporized and inhaled in e-cigarettes and other devices (liquid incense) (NIDA, 2015).

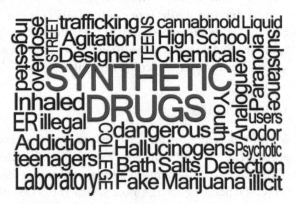

© Rob Wilson/Shutterstock.com

These chemicals are called *cannabinoids* because they are related to chemicals found in the marijuana plant. Because of this similarity, synthetic cannabinoids are sometimes misleadingly called "synthetic marijuana" (or "fake weed"), and are often marketed as "safe," legal alternatives to that drug. In fact, they may affect the brain much more powerfully than marijuana; their actual effects can be unpredictable and, in some cases, severe or even life-threatening.

Manufacturers sell these herbal incense products in colorful foil packages and sell similar liquid incense products, like other e-cigarette fluids, in plastic bottles. They market these products under a wide variety of specific brand names; in past years, K2 and Spice were common. Hundreds of other brand names now exist, such as Joker, Black Mamba, Kush, and Kronic.

Did you know . . .

According to the National Institute on Drug Abuse:

- Marijuana, including synthetic cannabinoids, can be addictive.
- After alcohol, marijuana is the drug most often linked to car accidents, including those involving deaths.
- Marijuana is linked to school failure.
- High doses of marijuana can cause psychosis or panic when you're high.
- The effects of synthetic cannabinoids can be unpredictable and life-threatening.

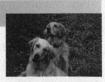

Courtesy of Shelley Hamill

Opioids

While this section will provide an overview about the types of opioids, it must start off discussing the staggering opioid epidemic the United States is dealing with in 2019. Every year, millions of adults are given opioids to manage pain. For some, those pills become addictive in a short amount of time. From 1999-2017, more than 700,00 people have died from a drug overdose. Of those, 68% involved opioids (CDC). On average, 130 Americans die every day from an opioid overdose.

This rise in opioid overdose deaths can be outlined in three distinct waves.

1. The first wave began with increased prescribing of opioids in the 1990s [3], with overdose deaths involving <u>prescription opioids</u> (natural and semi-synthetic opioids and methadone) increasing since at least 1999.

2. The second wave began in 2010, with rapid increases in overdose deaths involving <u>heroin</u>.

3. The third wave began in 2013, with significant increases in overdose deaths involving synthetic opioids – particularly those involving illicitly-manufactured <u>fentanyl</u> (IMF). The IMF market continues to change, and IMF can be found in combination with heroin, counterfeit pills, and cocaine.

While laws are efforts in education, law and policies are being put into place, we still have a long way to go before we truly get a handle on this crisis. "Derived from poppy seeds, **opium** is the base compound used for all narcotics. Opiates, which are narcotics, include opium and other drugs derived from opium, such as morphine, codeine, and heroin. Methadone is a synthetic chemical that has a morphine-like action, and also falls into this category of drugs."[1]

Heroin

Heroin is derived from a naturally occurring substance in the Oriental poppy plant called opium. It is a highly effective, fast-acting analgesic (painkiller) if injected when used medicinally; however, its benefits are outweighed by its risk of toxicity and high dependence rate. Heroin can be injected, snorted, or smoked. When heroin enters the brain it produces a dream-like euphoria. Abuse is common because this drug creates a strong physical and psychological dependence and tolerance. Recently heroin has become more popular among young people. The risks of heroin use are increased due to the use of needles for injection. There is an increased likelihood of transmission of communicable diseases like HIV and hepatitis due to the practice of sharing needles. Although abrupt withdrawal from heroin is rarely fatal, the discomfort associated with going 'cold turkey' is extremely intense.

Heroin users are at high risk for addiction. It is estimated that approximately 23% of heroin users become dependent. Anyone can become dependent, and life expectancy of the heroin addict who injects the drug intravenously is significantly lower than that of one who does not. Overdosing on heroin can result in death within minutes.

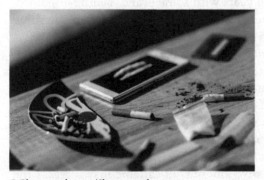

© Photographee.eu/Shutterstock.com

Heroin use has increased across the US among men and women, most age groups, and all income levels. Some of the greatest increases occurred in demographic groups with historically low rates of heroin use: women, the privately insured, and people with higher incomes. Not only are people using heroin, they are also abusing multiple other substances, especially cocaine and prescription opioid painkillers. As heroin use has increased, so have heroin-related overdose deaths. In 2019, 19.8% overdose deaths involved heroin (NIDA, 2020).

Fentanyl is a powerful synthetic opioid **analgesic** that is similar to morphine but is 80 to 100 times more potent. It is a schedule II prescription drug, and it is typically used to treat patients with severe pain or to manage pain after surgery. It has the potential to be easily abused and easily deadly especially if mixed with other substances including alcohol. Because of its powerful opioid properties, Fentanyl is also diverted for abuse. Fentanyl is added to heroin to increase its potency, or be disguised as highly potent heroin. Many users believe that they are purchasing heroin and actually don't know that they are purchasing fentanyl – which often results in overdose deaths. Clandestinely-produced fentanyl is primarily manufactured in Mexico. Fentanyl and other synthetic opiods are the most common drugs involved in overdose deaths. Even in small does, it can be deadly. Over 150 people die every day from overdoses related to synthetic opioids like Fentanyl (CDC, 2022).

Hydrocodone, codeine, and oxycodone also play a role in the addiction crisis and have come under much stricter regulation,

STIMULANTS

Caffeine

"**Caffeine** is a stimulant as well as a psychotropic (mind affecting) drug. Caffeine is generally associated with coffee, tea, and cola, but can also be found in chocolate, cocoa, and other carbonated beverages, as well as some medications, both prescription and non-prescription, i.e., Excedrin®. Approximately 65–180 milligrams of caffeine is found in one cup of coffee, compared to tea, which contains 40–100 mg per cup, and cola, which contains 30–60 mg per twelve ounce serving. Caffeine is readily absorbed into the body and causes stimulation of the cerebral cortex and medullary centers in the brain, resulting in mental alertness. Moderation is the key when using

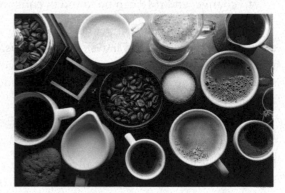

© Africa Studio/Shutterstock.com

caffeine. Researchers agree that 300 milligrams of caffeine is considered moderate intake, which is equivalent to approximately three cups of coffee. Some individuals are more sensitive to caffeine than others and may feel the effects at smaller doses. According to research, caffeine in beverage form is not dehydrating, but if ingesting caffeine from food or tablets, be sure to rehydrate from the drug's diuretic action.

"Excessive consumption of caffeine increases plasma levels of epinephrine, norepinephrine, and renin. It can also cause serious side effects, such as tremors, nervousness, irritability, headaches, hyperactivity, arrhythmia, dizziness, and insomnia. It can elevate the blood pressure and body temperature, increase the breathing rate, irritate the stomach and bowels, and dehydrate the body."[1]

Energy drink use has grown steadily over that past several years with some brands selling billions of dollars' worth of product. While some may use them as an energy boost, the amount of caffeine in some drinks can create some of the side effects listed above. Energy drinks are beverages like Red Bull, Rock Star, and Monster contain large doses of caffeine and other legal stimulants like guarana and ginseng. The amount of caffeine in an energy drink can range from 75 milligrams to over 200 milligrams per serving. This compares to 34 milligrams in Coke and 55 milligrams in Mountain Dew (Brown.edu).

"Excessive amounts of caffeine may increase the incidence of premenstrual syndrome (PMS) in some

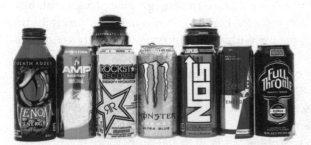

© Keith Homan/Shutterstock.com

women and may increase fibrocystic breast disease (noncancerous breast lumps) as well. The U.S. Surgeon General recommends that women avoid or restrict caffeine intake during pregnancy. Withdrawal symptoms from caffeine may include headaches, depression, drowsiness, nervousness, and a feeling of lethargy.

"College students have been known to use caffeinated products like these for extra energy when studying, driving long distances, or needing more energy in general. A common practice of mixing energy drinks and alcohol is of special concern. Drinking large amounts of caffeine (a stimulant) combined with large amounts of alcohol (a depressant) can cause people to misjudge their level of intoxication. The combination of drugs may mask symptoms such as headache, weakness, and muscle coordination, but in reality visual reaction time and motor coordination are still negatively affected by alcohol. Driving or making any other important decisions under these circumstances can be extremely dangerous."[1]

Cocaine

Cocaine is a powerfully addictive stimulant drug made from the leaves of the coca plant native to South America. It produces short-term euphoria, energy, and talkativeness in addition to potentially dangerous physical effects like raising heart rate and blood pressure.

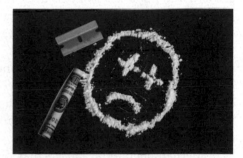

The powdered form of cocaine is either inhaled through the nose (snorted), where it is absorbed through the nasal tissue, or dissolved in water and injected into the bloodstream.

Crack is a form of cocaine that has been processed to make a rock crystal (also called "freebase cocaine") that can be smoked.

© Christopher Slesarchik/Shutterstock.com

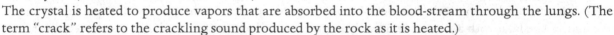

The crystal is heated to produce vapors that are absorbed into the blood-stream through the lungs. (The term "crack" refers to the crackling sound produced by the rock as it is heated.)

The intensity and duration of cocaine's pleasurable effects depend on the way it is administered. Injecting or smoking cocaine delivers the drug rapidly into the bloodstream and brain, producing a quicker and stronger but shorter-lasting high than snorting. The high from snorting cocaine may last 15 to 30 minutes; the high from smoking may last 5 to 10 minutes.

Cocaine affects the body in a variety of ways. It constricts blood vessels, dilates pupils, and increases body temperature, heart rate, and blood pressure. It can also cause headaches and gastrointestinal complications such as abdominal pain and nausea. Because cocaine tends to decrease appetite, chronic users can become malnourished as well.

Most seriously, people who use cocaine can suffer heart attacks or strokes, which may cause sudden death. Cocaine-related deaths are often a result of the heart stopping (cardiac arrest) followed by an arrest of breathing.

Cocaine is more dangerous when combined with other drugs or alcohol (poly-drug use). For example, the combination of cocaine and heroin (known as a "speedball") carries a particularly high risk of fatal overdose.

Amphetamines

"Amphetamines are drugs that speed up the nervous system. They do not occur naturally and must be manufactured in a laboratory. When used in moderation, amphetamines stimulate receptor sites for two naturally occurring neurotransmitters, having the effect of elevated mood, increased alertness, and feelings of well-being. In addition, the activity of the stomach and intestines may be slowed and appetite suppressed. When amphetamines are eliminated from the body, the user becomes fatigued.

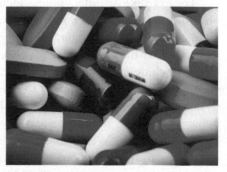

© Nenov Brothers Images/Shutterstock.com

With abuse, the user will experience rapid tolerance and a strong psychological dependence, along with the possibility of impotence and episodes of psychosis. When use stops, the abuser may experience periods of depression."[1]

Methamphetamines

"An extremely addictive and powerful drug that stimulates the central nervous system is commonly known as 'meth.' In its smoked form, it is called 'crystal,' 'crank,' or 'ice.' It is chemically similar to amphetamines, but much stronger. The effects from methamphetamine can last up to eight hours or in some cases even longer. It comes in many forms and can be injected, inhaled, orally ingested, or snorted. Methamphetamine is considered to be the fastest growing drug in the United States. According to the director of the Substance Abuse and Mental Health Services Administration (SAMHSA), the growth and popularity of this drug is because of its wide availability, easy production, low cost, and highly addictive nature. Methamphetamine is a psychostimulant but different than others like cocaine or amphetamine. Methamphetamine, like cocaine, results in an accumulation of dopamine. Dopamine is a neurotransmitter in regions of the brain that deal with emotion, movement, motivation, and pleasure. The large release of dopamine is presumed to help the drug's toxic effects on the brain. However, unlike cocaine, which is removed and metabolized quickly from the body, methamphetamine has a longer duration of action, which stays in the body and brain longer, leading to prolonged stimulant effects. Chronic methamphetamine abuse significantly changes the way the brain functions (NIDA, 2019).

"Methamphetamine abusers may display symptoms that include violent behavior, confusion, hallucinations, and possible paranoid or delusional feelings, also causing severe personality shifts. These feelings of paranoia can lead to homicidal or suicidal thoughts or tendencies. Methamphetamines are highly addictive and can be fatal with a single use. Deadly ingredients include antifreeze, drain cleaner, fertilizer, battery acid, or lantern fuel. The results when overused can cause heart failure and death. Long-term physical effects can lead to strokes, liver, kidney, and lung damage. Abuse can also lead to permanent and severe brain and psychological damage."[1]

Club Drugs /Street Drugs

The evolution of chemical substances to create an altered effect on the body or mind is ongoing. New combinations appear regularly with some causing catastrophic effects. Even substances designed for other uses, (remember bath salts?) can be used inappropriately leading to death. Some are given "friendly" street names masking their potentially harmful effects.

For example, "Smiles" is a hallucinogen whose effects are not immediately felt, increasing the risk of overdose. It can be taken as small tables, on blotter paper, or in powder form, often mixed with something else—chocolate, for instance. Side effects include loss of control, panic, heart palpitations and memory loss. "Wet" can refer to a marijuana cigarette dipped in liquid PCP, or to the PCP itself. Side effects include hostile behavior, feelings of detachment from reality, and distorted body perception. "Weed candy" is just what it sounds like— ordinary candy that's laced with marijuana, and oftentimes other dangerous ingredients (NIDA, 2015).

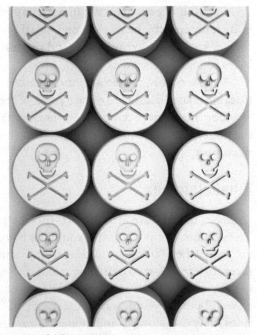

© ancroft/Shutterstock.com

MDMA

"**MDMA**, also known as **ecstasy**, has a chemical structure similar to methamphetamines and mescaline, causing hallucinogenic effects. As a result, it can produce both stimulant and psychedelic effects. In addition to its euphoric effects, MDMA can lead to disruptions in body temperature and cardiovascular regulation causing panic, anxiety, and rapid heart rate. It also damages nerves in the brain's serotonin system and possibly produces long-term damage to brain areas that are critical for thought and memory (NIDA, 2021). Physical effects can include muscle tension, teeth clenching, nausea, blurred vision, and faintness. The psychological effects can include confusion, depression, sleep disorders, anxiety, and paranoia that can last long after taking the drug. It is most often available in tablet form and usually taken orally. Occasionally it is found in powder form and can be snorted or smoked, but it is rarely injected. An overdose can be lethal, especially when taken with alcohol or other drugs, such as heroin ("H-bomb")."[1]

Rohypnol

"Flunitrazepam is an illegal drug in the United States, but an approved medicine in other parts of the world where it is generally prescribed for sleep disorders. A 2-mg tablet is equal to the potency of a six-pack of beer. Rohypnol is a tranquilizer, similar to Valium, but ten times more potent, producing sedative effects including muscle relaxation, dizziness, memory loss, and blackouts. The effects occur twenty to thirty minutes after use and lasts for up to eight hours. Rohypnol, more commonly known as "roofies," is a small, white, tasteless, pill that dissolves in food or drinks. It is most commonly used with other drugs, such as alcohol, ecstasy, heroin, and marijuana to enhance the feeling of the other drug. Although Rohypnol alone can be very dangerous, as well as physically addicting, when mixed with other

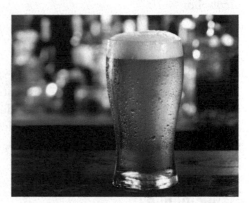

© Nitr/Shutterstock.com

drugs it can be fatal. It is also referred to as the "date rape" drug because there have been many reported cases of individuals giving Rohypnol to someone without their knowledge. The effects incapacitate the victim, and therefore they are unable to resist a sexual assault. It produces an 'anterograde amnesia,' meaning they may not remember events experienced while under effects of the drug (NIDA, 2010)."[1]

Gamma Hydroxybutyrate (GHB)

"GHB is a fast-acting, powerful drug that depresses the nervous system. It occurs naturally in the body in small amounts. Commonly taken with alcohol, it depresses the central nervous system and induces an intoxicated state. GHB is commonly consumed orally, usually as a clear liquid or a white powder. It is odorless, colorless, and slightly salty to taste. Effects from GHB can occur within fifteen to thirty minutes. Small doses (less than 1 g) of GHB act as a relaxant with larger doses causing strong feelings of relaxation, slowing heart rate, and respiration. There is a very fine line to cross to find a lethal dose, which can lead to seizures, respiratory distress, low blood pressure, and comas.

"According to the Drug Abuse Warning Network, The Drug Induced Rape Prevention and Punishment Act of 1996 was enacted into federal law in response to the abuse of Rohypnol. This law makes it a crime to give someone a controlled substance without his/her knowledge and with the intent to commit a crime. The law also stiffens the penalties for possession and distribution of Rohypnol and GHB. Used in Europe as a general anesthetic and treatment for insomnia, GHB is growing in popularity and is widely available underground. Manufactured by non-professional "kitchen" chemists, concerns about quality and purity should be considered."[1]

DISSOCIATIVE DRUGS

Ketamine Hydrochloride

"'Special K' or 'K' was originally created for use in a medical setting on humans and animals. Ninety percent is legally sold for veterinary use. Ketamine usually comes in liquid form and is cooked into a white powder for snorting. Higher doses produce a hallucinogenic effect and may cause the user to feel far away from his or her body. This is called a "K-hole" and has been compared to near-death experiences. Low doses can increase heart rate and numbness in the extremities with higher doses depressing consciousness and breathing. This makes it extremely dangerous if combined with other depressants such as alcohol or GHB."[1]

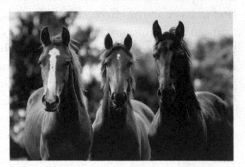

© Rita Kochmarjova/Shutterstock.com

Phencyclidine Hydrochloride

"Also known as PCP or angel dust, phencyclidine hydrochloride is sometimes considered a hallucinogen, although it does not easily fit into any category. First synthesized in 1959, it is used intravenously and as an anesthetic that blocks pain without producing numbness. Taken in small doses, it causes feelings of euphoria. The harmful side effects include depression, anxiety, confusion, and delirium. High doses of PCP causes mental confusion, hallucinations, and can cause serious mental illness and extreme aggressive and violent behavior, including murder."[1]

Hallucinogens

"**Hallucinogens**, also called psychedelics, are drugs that affect perception, sensation, awareness, and emotion. Changes in time, space, and hallucinations may be mild or extreme depending on the dose, and may vary on every occasion. There are many synthetic as well as natural hallucinogens in use. Synthetic groups include LSD, which is the most potent; mescaline, which is derived from the peyote cactus, and psilocybin, derived from mushrooms, have similar effects."[1]

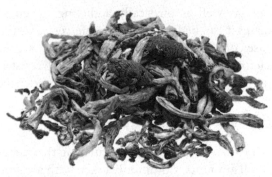

© robtek/Shutterstock.com

"Magic" Mushrooms

Psilocybin, also more widely known as magic mushrooms, is a psychedelic compound that is produced by a wide range of mushroom species. The more than 200 species of mushrooms that are responsible for the production of psilocybin are collectively known on the streets to recreational drug users as magic mushrooms. These psychedelic hallucinogens produce mind-altering effects when they are consumed.

Like other types of hallucinogenic drugs, psilocybin can produce a wide range of euphoric and psychedelic effects. Psilocybin can produce euphoria, hallucinations, and a distorted sense of time for the user. It is very common for those under the influence of magic mushrooms to act erratically and irrationally. Behavior may include odd reactions to normal events, distinct outbursts and panic attacks.

Lysergic Acid Diethylamide (LSD)

According to the National Survey on Drug Use and Health conducted in 2018, 5.6 million people aged 12 or older had used a hallucinogenic substance (SANSHA, 2019). "LSD is a colorless, odorless, and tasteless liquid that is made from lysergic acid, which comes from the ergot fungus. It was first converted to lysergic acid diethylamide (LSD) in 1938. In 1943, its psychoactive properties accidentally became known (NIDA, 2009). Hallucinations and illusions often occur, and effects vary according to the dosage, personality of the user, and conditions under which the drug is used. A flashback is a recurrence of some hallucinations from a previous LSD experience days or months after the dose. Flashbacks can occur without reason, occurring to heavy users more frequently. After taking LSD, a person loses control over normal thought process.

OTHER DRUGS

"**Inhalants** are poisonous chemical gases, fumes, or vapors that produce psychoactive effects when sniffed."[1] They are easy to access and inexpensive to purchase. Inhalants are often among the first drugs that young adolescents use. In fact, they are one of the few classes of drugs that are used more by younger adolescents than older ones. Inhalant use can become chronic and continue into adulthood. "When inhaled, the fumes take away the body's ability to absorb oxygen. Inhalants are considered deleriants, which can cause permanent damage to the heart, brain, lungs, and liver. Common inhalants include model glue, acetone, gasoline, kerosene, nail polish, aerosol sprays, Pam™ cooking spray, Scotchgard™ fabric protectant, lighter fluids,

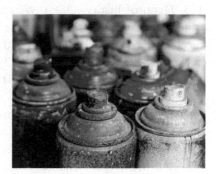

© dimbar76/Shutterstock.com

butane, and cleaning fluids, as well as nitrous oxide (laughing gas). These products were not created to be inhaled or ingested. They were designed to dissolve things or break things down, which is exactly what they do to the body."[1]

"Inhalants reach the lungs, bloodstream, and other parts of the body very quickly. Intoxication can occur in as little as five minutes and can last as long as nine hours. Inhaled lighter fluid/butane displaces the oxygen in the lungs, causing suffocation. Even a single episode can cause asphyxiation or cardiac arrhythmia and possibly lead to death. The initial effects of inhalants are similar to those of alcohol, but they are very unpredictable. Some effects include dizziness and blurred vision, involuntary eye movement, poor coordination, involuntary extremity movement, slurred speech, euphoric feeling, nosebleeds, and possible coma.

"Health risks involved with the use of inhalants may include hepatitis, liver and/or kidney failure, as well as the destruction of bone marrow and skeletal muscles. Respiratory impairment and blood abnormalities, along with irregular heartbeat and/or heart failure, are also serious side effects of inhalants. Regular use can lead to tolerance, the need for more powerful drugs, and addiction (NIDA, 2011)."[1]

Prescription Drugs

According to NIDA, in 2020 over 41 million people over the age of 12 have used prescription drugs non-medicinally. Prescription drugs were developed to help treat varying conditions and diseases and are very beneficial when used as

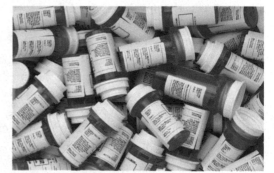

© David Smart/Shutterstock.com

directed. The problem occurs when people misuse them in ways they were not intended to be used. The following are some of the more common prescription drugs that are misused or abused.

Stimulants

"According to recent reports from the FDA, a highly abused stimulant among middle and high school students is methylphenidate, commonly known as **Ritalin**. This drug is more powerful than caffeine but not as potent as amphetamines and is prescribed for individuals with attention-deficit/hyperactivity disorders, ADHD, and sometimes to treat narcolepsy. Researchers speculate that Ritalin increases the slow and steady release of dopamine, therefore improving attention and focus for those in need of the increase. 'Individuals abuse Ritalin to lose weight, increase alertness and experience the euphoric feelings resulting from high doses' (U.S. Dept. of Justice, 2006). When abused, the tablets are either taken orally or crushed and snorted; some even dissolve the tablets in water and inject the mixture. Addiction occurs when it induces large and fast increases of dopamine in the brain (DOJ, 2006).

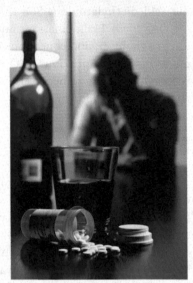

© Burlingham/Shutterstock.com

Adderall is a stimulant medication used to treat attention-deficit hyperactivity disorder (ADHD) and narcolepsy. It contains a mixture of both amphetamine and dextroamphetamine. While many people take Adderall with a doctor's prescription following a diagnosis of ADHD or narcolepsy, it is a commonly misused drug. In addition, non-medical use of stimulants, including Adderall and Ritalin, has more than doubled in the past few year (NIDA, 2016).

Depressants

"Depressants are sedatives or anxiolytic (anti-anxiety) drugs that depress the central nervous system. Benzodiazepines such as Valium and Xanax and barbiturates like Nembutal, Secobarbital, and Phenobarbital can be prescribed to relieve tension, induce relaxation and sleep, or treat panic attacks. All of these differ in action, absorption, and metabolism, but all produce similar intoxication and withdrawal symptoms. Depressants can produce both a physical and psychological dependence within two to four weeks. Those with a prior history of abuse are at greater risk of abusing sedatives, even if prescribed by a physician. If there is no previous substance abuse history, one rarely develops problems if prescribed and monitored by a physician. Depressants can be very dangerous, if not lethal, if used in combination with alcohol, leading to respiratory depression, respiratory arrest, and death. Some of the physiological effects of depressants include drowsiness, impaired judgment, poor coordination, slowed breathing, confusion, weak and rapid heartbeat, relaxed muscles, and pain relief. A major health risk associated with the use of depressants is the development of dependence to the drug, leading to serious side effects, such as stupors, coma, and death.

"The danger from prescription and over-the-counter drugs is often underestimated by students. Many assume that if the drug is legal and prescribed by a physician, even if for someone else, it must be safe. However, what they fail to realize is that medications and dosages are tailored to each patient and may not be appropriate in the manner they intend to use them."[1]

The proper disposal of prescription drugs is also important. They should not be discarded in the trash or flushed down the toilet. Many communities have designated dates when unused or expired prescription drugs can be brought in for proper disposal.

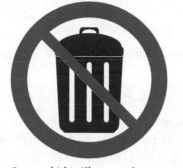

© veronchick84/Shutterstock.com

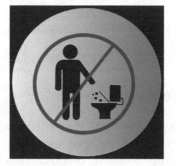

© Mukesh Kumar/Shutterstock.com

ANABOLIC STEROIDS

Steroids are synthetic substances similar to the male sex hormone testosterone. They do have legitimate medical uses. Sometimes doctors prescribe anabolic steroids to help people with certain kinds of anemia and men who don't produce enough testosterone on their own. Doctors also prescribe a different kind of steroid, called corticosteroids, to reduce swelling. Corticosteroids are not anabolic steroids and do not have the same harmful effects.

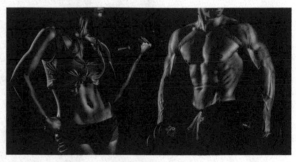

© Lebedev Roman Olegovich/Shutterstock.com

But doctors never prescribe anabolic steroids to young, healthy people to help them build muscles. Without a prescription from a doctor, steroids are illegal.

While a banned substance in athletics, some people may use these substances to enhance body image, build muscle mass and/or reduce body fat. There are many ways to take steroids whether by mouth, injection or topical.

There can be many side effects from anabolic steroid use and may include:

- severe acne, oily skin and hair
- hair loss
- **liver disease**, such as liver tumors and cysts
- kidney disease
- heart disease, such as heart attack and stroke
- altered mood, irritability, increased aggression, depression or suicidal tendencies
- alterations in cholesterol and other blood lipids
- high blood pressure
- gynecomastia (abnormal development of mammary glands in men causing breast enlargement)
- shrinking of testicles
- azoospermia (absence of sperm in semen)
- menstrual irregularities in women
- infertility
- **excess facial or body hair** (hirsutism), deeper voice in women

- stunted growth and height in teens
- risk of viral or bacterial infections due to unsterile injections

Unless prescribed by a physician, these and other medications should only be used as prescribed.

Are You a Wise Consumer?

Have you ever used a prescription medication that was not your own? If so, did you consider the possible side effects? Not everyone has the same body chemistry and if you were taking any other medication, even an over the counter drug, how would you know what the effects might be? Health literate individuals and wise consumers make informed decisions to avoid negative consequences.

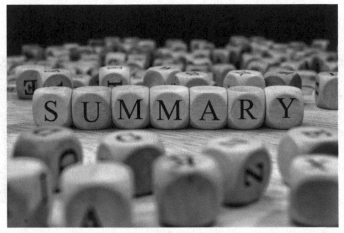

© Fabrik Bilder/Shutterstock.com

Students are faced with many decisions throughout their college experience. Social pressures can create instances where individuals feel that if they do not participate in certain behaviors, they might not be accepted. Knowing the potential consequences and making informed choices can not only prevent serious problems, it can also support long term goals. The improper use of drugs and alcohol can derail future plans and create significant health issues.

PERSONAL REFLECTIONS . . . SO, WHAT HAVE YOU LEARNED?

1. What is binge drinking and why is it so dangerous? If one of your friends was at a party and collapsed from drinking too much alcohol, what would you do?

2. What is the Good Samaritan law and why is it important?

3. What is changing about craft beer and why is it important for consumers to know?

4. Are E-cigarettes really safer? Why or why not? How do you feel when a person is smoking an E-cigarette next to you?

5. Should people who smoke pay more for insurance? Why or why not?

6. What about people who drink alcohol? Why or why not?

NOTES

RESOURCES ON CAMPUS FOR YOU!

Student Conduct

There are numerous campus resources available to students, as well as policies that outline university expectations across many areas. Listed in your Student Handbook are policies with respect to alcohol and tobacco use on campus. Additionally, students wishing to talk with a counselor concerning substance use will find the information at Health and Counseling services.

REFERENCES

American Heart Association (AHA). (2006). *Annual report.*

https://www.alcohol.org/statistics-information/

B-Well Health Promotion, Brown University. *Energy Drinks.* Retrieved 2016 from http://www.brown .edu/campus-life/health/services/promotion/nutrition-eating-concerns-eating-well-brown/ energy-drinks.

Caldwell, F. (2019). *Emerging issues with marijuana legalization.* SAMHSA. Retrieved April 2022, from https://www.samhsa.gov/sites/default/files/meeting/documents/emerging-issues-marijuana-legalization-06112019.pdf

Center on Addiction and Substance Abuse at Columbia University. Commission on Substances Abuse at Colleges and Universities.

Centers for Disease Control and Prevention. (2014). *Alcohol use in pregnancy.* Retrieved 2016 from http://www.cdc.gov/ncbddd/fasd/alcohol-use.html

Center for Disease Control and Prevention, 2022. Health Effects of Cigarette Smoking. Retrieved April, 2022 from https://www.cdc.gov/tobacco/data_statistics/fact_sheets/adult_data/cig_smoking/ index.htm#:~:text=Cigarette%20smoking%20remains%20the%20leading,about%201%20in%20 5%20deaths.&text=In%202020%2C%20nearly%2013%20of,12.5%25(%20currently*%20smoked%20 cigarettes

CDC. (2022). Youth and Tobacco Use. Retrieved April 2022 from https://www.cdc.gov/tobacco/data_ statistics/fact_sheets/youth_data/tobacco_use/index.htm#:~:text=Tobacco%20product%20 use%20is%20started%20and%20established%20primarily%20during%20 adolescence.&text=Nearly%209%20out%20of%2010,try%20smoking%20by%20age%20 26.&text=Each%20day%20in%20the%20U.S.,youth%20start%20smoking%20every%20day.

CDC. (2021). Notes from the field: E-cigarette use among middle and high school students. Retrieved April 2022, from https://www.cdc.gov/mmwr/volumes/70/wr/mm7039a4.htm#:~:text =Among%20current%20e%2Dcigarette%20users,middle%20school%20e%2Dcigarette%20users.

CDC. (2021). Hookah Use. Retrieved April 2022, from https://www.cdc.gov/tobacco/data_statistics/fact_ sheets/tobacco_industry/hookahs/index.htm#:~:text=Hookah%20Use,-Hookah%20use%20 began&text=Nearly%201%20in%20every%2013,tobacco%20during%20the%20previous%20year.

CDC. (2022). *Fentanyl facts.* Retrieved April 2022, from https://www.cdc.gov/stopoverdose/fentanyl/ index.html#:~:text=Pharmaceutical%20fentanyl%20is%20prescribed%20by,for%20its%20 heroin%2Dlike%20effect.

Centers for Disease Control and Prevention. (2015). *Today's heroin epidemic.* Retrieved 2016 from www.cdc.gov/vitalsigns/heroin/index.html,

Center for Disease Control and Prevention. (2015). *Youth risk behavior survey.* Retrieved December 2015 from www.cdc.gov/healthyyouth/data/yrbs/index.htm.

Cobb, N.K., Byron, M.J., Abrams, D.B., & Shields, P. G. (2010). Novel nicotine delivery systems and public health: the rise of the "e-cigarette." *Am J Public Health*, 100, 2340–2.

Dennis, M. E., & Texas Commission on Alcohol and Drug Abuse. (2005). *Instructor manual, alcohol education program for minors.* Austin: TCADA.

Department of Health and Counseling Services, Winthrop University. *Influenza update.* Retrieved 2016 from http://www.winthrop.edu/hcs/default.aspx?id=22925

Department of Health and Counseling Services, Winthrop University. Retrieved 2016 from http://www .winthrop.edu/student-affairs/

Department of Health and Human Services, www.hhs.gov

Department of Justice, & National Drug Intelligence Center. (2006). *Ritalin fast facts.*

Everett, S. A., Lowry, R., Cohen, L. R., Dellinger, A. M. (1999). Unsafe motor vehicle practices among substance-using college students. *Accident Analysis.*

Ewing, J. (1984). Detecting alcoholism: the CAGE questionnaire. *Journal of the American Medical Association.*

Fentanyl. Retrieved, April, 2022. https://www.dea.gov/factsheets/fentanyl

Hallucinogens.com. *Psilocybin.* Retrieved 2016 from http://hallucinogens.com/psilocybin/

Hoeger, W. and Hoeger, S. (1999). *Principles and labs for fitness and wellness* (5th ed). Englewood, CO: Morton Publishing Company.

Johnston, L.D., O'Malley, P.M., Miech, R.A., Bachman, J.G., Schulenberg, J.E. (2014). Monitoring the future national results on drug use: 1975–2014: Overview, key findings on adolescent drug use. Ann Arbor, MI: Institute for Social Research, The University of Michigan.

King, B.A., Alam, S. Promoff, G., Arrazola, R., & Dube, S.R. (2013). Awareness and ever use of electronic cigarettes among U.S. adults, 2010–2011. *Nicotine Tob*, 15, 1623–7.

National Institute on Alcohol Abuse and Alcoholism, & National Institutes of Health. *Statistics Snapshot of college drinking.*

National Institute on Alcohol Abuse and Alcoholism. Retrieved from 2016 http://niaaa.nih.gov/alcohol-health/special-populations-co-occurring-disorders/college-drinking

National Highway Traffic Safety Administration (NHTSA). (2019). *Drunk driving.* Retrieved April 2022, from https://www.nhtsa.gov/risky-driving/drunk-driving

National Institute on Alcohol Abuse and Alcoholism (NIAAA). (2021). *College drinking.* Retrieved April 2022, from https://www.niaaa.nih.gov/publications/brochures-and-fact-sheets/college-drinking#:~:text=The%20most%20recent%20statistics%20from,injuries%2C%20including%20motor%20vehicle%20crashes.

NIAAA. (2021). Fall semester – *A time for parents to discuss the risks of college drinking.* Retrieved April 2022, from https://www.niaaa.nih.gov/publications/brochures-and-fact-sheets/

time-for-parents-discuss-risks-college-drinking#:~:text=According%20to%20the%202019%20 National,drinking%20in%20the%20past%20month.

NIAAA. (2022). *Alcohol facts and statistics.* Retrieved April 2022, from https://www.niaaa.nih.gov/ publications/brochures-and-fact-sheets/alcohol-facts-and-statistics#:~:text=Prevalence%20of%20 Drinking%3A%20According%20to,in%20this%20age%20group%20and

National Institute on Alcohol Abuse and Alcoholism, & National Institutes of Health. (2008). *Integrative genetic analysis of alcohol dependence using the genenetwork web resources.*

National Institute on Drug Abuse. Retrieved 2016 from http://www.drugabuse.gov/

National Institute on Drug Abuse. (2013). *Drug facts: cocaine.* Retrieved 2016 from http://www.drugabuse .gov/publications/drugfacts/cocaine,

National Institute on Drug Abuse. (2014). *Hallucinogens.* Retrieved 2016 from http://www.drugabuse.gov /drugs-abuse/hallucinogens

National Institute of Drug Abuse (NIDA), & U.S. Dept. of Health and Human Services. (2008).

National Beer Sales and Production Data. https://www.brewersassociation.org/statistics-and-data/ national-beer-stats/

NIAAA. (2021). *Alcohol's effects on the body.* Retrieved April 2022, from https://www.niaaa.nih.gov/ alcohols-effects-health/alcohols-effects-body

National Institute on Drug Abuse (NIDA). (2020). *Heroin.* Retrieved April 2022, from https://nida.nih. gov/drug-topics/heroin

NIDA. (2022). *What are the long-term effects of methamphetamine misuse.* Retrieved April 2022, from https:// nida.nih.gov/publications/research-reports/methamphetamine/what-are-long-term-effects- methamphetamine-misuse#:~:text=Studies%20in%20chronic%20methamphetamine%20 users,problems%20observed%20in%20these%20individuals.

NIDA. (2021). *What are MDMA's effects on the brain?* Retrieved April 2022, from https://nida.nih.gov/ publications/research-reports/mdma-ecstasy-abuse/what-are-mdmas-effects-on-brain

NIDA. (n.d.). *NIDA highlights drug use trends among college-age and young adults in new online resource.* Retrieved April 2022, from https://archives.drugabuse.gov/es/category/drugs-abuse/ritalin

NIDA for Teens. *Inhalants.* Retrieved 2016 from http://teens.drugabuse.gov/drug-facts/inhalants

Public Media. (2013). *DEA warns of new street drugs with friendly-sounding nicknames.* Retrieved 2016 from http:// wusfnews.wusf.usf.edu/post/dea-warns-new-street-drugs-friendly-sounding-nicknames#stream/0

Ray, O., Ksir, C. (1999). *Drugs, society, and human behavior* (8th ed). New York: WCB McGraw-Hill.

SAMHSA. (2019). *Key substance use and mental health indicators in the United States: Results from the 2018 National Survey on Drug Use and Health.* Retrieved April 2022, from https://www.samhsa.gov/data/ sites/default/files/cbhsq-reports/NSDUHNationalFindingsReport2018/NSDUHNational FindingsReport2018.pdf

SAMHSA. (2020). *Key substance use and mental health indicators in the United States: Results from the 2019 National Survey on Drug Use and Health.* Retrieved April 2022, from https://www.samhsa.gov/data/ sites/default/files/reports/rpt29393/2019NSDUHFFRPDFWHTML/2019NSDUHFFR090120.htm

Substance Abuse and Mental Health Service Administration. Retrieved 2016 from www.samhsa.gov.

Traffic Safety Facts 2013 Data. *Alcohol-impaired driving.* Retrieved 2016 from http://www-nrd.nhtsa.dot.gov/Pubs/812102.pdf

U.S. Food and Drug Administration, & Department of Health and Human Services. FDA issues regulation prohibiting sale of dietary supplements containing ephedrine alkaloids and reiterates its advice that consumers stop using these products.

www.alcohol.org/effects/sexual-assault-college-campus/

CREDITS

NOTES

Chapter 9

Human Diseases +

OBJECTIVES

Students will be able to:

- Differentiate between communicable and non-communicable diseases.
- Discuss the major hypokinetic diseases afflicting Americans.
- List the six major cardiac risk factors and the three unalterable cardiac risk factors.
- Know the warning signs for a heart attack and stroke.
- Discuss three ways to combat obesity.
- Recognize the risk factors for cancer and describe the cancer warning signs.
- Identify four cancers that affect young adults; discuss prevention and risk factors.
- Differentiate between Type I and Type II diabetes and define the risk factors for each.
- Discuss ways to prevent other chronic illnesses, such as osteoporosis, asthma, anemia, lupus, and gastrointestinal disorders.
- Discuss strategies to avoid contraction of communicable diseases and identify the symptoms and treatment for each disease.

American Heart Association's (AHA) Risk for Disease Questionnaire

History

"You have had:

____ Heart attack

____ Heart surgery

____ Cardiac catheterization

____ Coronary angioplasty (PTCA)

____ Pacemaker/implantable cardiac defibrillator/rhythm disturbance

____ Heart valve disease

____ Heart Failure

____ Heart transplantation

____ Congenital heart disease

Symptoms

____ Chest discomfort from exertion

____ Unreasonable breathlessness

____ Dizziness, fainting, blackouts

____ Take heart medications

If you marked any of these statements in this section, AHA recommends you get a physician's clearance before activity.

Other health issues

____ Diabetes

____ Asthma or another lung disease

____ Burning or cramping in lower legs when walking short distances.

____ Musculoskeletal problems that limit physical activity

____ Concerns about the safety of exercise.

____ Take prescription medication(s)

____ Pregnancy

Cardiovascular risk factors

You are a man older than 45 years.

You are a woman older than 55 years, you have had a hysterectomy, or you are postmenopausal.

You smoke, or quite within the previous 6 mo.

Your blood pressure is greater than 140/90.

You don't know your blood pressure.

You take blood pressure medication.

____ Your blood cholesterol level is >200 mg/dL.

____ You don't know your cholesterol level.

____ You have a close blood relative who had a heart attack before age 55 (father or brother) or age 65 (mother or sister).

____ You are physically inactive (i.e., you get less than 30 min. of physical activity on at least three days per week).

____ You are more than 20 pounds overweight

If you marked two or more of the statements in this section, AHA recommends checking with your doctor before starting a regular exercise program.

____ None of the above is true."[3]

You should be able to exercise safely without consulting your physician or other healthcare provider in a self-guided program or almost any facility that meets your exercise program needs.

Source: American Heart Association, Inc.

NON-COMMUNICABLE DISEASES

Non-communicable diseases are not transmitted person to person. These diseases can develop from many sources, some of which include genetic predisposition, behaviors such as excessive sun exposure, smoking, unhealthy eating habits, and/or lack of exercise.

Cardiovascular Disease (CVD)

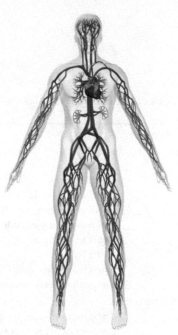

"The cardiovascular system is responsible for delivering oxygen and other nutrients to the body. The major components of the cardiovascular system are the heart, blood, and the vessels that carry the blood. Cardiovascular disease (CVD) is a catch-all term that includes several disease processes including various diseases of the heart, stroke, high blood pressure, congestive heart failure, and atherosclerosis. The heart muscle may become damaged or lose its ability to contract effectively. The vessels that supply the heart with oxygen may become blocked or damaged and subsequently compromise the heart muscle. Finally, the peripheral vascular system (all of the vessels outside the heart) may become damaged and decrease the ability to provide oxygen to other parts of the body. The great news is that from 1998 to 2008, deaths due to cardiovascular disease declined 30.6% (AHA, 2012). Americans are also on the whole, living longer, as life expec-

© Sebastian Kaulitzki/Shutterstock.com

tancy increases. The bad news is that many of the risk factors for CVD are lifestyle-related and therefore preventable, and Americans are much more likely to die from CVD than anything else. MyLifeCheck.org is a part of a campaign to increase awareness of positive attributes of health.

"CVD and stroke are largely preventable for a significant part of the lifespan. High blood pressure, high cholesterol, and smoking continue to put people at risk of heart attack and stroke. To address these risk factors, the Centers for Disease Control and Prevention is focusing many of its efforts on the 'A B C's' of heart disease and stroke prevention: appropriate Aspirin therapy, Blood pressure control, Cholesterol control, and support for Smoking cessation for those trying to quit and, even more generally, comprehensive tobacco prevention and control efforts. (CDC, 2012)."[1]

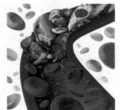

© Lightspring /Shutterstock.com

WHAT ARE THE RISK FACTORS OF CARDIOVASCULAR DISEASE?

"A risk factor for a disease is something that increases your risk of developing that disease. Risk factors can be behavioral, environmental, or genetic. See Figure 9.1 for the risk factors for cardiovascular disease.

- **Cigarette Smoking**—Smokers have two to four times the risk of developing cardiovascular disease than do nonsmokers (AHA, 2014). Cigarette smoking is the most 'potent' of the preventable risk factors. Former U.S. Surgeon General C. Everett Koop claims that cigarette *smoking is the number one preventable cause of death and disease in the United States* and the most important health issue of our time. Smoking accounts for 50 percent of female deaths due to heart attack before the age of 55 (Rosato, 1994).

- **Hypertension (High Blood Pressure)**—The AHA (2015) reports that approximately 80 million American adults have high blood pressure. *Hypertension is the most important modifiable risk factor for stroke.*

- **Cholesterol**—Dietary cholesterol contributes to blood serum cholesterol (cholesterol circulating in the blood), which can contribute to heart disease. Every 1 percent reduction in serum cholesterol can result in a 2–3 percent reduction in the risk of heart disease (AHA, 2014). To lower cholesterol, reduce intake of dietary saturated fat, increase consumption of soluble fiber, maintain a healthy weight, do not smoke, and exercise regularly.

- **Inactivity**—Aerobic exercise on a regular basis can favorably influence the other modifiable risk factors for heart disease. Consistent, moderate amounts of physical activity can promote health and longevity. The Surgeon General's report (Satcher, 1996) states that as few as 150 extra calories expended daily exercising can dramatically decrease CVD risk.

- **Obesity**—Highly correlated to heart disease, mild to moderate obesity is associated with an increase in risk of CVD. Fat distribution around the mid-section produces a higher risk than fat distribution around the hips and lower body.

- **Diabetes**—At least 65 percent of diabetics die of some form of CVD (CDC, 2012). Exercise is critical to help increase the sensitivity of the body's cells to insulin. 18.3 million Americans have diabetes (AHA, 2012.)

- **Stress**—Although difficult to measure in concrete form, stress is considered a factor in the development and acceleration of CVD. Without stress-management techniques, constant stress can manifest itself in a physical nature in the human body. Stress contributes to many of today's illnesses.

- **Age**—Risk of CVD rises as a person ages.

- **Gender**—Men have a higher risk than women until women reach postmenopausal age.

- **Heredity**—A family history of heart disease will increase risk."[1]

What is your risk? Mark any of the following that apply to you.

 Smoking - Current smoker or those that quit within the past 6 months

 Hypertension - Currently taking medication for hypertension or blood pressure > 140/90 on at least 2 occasions

 High Cholesterol - Currently taking cholesterol lowering medications or:
1. Total Cholesterol > 200 ml/dL
2. LDL Cholesterol > 130 ml/dL
3. HDL Cholesterol < 40 ml/dL

 Sedentary Lifestyle/Inactivity - Not participating in a regular physical activity program or < 150 accumulated minutes of moderate physical activity in a week

 Obesity -
1. Body Mass Index (BMI) > 30 or
2. Waist-to-hip ratio > 1.0 for men or .95 for women or
3. Waist circumference > 102 cm for men or 88 cm for women

 Prediabetes (High Blood Sugar) - fasting blood glucose > 100 on at least 2 occasions

 Age - men > 45 years of age; women > 55 years of age

Family History - 1st degree (or immediate) family members that have had a heart attack, heart surgery, or heart-related death before the age of 55 in the male family member or before the age of 65 in female family member

Illustrations © Arak Rattanawijittakorn/Shutterstock.com
Figure 9.1 The Risk Factors for Cardiovascular Disease

Measuring your risk: If you said yes to two or more of the above risk factors, you have a moderate-high risk of developing CVD over your lifetime. It's time to make some changes!!

WHO IS AT RISK FOR CVD?

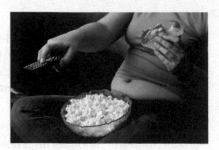

© esolla/Shutterstock.com

"There are an estimated 82,600,000 Americans that have some form of CVD. Many factors can predispose a person to be at risk for CVD. Sedentary living, habitual stress, smoking, poor diet, high blood pressure, diabetes, obesity, high cholesterol, and family history can all increase risk. Advancing age increases risk. Males typically have a higher risk than women until women are post-menopausal, then risk evens out. Misconceptions still exist that CVD is not a real problem for women. Because more women have heart attacks when they are older, the initial heart attack is more likely to be fatal. It is important for women to realize that CVD is an equal opportunity killer. Just like men, more women die from heart disease than anything else.

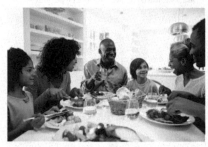

© Monkey Business Images/Shutterstock.com

"Certain populations have an inherently higher health risk such as African Americans and Hispanics. Genetic predisposition is a strong factor; familial tendencies toward elevated triglycerides, fat distribution (abdominal fat accumulation denotes a higher health risk than hip/thigh accumulation of fat), and high low-density lipoprotein cholesterol (LDL-C) levels increase risk. LDL-C is a blood lipid that indicates a higher cardiac risk. Saturated fat intake tends to increase LDL cholesterol. Dr. William Franklin of Georgetown University Medical School in Washington claims that anyone who has a close relative who has had a heart attack should begin monitoring his heart with regular stress tests when he is 45. If your father died in his 40's of a heart attack, then you should be concerned a decade earlier in your 30's. Variables such as age, gender, race, and genetic makeup may place you at a higher or lower risk but cannot be changed. These can be termed unalterable risk factors."[1]

Does Exercise Help?

"A growing body of evidence, however, indicates physical inactivity is more critical than excess weight in determining health risk. Longitudinal studies such as the ongoing research by epidemiologist Steven Blair, previously of the Cooper Institute in Dallas, Texas, and information from the ongoing Harvard alumni study indicate that lifestyle is more significant than weight. **Fitter people have lower death rates regardless of weight.** Indeed, the mortality rate for low fit males is more than 20% higher than for those that are

Spotlight on . . .

Family History

It is critically important that every person know and understand as much about their family history as they can. Family history is not exclusive to blood relatives. Looking closely at genes, habits, and environment of you and your family can help you to identify areas of concern for your health. Start with the immediate family members, move to grandparents, and finally to aunts, uncles, and cousins. Don't rule out your close friends with whom you spend a great amount of time. Realize that habits and environments can include those that we spend time with beyond our family members.

Check out the Web-based tool "My Family Health Portrait" at https://familyhistory.hhs .gov/FHH/html/index.html?_ga=1.135790840.878283.1456872088

high fit. While this effect is smaller for women, the decrease in mortality rate for high fit females is more than 6% compared to those who are lower fit. Increasing lifestyle activity and walking regularly, spending less time on the couch, and doing something active daily can have a positive impact on health."[1]

TYPES OF CARDIOVASCULAR DISEASE

Arteriosclerosis & Atherosclerosis

"**Arteriosclerosis** is a term used to describe the thickening and hardening of the arteries. Healthy arteries are elastic and will dilate and constrict with changes in blood flow, which allows proper maintenance of blood pressure. Hardened, non-elastic arteries do not expand with blood flow and can increase intra-arterial pressure causing high blood pressure. Both high blood pressure and arteriosclerosis increase the risk of an **aneurysm**. With an aneurysm, the artery loses its integrity and balloons out under the pressure created by the pumping heart, in much the same way as an old garden hose might if placed under pressure. If an aneurysm occurs in the vessels of the brain, a stroke might occur. Aneurysms in the large vessels can place a person at risk of sudden death. Maintaining normal elasticity of the arteries is very important for good health. Exercise helps to manage symptoms and the factors that contribute to cardiac risk.

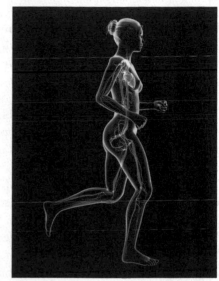

© Sebastian Kaulitzki/Shutterstock.com

"**Atherosclerosis** is a type of arteriosclerosis. Atherosclerosis is the long-term buildup of fatty deposits and other substances such as cholesterol, cellular waste products, calcium, and fibrin (clotting material in the blood) on the interior walls of arteries (see Figure 9.2). This may create a partial or total blockage (called an occlusion) that may cause high blood pressure, a heart attack, or stroke. This process can occur in any vessel of the body. If it occurs outside of the brain or heart, it is termed **peripheral vascular disease**. Within the heart the gradual narrowing of the coronary arteries to the myocardium, or heart muscle, is called **coronary artery disease**. *Atherosclerosis is a disease that can start early in childhood.* The rate of progression of the disease depends on family history and lifestyle choices. Exercise helps manage symptoms as well as increase coronary collateral circulation."[1]

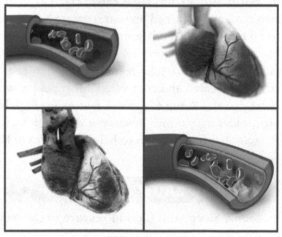

© Giovanni Cancemi/Shutterstock.com

Figure 9.2 Healthy Arteries (Top) vs. Unhealthy Arteries (Bottom)

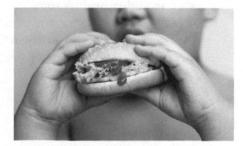

© kwanchai.c/Shutterstock.com

Hypertension

"**Hypertension,** or high blood pressure, is often called the "silent killer" because typically there are no symptoms. Because hypertension is asymptomatic, it is important to get your blood pressure checked on a regular basis. In 2009, the estimated prevalence of hypertension (a blood pressure reading of 140/90 mm or higher) was one in 3 adults. High blood pressure is associated with a shortened life span. A higher percentage of men than women have HBP until 45 years of age. From ages 45 to 54 and 55 to 64, the percentages of men and women with HBP are similar. After that, a much higher percentage of women have HBP than men (AHA, 2014). High blood pressure causes the heart to work harder. Chronic, untreated hypertension can lead to aneurysms in blood vessels, heart failure from an enlarged heart, kidney failure, atherosclerosis, and blindness.

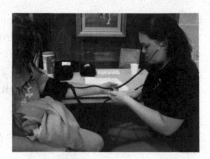

© Winthrop University

"The top number is the **systolic** reading, which represents the arterial pressure when the heart is contracting and forcing the blood through the arteries. The bottom number is the diastolic reading, which represents the force of the blood on the arteries while the heart is relaxing between beats. In 2017 new blood pressure guidelines were issued. Based on readings, the blood pressure categories are normal, elevated, or hypertension (stage 1 or stage 2). Normal blood pressure is less than 120/80 mm Hg. Elevated blood pressure includes a reading from 120–129/<80 mm Hg. Blood pressure readings of 130–139 (systolic) mm Hg or 80–89 (diastolic) mm Hg is categorized as Stage 1 hypertension, and readings of >140 (systolic) or >90 (diastolic) mm Hg is categorized as Stage 2 hypertension. Classifications are determined by at least two readings obtained on two separate occasions. If you are considered elevated or hypertensive, it is time to take action by modifying your lifestyle. Any reading consistently over 120/80 mm Hg could indicate a high risk. With persons over 50 years old, a systolic reading of 140 or above is a more important CVD risk factor than the diastolic reading (Whelton et al., 2017). Hypertension cannot be cured, but it can be successfully treated and controlled. Most people with hypertension have additional risk factors for cardiovascular disease. Some of the risk factors for high blood pressure include Hispanic or African American heritage, older age, family history, a diet high in fat and sodium, alcoholism, stress, obesity, and inactivity. Exercise has been shown to help symptoms of high blood pressure in mild to moderate hypertension."[1]

Did you know . . .

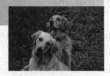

Teens, Sleep, and Blood Pressure in the News

A new study finds that teens who get too little sleep or erratic sleep may elevate their blood pressure. "Our study underscores the high rate of poor quality and inadequate sleep in adolescence coupled with the risk of developing high blood pressure and other health problems which may lead to cardiovascular disease," says Susan Redline, M.D., professor of medicine and pediatrics and director of University Hospital's Sleep Center at Case Western Reserve University in Cleveland, Ohio. Researchers say technology in bedrooms (phone, games, computers, and music) may be part of the problem (AHA, 2016).

Courtesy of Shelley Hamill

HEART ATTACK

"A heart attack or **myocardial infarction** occurs when an artery that provides the heart muscle with oxygen becomes blocked or flow is decreased. The area of the heart muscle served by that artery does not receive adequate oxygen and becomes injured and may eventually die (see Figure 9.3). The heart attack may be so small as to be imperceptible by the victim, or so massive that the victim will die. It is often reported that heart attack victims delay seeking medical help with the onset of symptoms. Every minute counts! In one study, men waited an average of three hours before seeking help. Women waited four hours.

It is important to seek medical help at the first sign of a heart attack. Women who smoke and take oral contraceptives are ten times more likely to have a heart attack (Payne and Hahn, 2000). In addition to the classic symptoms of heart attack, women were more likely than men to report throat discomfort, pressing on the chest, and vomiting."[1]

Women & Heart Attacks

We now understand that men and women can experience heart attacks differently. Women, especially those under the age of fifty-five, who suffer a heart attack are less likely to feel the classic chest pain or pressure that their male counterparts. Women report more atypical symptoms, such as shortness of breath or pain in the neck, shoulder, arms, back, abdomen, or stomach. Women are also less likely to seek medical attention immediately following a heart attack, which increases their chance of heart damage and death from a heart attack. For these reasons, women have lower survival rates from a heart attack than males of the same age.

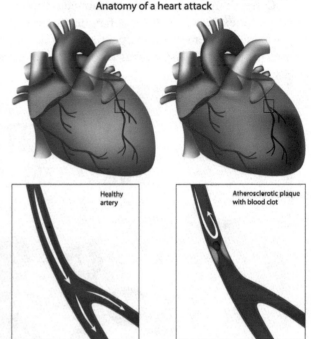

Anatomy of a heart attack

Healthy artery

Atherosclerotic plaque with blood clot

© Alila Medical Media/Shutterstock.com

Figure 9.3 Anatomy of a Heart Attack

Spotlight on . . .

Heart Attack Symptoms and Warning Signs

If you think you're having a heart attack, call 911 or your emergency medical system immediately.

Some heart attacks are sudden and intense—the "movie heart attack," where no one doubts what's happening—but most heart attacks start slowly, with mild pain or discomfort. Often people affected aren't sure what's wrong and wait too long before getting help. Here are signs that can mean a heart attack is happening:

- **Chest discomfort.** Most heart attacks involve discomfort in the center of the chest that lasts more than a few minutes, or that goes away and comes back. It can feel like uncomfortable pressure, squeezing, fullness, or pain.
- **Discomfort in other areas of the upper body.** Symptoms can include pain or discomfort in one or both arms, the back, neck, jaw, or stomach.
- **Shortness of breath.** This feeling often comes along with chest discomfort. But it can occur before the chest discomfort.
- **Other signs:** These may include breaking out in a cold sweat, nausea, or lightheadedness.

If you or someone you're with has chest discomfort, especially with one or more of the other signs, don't wait longer than a few minutes (no more than five) before calling for help. Call 911 and get to a hospital right away.

Calling 9-1-1 is almost always the fastest way to get lifesaving treatment.

Other than the previously mentioned symptoms, women may experience chest pressure or pain, dizziness, and unexplained feelings of fatigue, anxiety, or weakness (see Figure 9.4). If someone is experiencing any of these signs or symptoms, get them to a doctor quickly. Additionally, have the person take full strength aspirin immediately. Aspirin has blood-thinning properties that can help prevent fatal clots from forming (AHA, 2012).

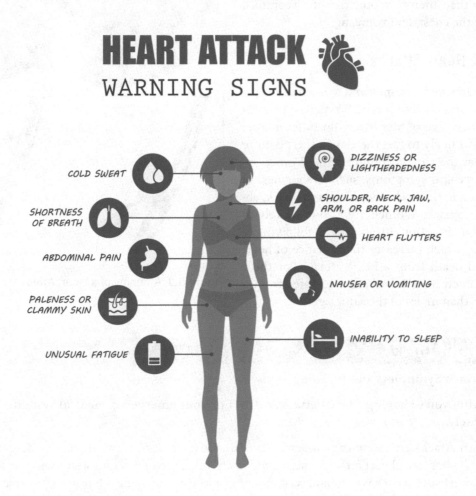

© eveleen/Shutterstock.com

Figure 9.4 Warning Signs of a Heart Attack for Women May Look Different Than for Men

Did you know . . .

The "ABCs" of heart disease and stroke prevention

Aspirin therapy

Blood pressure control

Cholesterol control

Smoking cessation

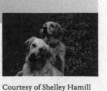

Courtesy of Shelley Hamill

The American Heart Association projects that by 2030, 40.5% of the U.S. population will have some form of CVD, costing the healthcare system an estimated $1 trillion every year. (AHA, 2012).

ISCHEMIC STROKE
UNSTABLE PLAQUE IN THE CEREBRAL ARTERY
ATHEROSCLEROSIS

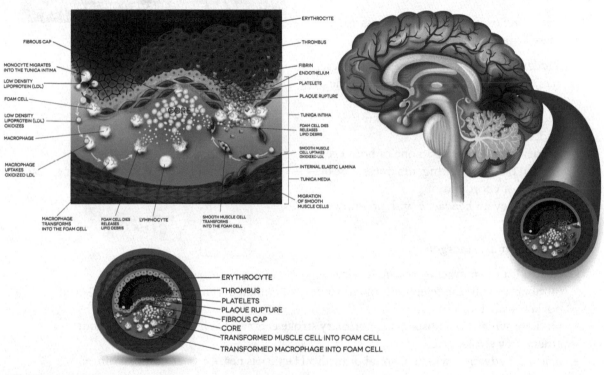

© Tefi/Shutterstock.com

Figure 9.5 Plaque Buildup in Arteries That Can Lead To Stroke or Heart Attack

Stroke

"Do you know the warning signs of a stroke? There is a public awareness campaign to increase knowledge of stroke warning signs and symptoms. Stroke, or more recently called **'brain attack,'** is the third leading cause of death affecting 795,000 Americans per year (AHA, 2015). As shown in Figure 9.5, vessels that supply the brain with nutrients become damaged or occluded and the brain tissue dies because of insufficient oxygen. The cerebral artery, the main supply of nutrients to the brain, can be narrowed due to atherosclerosis. The conditions that precipitate stroke may take years to develop. Stroke has the same risk factors as heart disease. African-Americans have nearly twice the risk for a first-ever stroke than Caucasians and a much higher death rate from stroke (AHA, 2015). African Americans also have a high incidence of stroke risk factors such as high blood pressure. On the average, someone in the United States has a stroke every forty seconds, and every three to four minutes someone dies of a stroke (AHA, 2015). One-third of all stroke victims die, one-third of stroke victims suffer permanent disability, and one-third of stroke victims gradually return to their normal daily routines (Bishop and Aldana, 1999). Stroke is also a leading cause of serious disability. Various studies have shown significant trends toward lower stroke risk with moderate and high levels of leisure time physical activity."[1]

Spotlight on . . .

Stroke Symptoms/Warning Signs (see Figure 9.6).

If you notice one or more of these signs, don't wait. Stroke is a medical emergency. Call 911 or your emergency medical services. Get to a hospital right away!

The American Stroke Association wants you to learn the warning signs of stroke:

- Sudden numbness or weakness of the face, arm, or leg, especially on one side of the body
- Sudden confusion, trouble speaking or understanding
- Sudden trouble seeing in one or both eyes
- Sudden trouble walking, dizziness, loss of balance or coordination
- Sudden, severe headache with no known cause

Be prepared for an emergency.

- Keep a list of emergency rescue service numbers next to the telephone and in your pocket, wallet, or purse.
- Find out which area hospitals are primary stroke centers that have twenty-four-hour emergency stroke care.
- Know (in advance) which hospital or medical facility is nearest your home or office.

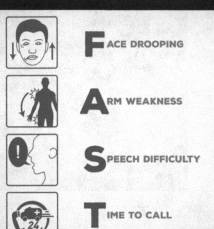

STROKE WARNING SIGNS AND SYMPTOMS

FACE DROOPING

ARM WEAKNESS

SPEECH DIFFICULTY

TIME TO CALL

© iLoveCoffeeDesign/Shutterstock.com

Figure 9.6 The Warning Signs of a Stroke

Take action in an emergency.

- Not all the warning signs occur in every stroke. Don't ignore signs of stroke, even if they go away!
- Check the time. When did the first warning sign or symptom start? You'll be asked this important question later.
- If you have one or more stroke symptoms that last more than a few minutes, don't delay! Immediately call 911 or the emergency medical service (EMS) number so an ambulance (ideally with advanced life support) can quickly be sent for you.
- If you're with someone who may be having stroke symptoms, immediately call 911 or the EMS. Expect the person to protest—denial is common. Don't take "no" for an answer. Insist on taking prompt

For stroke information, call the American Stroke Association at 1-888-4-STROKE. For information on life after stroke, ask for the Stroke Family Support Network.

OBESITY

"Since 1979 the World Health Organization (WHO) has classified obesity as a disease. 'Obesity is a complex condition, one with serious social and psychological dimensions, that affects virtually all age and

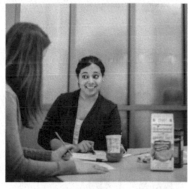

© Winthrop University

socioeconomic groups and threatens to overwhelm both developed and developing countries. As of 2000, the number of obese adults has increased to over 300 million' (WHO, 2008). 'Globesity' may be the new term coined for the world's heavy populations. While malnutrition still contributes to an estimated 60 percent of deaths in children ages five and under globally, in the United States the excess body weight and physical inactivity that leads to obesity cause more than 112,000 deaths each year, making it the second leading cause of death in our county (see figure 9.7).

"Obesity causes, contributes to, and complicates many of the diseases that afflict Americans. Obesity is associated with a shortened life, serious organ impairment, poor self-concept, and a higher risk of cardiovascular disease and diabetes, as well as colon and breast cancer. Fat distribution is related to health risk (Canoy, 2007). 'Apples' describe male-fat patterned distribution with fat accumulating mostly around the torso. 'Pears' describe female-fat patterned distribution with fat accumulating mostly on the hips and upper thighs. Apples have a higher health risk especially if they have visceral fat located around internal organs."[1]

Causes of Obesity

"Is it your genes or your fast-food lunches every day? Most likely it is both. Since you cannot change who your parents are, change your lifestyle habits. Physical inactivity is certainly a major, if not the primary, cause of obesity in the United States today (Wilmore, 1994). Most often caloric intake exceeds caloric expenditure. Glandular disorders affect 2 percent of the obese population. Genetically we are predisposed to a certain somatotype, fat distribution, size, and weight. In every person, body weight is the result of many factors; genetic, metabolic, behavioral, environmental, cultural as well as socioeconomic influences (Surgeon General, 2005). An individual's lifestyle choices can help to

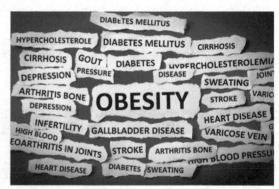

© Aliwak/Shutterstock.com

modify these tendencies. Nineteen out of twenty overweight teenagers will be overweight adults (Texas A&M University Human Nutrition Conference, 1998)."[1]

Did you know . . .

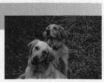

Courtesy of Shelley Hamill

Health Risks of Obesity

Each of the diseases listed below is followed by the percentage of cases that are caused by obesity.

Colon cancer 10%   Breast cancer 11%   Hypertension 33%

Heart disease 70%   Diabetes 90% (Type II, non-insulin-dependent)

As these statistics show, being obese greatly increases the risk of many serious and even life threatening diseases.

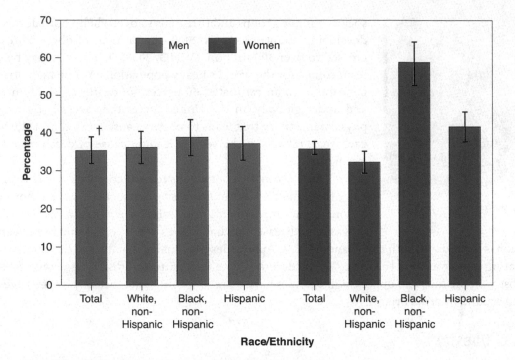

Figure 9.7 Prevalence of Obesity Among Adults Aged ≥20 Years, by Race/Ethnicity and Sex—National Health and Nutrition Examination Survey. United States, 2009—2010

Spotlight on . . .

Childhood Obesity

About one in three children and teens in the U.S. are overweight or obese. Overweight kids have a 70–80 percent chance of staying overweight their entire lives. Obese and overweight adults now outnumber those at a healthy weight; nearly seven in ten U.S. adults are overweight or obese. Excess weight at young ages has been linked to higher and earlier death rates in adulthood. Perhaps one of the most sobering statements regarding the severity of the childhood obesity epidemic came from former Surgeon General Richard Carmona, who characterized the threat as follows:

> "Because of the increasing rates of obesity, unhealthy eating habits, and physical inactivity, we may see the first generation that will be less healthy and have a shorter life expectancy than their parents."

Obesity has also risen dramatically in adults. Today over 144 million Americans, or 66 percent of adults age 20 and older, are overweight or obese (BMI at or above 25). That is nearly seven out of every 10 adults. Additionally, 33 percent (over 71 million) of adults are classified as obese (BMI at or above 30). Obese Americans now outnumber overweight Americans, which means that individuals who are above a healthy weight are significantly, not slightly, above a healthy weight. Some experts project that by 2015, 75 percent of adults will be overweight, with 41 percent obese.

Source: American Heart Association, Inc.

Physiological Response to Obesity

"For an obese person, more blood vessels are needed to circulate blood. The heart has to pump harder, therefore increasing blood pressure. Extra weight can be tough on the musculoskeletal joints, causing problems with arthritis, gout, bone and joint diseases, varicose veins, gallbladder disease, as well as complications during pregnancy. Obese individuals often are heat intolerant and experience shortness of breath during heavy exercise. Obesity increases most cancer risks (Bishops and Aldana, 1999)."[1]

CANCER

"Cancer is characterized by the spread of abnormal cells that serve no useful purpose (see Figure 9.8). Tumors can be either benign, having a slow and expanding type of growth rate, remaining localized, and being well differentiated; or malignant, growing rapidly, infiltrating (crowding out and replacing normal cells), metastasizing (spreading to other parts of the body via the circulatory or lymphatic system) and being poorly differentiated. There are four classifications of cancers according to the type of cell and organ of origination:

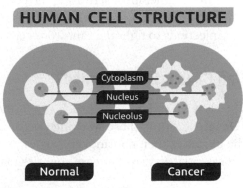

© Becris/Shutterstock.com

Figure 9.8 The Difference Between a Healthy Cell and a Cancerous Cell

1. Carcinoma cancers originate in epithelium (layers of cells that cover the body and line organs and glands). These are the most common.
2. Sarcomas begin in the supporting or connective tissues including bones, muscles, and blood vessels.
3. Leukemias arise in the blood-forming tissues of bone marrow and spleen.
4. Lymphomas form in the lymphatic system."[1]

Risk Factors

"Risk factors include a family history, race and culture, viruses, environmental and occupational hazards, cigarette smoking, alcohol consumption, poor dietary habits, and psychological factors that compromise the immune system. Heredity or family history is thought to account for 10 percent of all cancers with the most likely sites for inherited cancers involving the breast, brain, blood, muscles, bones, and adrenal gland.

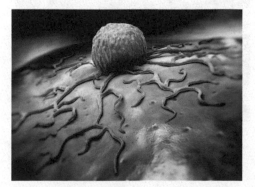

© Tatiana Shepeleva/Shutterstock.com

Research has revealed a variety of internal and external agents that are believed to cause cancer. These agents are termed carcinogens and include occupational pollutants (nickel, chromate, and asbestos), chemicals in food and water, certain viruses, and radiation (including the sun).

"Be certain to contact a physician if you experience any of these signs. With any cancer, early detection is the key to treatment and survival. A common misconception is that cancer is a death sentence. However, the forms of cancer with the highest incidence and mortality rates are those directly related to lifestyle factors that can be changed or eliminated. Due to dramatic improvements in diagnosis and treatment, more cancer patients are being cured and their quality of life is greatly improved. Treatment usually involves one or the combination of the following procedures:

- Surgery—removal of the tumor and surrounding tissue
- Radiation—X-rays that are aimed at the tumor to destroy or stop the growth
- Chemotherapy—an intravenous administration of fifty or more drugs combined to kill the cancerous cells
- Immunotherapy—activating the body's own immune system with interferon injections to fight the cancerous cells"[1]

"The seven warning signs of cancer are:

1. Change in bowel or bladder habits
2. A sore that does not heal
3. Unusual bleeding or discharge
4. Thickening or lump in the breast, testes, or elsewhere
5. Indigestion or difficulty swallowing
6. Obvious change in a wart or mole
7. Nagging cough or hoarseness."[1]

© martan
/Shutterstock.com

Can Cancer Be Prevented?

"Healthy lifestyle practices such as not smoking—30 percent of all cancer deaths are attributed to smoking (Donatelle, 2010); those smoking two or more packs a day are fifteen to twenty-five times more likely to die of cancer than nonsmokers (Hales, 2011)—exercising regularly, and avoiding sun exposure are simple yet essential ways to decrease your risk of cancer. A diet low in fat (less than 30 percent of total calories) but high in fruits, vegetables (at least five servings per day), and whole grains are the best nutritionally for reducing cancer risk. Avoid smoke-filled areas. Second hand or environmental tobacco smoke (ETS) can increase the risk among nonsmokers. Researchers have found the risk of cancer to increase threefold with as little as three hours of exposure per day. Avoid environmental carcinogens whenever possible. Follow safety precautions if employed in or living near factories that create smoke or dust.

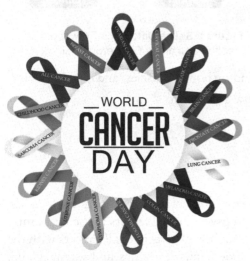

© suns design/Shutterstock.com

"It is theorized that 80 percent of cancers can be prevented with positive lifestyle choices. Avoiding tobacco and over-exposure to sunlight are two major examples. Eating a varied diet, consuming antioxidants, having a positive attitude, and participating in regular physical activity are simple choices that can have a large impact on cancer prevention. Thirty-five percent of the total cancer death toll is associated with diet (Rosato, 1994), and fit individuals may have a decreased risk of reproductive organ cancers (Bishop and Aldana, 1999). Cancer is the second leading cause of death in the United States, accounting for about 23 percent of all deaths yearly (Hoeger et al., 2009)."[1]

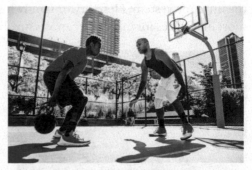

© oneinchpunch/Shutterstock.com

Does Exercise Help?

"Recognition of the potential of exercise to prevent cancer came in 1985 when the American Cancer Society began recommending exercise to protect against cancer. Regular activity has been shown to reduce risk of colon cancer. Active people have lower death rates from cancer than inactive people—50 to 250 percent lower. Colon, breast, rectal, and prostate cancers each have an established link with inactivity.

"It is also thought that exercise can boost immunity that can help kill abnormal cancer cells (Bishop and Aldana, 1999). Dr. Steven Blair at the Institute for Aerobics Research in Dallas, Texas, has done long-term epidemiological studies that show rate of death due to cancer is significantly lower in patients with elevated levels of fitness. It must also be noted that people who are active tend to also participate in other healthy behaviors, such as eating a varied diet low in fat and high in fiber. These other behaviors may also influence cancer risk and help those with cancer lead more fulfilling and productive lives. The American Cancer Society reports that people with healthy lifestyles (non-smokers, regular physical activity, and sufficient sleep) have the lowest cancer mortality rates. Table 9.1 provides information on how physical activity can effect different types of cancer.

TABLE 9.1 Physical Activity and Cancer

Cancer Type	Effect of Physical Activity
Colon	Exercise speeds movement of food and cancer-causing substances through the digestive system, and reduces prostaglandins (substances linked to cancer in the colon).
Breast	Exercise decreases the amount of exposure of breast tissue to circulating estrogen. Lower body fat is also associated with lower estrogen levels. Early life activity is deemed important for both reasons. Fatigue from therapy is reduced by exercise.
Rectal	Similar to colon cancer, exercise leads to more regular bowel movements and reduces "transit time."
Prostate	Fatigue from therapy is reduced by exercise.

TYPES OF CANCER

Lung Cancer

"Lung cancer is the number one cause of cancer deaths in the United States (CDC, 2015). The major cause of lung cancer is cigarette smoking, accounting for 85 percent of all lung cancer deaths, making it one of the most preventable forms of cancer. Smoking cessation decreases the death rate of lung cancer in half. Other risk factors include asbestos exposure, secondhand smoke, radiation exposure, and radon exposure. Early detection of lung cancer is difficult, resulting in only 15 percent of cases being discovered early. With early detection, there is a 43 percent chance of surviving twelve months; however, the overall five-year relative survival rate is only 16 percent. Symptoms include a nagging or persistent cough, blood in the sputum, chest pain, shortness of breath, recurring bronchitis or pneumonia, weight loss, loss of appetite, and/or anemia."[1]

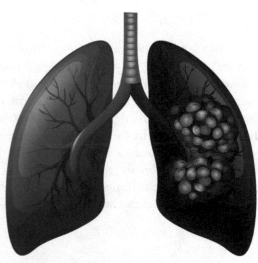

© BlueRingMedia/Shutterstock.com

Skin Cancer

"Overexposure to the ultraviolet (UV) rays of the sun is the primary culprit in these cases (see Figure 9.9). Ninety percent occur on parts of the body not usually covered with clothes, including the face, hands, forearms, and ears. The two most common types of skin cancers are basal cell carcinoma and squamous cell carcinoma (non-melanomas). Both are usually treated successfully with surgery, especially if detected early. Subsequent tumors are likely in persons previously treated for these types of cancer. The fatality rate for these cancers is less than one percent. Monthly skin self-exam (SSE) can reveal cancerous changes at an early stage. Use a systematic approach. During this exam, look for abnormal growth of cells. If you notice any of these warning signs see your physician immediately."[1]

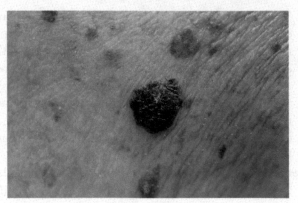

© charnsitr/Shutterstock.com

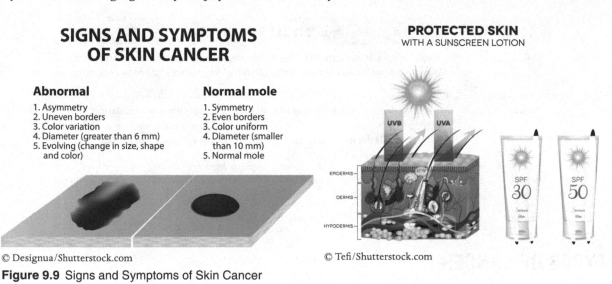

SIGNS AND SYMPTOMS OF SKIN CANCER

Abnormal
1. Asymmetry
2. Uneven borders
3. Color variation
4. Diameter (greater than 6 mm)
5. Evolving (change in size, shape and color)

Normal mole
1. Symmetry
2. Even borders
3. Color uniform
4. Diameter (smaller than 10 mm)
5. Normal mole

© Designua/Shutterstock.com

PROTECTED SKIN
WITH A SUNSCREEN LOTION

UVB   UVA

EPIDERMIS
DERMIS
HYPODERMIS

SPF 30   SPF 50

© Tefi/Shutterstock.com

Figure 9.9 Signs and Symptoms of Skin Cancer

Breast Cancer

"One in eight women will develop breast cancer in her lifetime (American Cancer Society, 2016). Risk factors include: age 40 years or older, family history or personal history of breast cancer, early onset of menstruation (before age 12), having no children, having a first child at a late age (after age 30), late menopause (after age 55), exposure to radiation, obesity, and certain types of benign breast disease (premenopausal women). Early detection is the best way to reduce the mortality rate among breast cancer patients. It is recommended by the American Cancer Society that women 20 years of age and older perform a breast self-examination once a month. As shown in Figure 9.10, any persistent lumps, swelling, thickening or distortion of the breast, pain or tenderness of the nipple, or discharge of blood or fluid from the nipple should be reported immediately. A diagnostic X-ray, called a mammogram, can detect a tumor two or three years before it can be detected by a self-exam. The American Cancer Society recommends all women begin routine mammograms by the age of 40, and physicians recommend that women at high risk (with a family history) have mammograms every six to twelve months beginning between the ages of 25 and 35. With early diagnosis and a localized tumor, there is an 89 percent chance of surviving five years."[1]

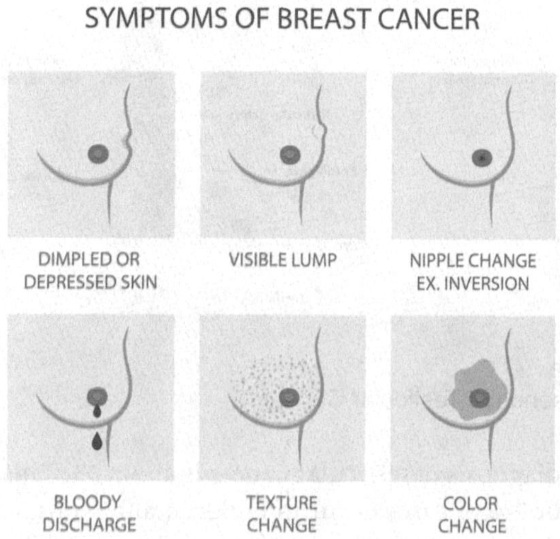

SYMPTOMS OF BREAST CANCER

DIMPLED OR
DEPRESSED SKIN

VISIBLE LUMP

NIPPLE CHANGE
EX. INVERSION

BLOODY
DISCHARGE

TEXTURE
CHANGE

COLOR
CHANGE

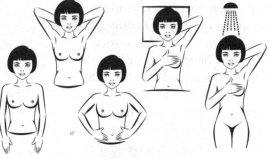

© eveleen/Shutterstock.com

Figure 9.10 Symptoms of Breast Cancer

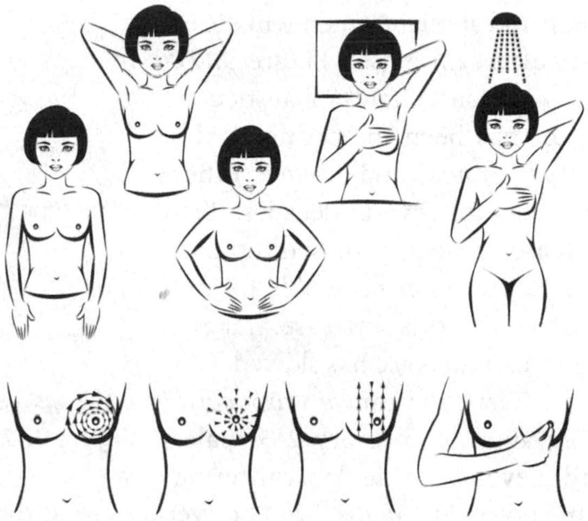

© eveleen/Shutterstock.com

Figure 9.11 Self-Evaluation Can Detect
Abnormalities Early

"Breast self-exam (BSE) is a method utilized in an effort to promptly detect lumps located in the breast. Early detection increases survival. During this exam, one looks for masses within the soft tissue of the breast or changes in the breast appearance. Due to the varying texture, size, and sensitivity of one's breast, it is important to do the self-exam at the same time each month. Figure 9.11 provides illustrations on how to complete a self-exam. The following is a guideline to determine the proper timing:

- Women with menstrual cycles—one week after the beginning of the menstrual period when the breasts are usually not tender
- After menopause or hysterectomy—choose a day that is easy to remember, such as the first day of the month."[1]

Cervical Cancer

"Cervical cancer is representative of abnormal growth and maturation of the cervical squamous epithelium. Typically there are no symptoms in the early stages. Eventually individuals with cervical cancer will have uterine bleeding, cramps, infections, and pain in the abdominal region. Risk factors include: first vaginal intercourse at an early age, multiple sexual partners, cigarette smoking, and infections with certain types of human papilloma viruses. Due to early detection with the Pap smear, cancer of the cervix is rare and easily treated in women who have regular exams. It is recommended that all women begin Pap tests no later than three years after first intercourse or starting at age 21, whichever comes first. This procedure should continue until an individual reaches the age of 70, at which point the physician may recommend discontinuing Pap smears."[1]

Testicular Cancer

Testicular Cancer

"In 2016, the American Cancer Society estimated about 8,720 new cases of testicular cancer will be diagnosed and about 380 men will die of testicular cancer (see Figure 9.12). The incidence rate of testicular cancer has been increasing in the United States and many other countries for several decades. The increase is mostly in seminomas. Experts have not been able to find reasons for this increase. Lately, the rate of increase has slowed.

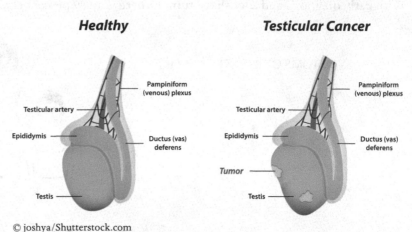

© joshya/Shutterstock.com

Figure 9.12 The Presence of Testicular Cancer

"Testicular cancer is not common; about 1 of every 263 males will develop testicular cancer at some point during his life. The average age at the time of diagnosis of testicular cancer is about 33. This is largely a disease of young and middle-aged men, but about 7% of cases occur in children and teens, and about 7% occur in men over the age of 55. Because testicular cancer usually can be treated successfully, a man's lifetime risk of dying from this cancer is very low: about 1 in 5,000 (American Cancer Society, 2016).

"Men with undescended testicles in childhood seem to be at greatest risk. Other risks may include: family history, inguinal hernia, testicular trauma, mumps orchitis, elevated testicular temperature, vasectomy, or exposure to electromagnetic fields. Testicular self-exams should be performed monthly to detect any enlargement or thickening of the testes. The cure rate if detected early is close to 80 percent. Testicular self-exam (TSE) can detect cancer in early stages when disease is more curable. Exams should begin at age 15. Self-examination should be performed every month in order to detect any changes. The best time to perform the exam is after taking a warm bath or shower when the skin of the scrotum is relaxed."[1]

Google Challenge!

How can the way we "potty" affect our risk for colon cancer?

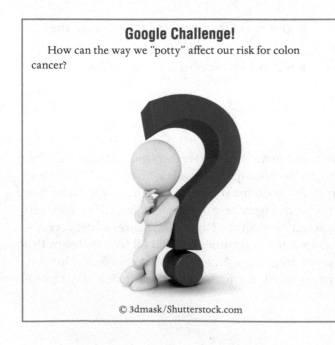

© 3dmask/Shutterstock.com

Colon and Rectum Cancers

"Colon and rectum cancers are the third leading types of cancer in men and women, claiming about 100,000 lives a year (American Cancer Society, 2016). The majority of cases occur in men and women over the age of 50. Risk factors include a family or personal history of colorectal cancer or polyps (growths) and ulcerative colitis. High fat, low-fiber diets have also been shown to increase the risk. Symptoms include bleeding from the rectum, blood in the stool, or a change in bowel habits (recurring constipation or diarrhea). Digital rectal exams, stool blood tests, and proctoscopic exams can detect early stages of colorectal cancer."[1]

Oral Cancers

"Each year, more than 48,330 new cases of cancer of the oral cavity and pharynx are diagnosed and over 9,570 deaths due to oral cancer occur. The five year survival rate for these cancers is only about 60 percent (ACS, 2016) http://www.cdc.gov/oralhealth/oral_cancer/. Oral cancer is related directly to a person's behavior. The major behavioral risk factors include cigarette, pipe, or cigar smoking, excessive alcohol use, and chewing tobacco use. Particularly vulnerable are persons who drink and smoke. Early symptoms include: a bleeding sore that will not heal, a lump or thickening, a red or white patch (lesion) that will not go away, a persistent sore throat, difficulty chewing, swallowing, or moving of the tongue or jaws. A cure is often achieved easily with early detection."[1]

TABLE 9.2 Preventing Cancer through Diet and Lifestyle

Type	Decreases Risk	Increases Risk	Preventable by Diet
Lung	Vegetables, fruits	Smoking; some occupations	33–50%
Stomach	Vegetables, fruits; food refrigeration	Salt and salted food	66–75%
Breast	Vegetables, fruits	Obesity; alcohol	33–50%
Colon/rectum	Vegetables; physical activity	Meat; alcohol; smoking	66–75%
Mouth/throat	Vegetables, fruits; physical activity	Salted fish; alcohol; smoking	33–50%
Liver	Vegetables	Alcohol; contaminated food	33–66%
Cervix	Vegetables, fruits	Smoking	10–20%
Esophagus	Vegetables, fruits	Deficient diet; smoking; alcohol	50–75%
Prostate	Vegetables	Meat or meat fat; dairy fat	10–20%
Bladder	Vegetables, fruits	Smoking; coffee	10–20%

Here are some tips issued by a panel of cancer researchers:
- Avoid being underweight or overweight, and limit weight gain during adulthood to less than eleven pounds.
- If you don't get much exercise at work, take a one-hour brisk walk or similar exercise daily, and exercise vigorously for at least one hour a week.
- Eat eight or more servings a day of cereals and grains (such as rice, corn, breads, and pasta), legumes (such as peas), roots (such as beets, radishes, and carrots), tubers (such as potatoes), and plantains (including bananas).
- Eat five or more servings a day of a variety of other vegetables and fruits.
- Limit consumption of refined sugar.
- Limit alcoholic drinks to less than two a day for men and one a day for women.
- Limit intake of red meat to less than three ounces a day, if eaten at all.
- Limit consumption of salted foods and use of cooking and table salt. Use herbs and spices to season foods.

Sources: World Cancer Research Fund; American Institute for Cancer Research, 2003, © Kendall Hunt Publishing Company

DIABETES

"**Diabetes** is a disorder that involves high blood sugar levels and inadequate insulin production by the pancreas or inadequate utilization of insulin by the cells (Wilmore, 1994). Diabetes is becoming more common in the United States. In 2008, CDC estimated that 23.6 million Americans, or 7.8 percent of the

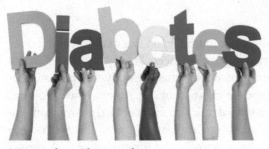

© Rawpixel.com/Shutterstock.com

population, had diabetes and another 57 million adults had prediabetes (CDC, 2011). There are three types of diabetes, Type I, Type II, and gestational.

"Type I or insulin-dependent diabetes is typically associated with childhood or adolescent onset. In this form of diabetes the pancreas does not produce insulin, and the individual requires regular injections. According to Figure 9.13, the signs and symptoms of Type I diabetes appear suddenly and dramatically. Symptoms include fatigue, irritability, abnormal hunger and thirst, frequent urination, and weight loss (Floyd et al., 2007). This type of diabetes is only seen in about 5 percent of all diabetics and is considered the more serious of the two forms.

"Type II or non-insulin-dependent diabetes is typically associated with adult onset and obesity. In this form of the disease the pancreas produces insulin, but the cells of the body are not able to use it effectively. The onset of Type II diabetes is more gradual than Type I. Some symptoms include drowsiness, blurred vision, itching, slow healing of cuts, skin infections, and numbness of fingers or toes (Floyd et al., 2007).

"Gestational diabetes is a form of glucose intolerance or insulin resistance that is typically diagnosed in some women late in pregnancy. This type of diabetes affects about 9.2 percent of all pregnant women in the United States each year (ADA 2014 or www.diabetes.org/gestational-diabetes.jsp.) Gestational diabetes can cause dangerously high blood sugar levels to occur in the pregnant female. This type of diabetes occurs more frequently among African Americans, Hispanic/Latino Americans, and Asians (Dabelea, Snell-Bergeon, Heartsfield, et al, 2005). It is also more common among obese women and women with a family history of diabetes.

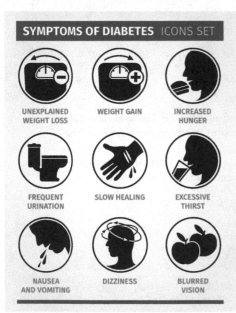

© Leyasw/Shutterstock.com

Figure 9.13 Symptoms of Diabetes

"If an individual suffering from diabetes is not treated, the illness can progress into a diabetic coma. If too much insulin is taken or inadequate food is eaten, an insulin reaction may occur, which, if serious, can result in a seizure (convulsions). Patients with diabetes have a higher incidence of arteriosclerosis and the associated complications such as strokes, heart attacks, and gangrene of the lower extremities due to poor circulation, as well as degenerative effects of the small blood vessels supplying oxygen to the retina of the eye, which can lead to blindness.

"The goal for those who have this condition is to balance blood sugar levels. Normal blood sugar ranges from 70 to 110 mg/dL. This can be done with insulin regimens, a structured diet, and regular exercise. With Type I diabetes, the individual usually can achieve this by monitoring the blood glucose level and adjusting the amount of insulin injected each day. In Type II diabetes, this can be accomplished with a controlled diet and regular exercise alone; in some instances oral hypoglycemic medication or insulin is required as well. The risk of developing diabetes can be reduced with regular activity, which reduces body weight and fat levels, and increases insulin

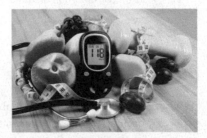

© ratmaner/Shutterstock.com

sensitivity and glucose tolerance. Healthy dietary habits also decrease the fat levels as well as obesity, therefore enhancing the body's ability to transport glucose into the muscles."[1]

Who Gets Diabetes?

"Eighty percent of the adults who develop Type II diabetes are obese (Surgeon General, 2005). The mortality rate is greater in diabetics with CVD—68% of people with diabetes die from some form of CVD. Each year, 1.6 million new cases of diabetes are diagnosed (AHA, 2012). Diabetes is the seventh leading cause of death in people over 40 (Corbin and Welk, 2009). Due to the surge in childhood obesity in the decade of the 90's, children are more at risk for diabetes. Diabetes is one of the most important risk factors for stroke in women. "[1]

Can Diabetes Be Prevented?

"Research shows that changing lifestyle habits to decrease risk for heart disease also decreases risk for diabetes. 'According to research, a seven percent loss of body weight and 150 minutes of moderate-intensity physical activity a week can reduce the chance of developing diabetes by 58 percent in those who are at high risk. These lifestyle changes cut the risk of developing Type II diabetes regardless of age, ethnicity, gender, or weight.' Type II diabetes may account for 90–95 percent of all diagnosed cases of diabetes (AHA, 2012). "[1]

Does Exercise Help?

"Exercise plays an important role in managing this disease, as exercise helps control body fat and improves insulin sensitivity and glucose tolerance. Exercise does not prevent Type II diabetes; however, exercise does help manage the disorder. "[1]

OSTEOPOROSIS

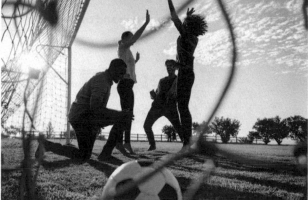

© Monkey Business Images/Shutterstock.com

"**Osteoporosis** is a disease characterized by low bone density and structural deterioration of bone tissue, which can lead to increased bone fragility and increased risk of fractures to the skeletal structure. Osteoporosis is sometimes called the 'silent disease' because there are often no symptoms as bone density decreases. "[1]

Who Gets Osteoporosis?

"For 53 million Americans, osteoporosis is a major public health threat (NIH, 2015). Considered to afflict mostly women, this disease can affect males as well. Of the women with osteoporosis, 80 percent are postmenopausal. One out of two women and one out of eight men over 50 will get osteoporosis in their lifetime. Risk increases with age. Have you observed older women who seem to slump? Many women with low bone density have kyphosis (also called dowager's hump), or a rounding of the upper back. The head tilts forward because often the cervical vertebrae in the upper spine actually suffer compression fractures. This keeps older women from being able to stand up straight or to get a full breath. Small, thin-boned women are at higher risk, and there may also be a genetic factor. If there are people in a family with weak, thin bones then relatives with the same body type may have an inherently higher risk. Post-menopausal Caucasian and Asian women are at the highest risk. It is unknown why these particular groups are more susceptible to osteoporosis. African Americans have bone that is 10 percent more dense than Caucasians. Others at risk include those with poor diets, especially if calcium and vitamin D are low over a long period of time. It is estimated that 75 percent of adults do not consume enough calcium on a daily basis. An inactive lifestyle contributes greatly. A history of excessive use of alcohol or cigarette smoking can also increase risk (see Figure 9.14). Another growing group of high-risk individuals is the eating disordered. Many active young women suffer stress fractures, which can be a sign of osteoporosis (NIH, 2015). "[1]

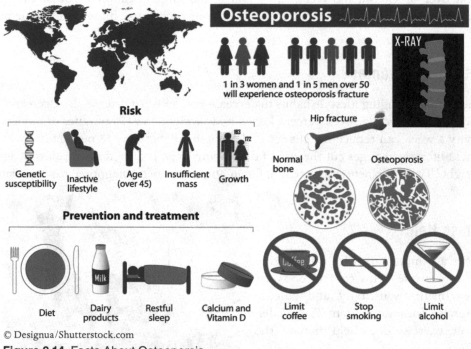

© Designua/Shutterstock.com

Figure 9.14 Facts About Osteoporsis

Can Osteoporosis Be Prevented?

"The good news is that osteoporosis can be both prevented and treated. Regular physical activity reduces the risk of developing osteoporosis. A lifetime of low calcium intake is associated with low bone mass (www.osteo.org). Adequate calcium intake is critical for optimal bone mass. Growing children, adolescents, and pregnant and breast-feeding women need more calcium. It is estimated by the National Institutes of Health that less than 10 percent of girls age 10–17 years are getting the calcium they need each day. A varied diet with green leafy vegetables and plenty of dairy will help ensure good calcium intake. Many calcium-fortified foods are now available. A varied diet will also ensure adequate intake of vitamin D, which aids in prevention. It is also advisable to limit caffeine and phosphate-containing soda, which may interfere with calcium absorption. Prolonged high-protein diets may also contribute to calcium loss in bone. A high-sodium diet is thought to increase calcium excretion through the kidneys. For post-menopausal women, some physicians consider hormone replacement therapy to help

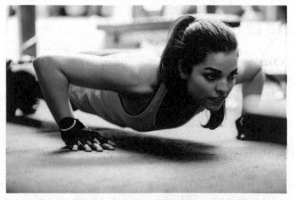

© antoniodiaz/Shutterstock.com

strengthen bones. Weight bearing exercise such as walking, running, tennis, and basketball is an excellent way to strengthen bones to help prevent osteoporosis."[1]

Did you know . . .

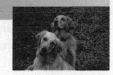

Courtesy of Shelley Hamill

Current Recommendations to Decrease Osteoporosis Risk

- Engage in daily weight-bearing aerobic activity
- Weight training (the ACSM recommends ten–twelve reps, two sets two times weekly)
- Vitamin D (well-balanced diet and adequate exposure to sunlight)
- Estrogen replacement therapy (for some women, especially post-menopausal women)

ASTHMA

"Asthma is a respiratory disorder that involves difficulty breathing, wheezing, and/or coughing due to the constriction of the bronchial tubes. An individual will typically notice a wheezing sound when they are trying to breathe, while coughing and/or when experiencing difficulty breathing (see Figure 9.15). In some cases those who suffer from asthma can stop an attack by simply removing themselves from an irritant such as cigarette smoke. Most of the time asthma attacks require some type of medical intervention, and, in rare cases, death can result from lack of treatment. Antihistamines, corticosteroids, and bronchodilation drugs are usually successful in reducing the bronchospasm."[1]

Pathology of Asthma

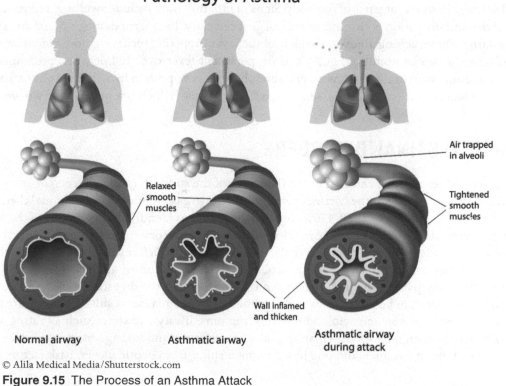

© Alila Medical Media/Shutterstock.com

Figure 9.15 The Process of an Asthma Attack

ANEMIA

"Anemia means 'without blood.' It is a condition in which the quantity or quality of red blood cells is insufficient. Normal red blood cells contain hemoglobin, which carries oxygen to organs and tissues. Anemic individuals have a reduced oxygen carrying capacity. Anemias can be the result of too little iron, loss of blood (including heavy menstrual bleeding or frequent blood donations), insufficient red cell production or genetic abnormalities. Symptoms include fatigue, infection, and/or trouble healing. There are four types of anemias known: iron-deficiency anemia, pernicious anemia, aplastic anemia, and sickle-cell anemia. "[1]

LUPUS

"Lupus is a chronic inflammatory disease that occurs when your body's immune system attacks your own tissues and organs. There are four different types of lupus. They are: systemic lupus erythematosus (SLE), cutaneous lupus erythematosus (CLE), drug-induced lupus, and neonatal lupus.

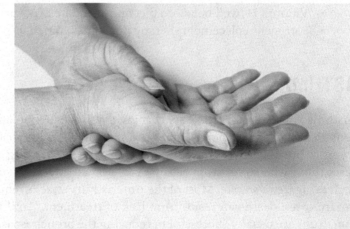

"With an autoimmune disease, the body cannot tell the difference between foreign substances such as viruses and bacteria and its own cells and tissues. When this happens the body begins attacking itself with auto-antibodies. This causes inflammation,

© blackboard1965/Shutterstock.com

pain, and damage in different parts of the body. Signs of inflammation include swelling, redness, pain, and warmth. If this inflammation is chronic, as with SLE, it can cause long-term damage. Signs and symptoms of a lupus flare include: aching all over, swollen joints, loss of appetite, recurring nose bleeds, sores on the skin, headache, nausea or vomiting, puffy eyelids, persistent fever over 100 degrees, prolonged fatigue, skin rashes, anemia, pain in the chest with deep breaths, excessive protein in urine, sensitivity to sun, hair loss, abnormal blood clotting problems, seizures, or mouth ulcers which last more than two weeks. "[1]

GASTROINTESTINAL DISORDERS

"Ulcers, which are open sores, can develop in the lining of the stomach (gastric ulcers) or small intestine (duodenal ulcers) and are due to the corrosive effect of excessive gastric juices. Conventional theory blames lifestyle factors such as stress and diet. However, new research has identified a link between the bacterium Helicobacter pylori (H. pylori) and the formation of ulcers. One theory suggests that an infection caused by this bacterium leads to an inflammation of the stomach lining, which results in increased susceptibility of the stomach to stressors such as smoking, alcohol, high-fat diets, and/or anxiety. The most prominent symptom is a burning pain in the upper abdomen that is related to the digestive cycle. A bleeding ulcer, although not common, can be fatal. Excessive weight loss and anemia can result from an untreated ulcer. Medications that reduce stomach acid and relieve symptoms, lifestyle changes such as eating small, frequent meals, avoiding high-fat foods, cigarettes, alcohol, caffeine, and taking antacids can all reduce the effects of ulcers. One in five men and one in ten women suffer from peptic ulcers. Risk factors include: a

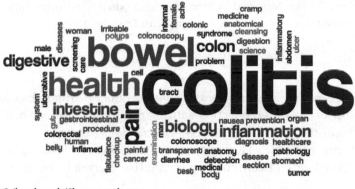

© ibreakstock/Shutterstock.com

stressful lifestyle, cigarette smoking, heavy use of alcohol, caffeine, or painkillers containing aspirin or ibuprofen, advanced age, and family history.

"Irritable bowel syndrome (IBS) (spastic colon or irritable colon) is a common problem resulting from intestinal spasms. Symptoms include episodes of abdominal cramping, nausea, pain, gas, loud gurgling bowel sounds, and disturbed bowel function. No biochemical or structural abnormalities have been identified as the cause; therefore, no standard medical treatment exists for IBS. Common interventions include reducing emotional stress, eating high- fiber diets, or taking stool softeners, laxatives, and drugs to reduce intestinal spasms. "[1]

COMMUNICABLE DISEASES

"Communicable diseases are those diseases that are transmitted from person to person. These diseases can be transmitted directly by physical contact, which can include coughing or sneezing, or indirectly by contaminated water or infected insects. "[1]

HIV/AIDS (Non-Sexual Contraction)

"HIV/AIDS can be contracted through blood transfusions, sharing needles, and/or the exchange of blood or breast milk from a mother to her unborn or newborn child. The groups that have been found to be at higher risk include IV drug users and those individuals who received a blood transfusion before 1985. More information on HIV/AIDs can be found in Chapter 7. "[1]

Mononucleosis

"Mononucleosis, also known as 'the kissing disease' because it is transmitted by saliva exchange, is primarily a self-limited (one that does not need treatment and will go away on its own) infection of young adults. The majority of cases occur in the 15 to 30 age range. This disease is most frequently caused by the Epstein-Barr virus (EBV); however, other viruses including cytomegalovirus (CMV) and the bacterium Toxoplasma gondii have been implicated (McCance and Huether, 2009). As shown in Figure 9.16, the virus attacks lymphocytes (cells found in blood and lymph tissues), which causes proliferation of cells in the immune system. This results in swelling of the lymph nodes, which is a prominent feature of this illness. After infection, there is an incubation period of thirty to fifty days (McCance and Huether, 2009). Initially,

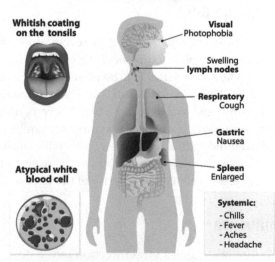

© Designua/Shutterstock.com

Figure 9.16 Signs and Symptoms of Mononucleosis

there are mild symptoms of headache and fatigue. This is followed by fever, lymph node enlargement (primarily those in the neck), and sore throat, which is the most common symptom and can be quite severe. "[1]

Hepatitis

"Hepatitis means 'inflammation of the liver.' There are various causes, such as alcohol or drug-induced inflammation; however, the most common cause of hepatitis is infection with a virus. At the current time, there are six types of viruses known to cause hepatitis (A, B, C, D, E, and G). Descriptions of hepatitis have been found by Hippocrates as far back as the fifth century BC. The first recorded cases were believed to be transmitted by the smallpox vaccine contaminated with infected human lymph tissue given to German shipyard workers in 1883.

"The course of hepatitis can vary from asymptomatic infection (which is completely cleared by the immune system and unknown to the infected person) to rapid liver failure and death, or a slower process with cirrhosis and/ or liver cancer. In early hepatitis there is an inflammation of the liver due to the response of the immune system in an attempt to eradicate the virus. The damaged liver produces scar tissue as it attempts to heal itself, which can lead to cirrhosis (causing the liver to shrink and harden). This makes the liver unable to perform its life-sustaining functions. The individual who is chronically infected with hepatitis B or C is at a higher risk for the development of liver cancer. Unfortunately, chronic hepatitis is often asymptomatic until irreversible liver damage has occurred. "[1]

Meningitis

"Meningitis is an inflammation of the membranes that cover the spinal cord and the brain. Meningitis is usually caused by a viral (the most common type) or bacterial infection. It is important to determine which type of infection is causing the meningitis. If the meningitis is from a viral source, typically it will be less severe and resolve on its own. The best course of action if you have contracted viral (aseptic) meningitis is bed rest, drink plenty of fluids, and take medicine to relieve fever and headaches. If the meningitis is from a bacterial source, it can result in blindness, deafness, permanent brain damage, learning disability, or even death. Most often bacterial meningitis can be treated successfully with antibiotics if caught early. "[1]

Common Cold

"The common cold is caused by several different viruses that are spread by droplets from sneezing or coughing, or touching surfaces where the virus is present such as hands, money, or door handles. Symptoms include congestion, sneezing, sore throat, coughing, and a low-grade fever. There is no treatment for the common cold; however, the symptoms can be treated to help the infected individual feel more comfortable until the virus has run its course. Gargle with saltwater at the onset to relieve symptoms and possibly reduce the severity of the illness. "[1]

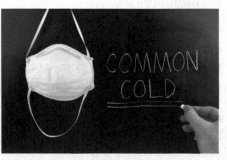
© simez78/Shutterstock.com

Influenza

"Influenza (flu) is a viral infection of the nose, throat, bronchial tubes, and lungs. The flu is spread in a similar manner as the common cold. Symptoms include high fever, chills, headache, muscle and joint ache, coughing, and fatigue. As with the common cold, there is no treatment for the flu; however, medication can be taken to ease the symptoms. The following reduce the risk of contracting colds and/or flu:

- Wash hands often.
- Keep hands away from your eyes, nose, and mouth.
- Drink at least eight glasses of water a day.
- Get enough rest (six to eight hours a night).
- Use Kleenex instead of handkerchiefs.
- Get enough vitamin C.
    - Receive a flu shot."[1]

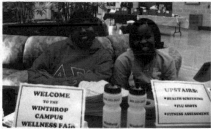

© Winthrop University

TABLE 9.3 Is It a Cold or the Flu?

Symptoms	Cold	Flu
Fever	Rare	Characteristic, high (102–104°F); lasts 3–4 days
Headache	Rare	Prominent
General Aches, Pains	Slight	Usual; often severe
Fatigue, Weakness	Quite mild	Can last up to 2–3 weeks
Extreme Exhaustion	Never	Early and prominent
Stuffy Nose	Common	Sometimes
Sneezing	Usual	Sometimes
Sore Throat	Common	Sometimes
Chest Discomfort, Cough	Mild to moderate; hacking cough	Common; can become severe
COMPLICATIONS	Sinus congestion or earache	Bronchitis, pneumonia; can be life-threatening
PREVENTION	None	Annual vaccination; antiviral medicines– see your doctor
TREATMENT	Only temporary relief of symptoms	Antiviral medicines–see your doctor

Source: From the National Institute of Allergy and Infectious Diseases, www.niaid.nih.gov Nov 2008.

Are you a healthy consumer?

Since we are so driven for survival, we sometimes consume products that we think might be beneficial in preventing disease. Most of the decisions of our consumer behavior is driven by ads, claims, and testimonies that are not often grounded in science or research support. While there are some products that are effective in helping prevent disease and improve health, make sure that your consumer behaviors are based on science and research rather than fads and false claims.

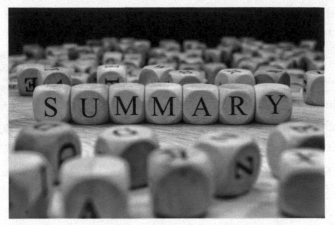

Throughout this chapter we have discussed many human diseases that can affect an individual's life. Chronic diseases, such as cardiovascular disease, stroke, obesity, cancer, diabetes, osteoporosis, and asthma, are common within America. We also discussed communicable diseases, such as colds and flu, among others. Being informed of your risk is important in your efforts to prevent disease. Understanding how quality of life is affected through disease can be a powerful motivator.

PERSONAL REFLECTIONS . . . SO, WHAT HAVE YOU LEARNED?

1. List the eight risk factors for cardiovascular disease. Do any apply to you currently? Are any risk factors within your family that you should be aware of and work to prevent?

2. What are the signs and symptoms of a heart attack in men and women? What are the signs and symptoms of a stroke?

3. How is obesity related to chronic disease?

4. What are the seven warning signs of cancer? What are three methods of cancer prevention that you practice regularly? What is at least one other cancer prevention strategy you could employ?

5. What are three differences between a cold and a flu?

NOTES

RESOURCES ON CAMPUS FOR YOU!

Health & Counseling Services

Follow these Centers for Disease Control and Prevention tips to stay healthy

- Avoid touching your eyes, nose, or mouth. Germs spread this way.
- Cover your nose and mouth with a tissue when you cough or sneeze. Throw the tissue in the trash after you use it.
- Try to avoid close contact with sick people.
- Wash your hands often with soap and water, especially after you cough or sneeze. Alcohol-based hand cleaners are also effective.

More information on Human Diseases can be found at:

Centers for Disease Control (CDC)   American Heart Association (AHA)

American Cancer Society (ACS)   American Diabetes Association (ADA)

World Health Organization (WHO)   U.S. Department of Health and Human Services

National Breast Cancer Foundation

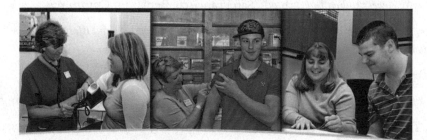

© Winthrop University

REFERENCES

American Cancer Society. (2016). Retrieved from www.cancer.org

American Diabetes Association (ADA). (2005). Retrieved from www.diabetes.org/gestational-diabetes.jsp

American Heart Association (AHA). (2015). *About high blood pressure.* Retrieved from http://www.heart .org/HEARTORG/Conditions/HighBloodPressure/AboutHighBloodPressure/About-High-Blood -Pressure_UCM_002050_Article.jsp#.Vtb7gH-LdHQ

American Heart Association (AHA). (2016). *Poor teen sleep habits may raise blood pressure, lead to CVD.* Retrieved from http://heartinsight.heart.org/Spring-2016/The-Importance-of-Sleep/

American Heart Association (AHA). (2015). *Heart disease and stroke statistics–2012 update.* Retrieved from www.aha.com

American Heart Association (AHA). (2015). *My life check- Life's simple 7.* Retrieved from www.mylifecheck.org

American Heart Association (AHA). (2014). *Understand your risk for high blood pressure.* Retrieved from http://www.heart.org/HEARTORG/Conditions/HighBloodPressure /UnderstandYourRiskforHighBloodPressure/Understand-Your-Risk-for-High-Blood-Pressure _UCM_002052_Article.jsp#.VtcM5X-LdHQ

Canoy, M.P. et al. (2007). Abdominal fat distribution predicts heart disease, *Circulation.*

Centers for Disease Control (CDC). (2015). *Lung cancer statistics.* Retrieved from http://www.cdc.gov /cancer/lung/statistics/index.htm

Centers for Disease Control and Prevention (CDC). (2014). *Number of Ccvilian, non-institutionalized persons with diagnosed diabetes, United States, 1980–2014.* Retrieved from www.cdc.gov/diabetes/statistics /prev/national/figpersons.htm

Centers for Disease Control and Prevention (CDC). (2013). *Oral cancer.* Retrieved from www.cdc.gov /oralhealth/topics/cancer.htm

Corbin, C. and Welk, G. (2009). *Concepts of physical fitness* (15th ed). New York: McGraw-Hill.

Dabelea, D., Snell-Bergeon, J.K., Heartsfield, C.L. et al. (2005). Increasing prevalence of gestational diabetes mellitus (GDM) over time and by birth cohort. *Diabetes Care,* 28, 579–584.

Donatelle, R.J. and Davis, L.G. (2007). *Access to health* (10th ed). Boston: Benjamin Cummings.

Donatelle, R.J. (2010). *Access to health* (12th ed). San Francisco: Benjamin Cummings.

Floyd, P., Mimms, S., and Yelding, C. (2007). *Personal health: perspectives and lifestyles* (4th ed). Englewood, CO: Morton Publishing Company.

Greenberg, J. et al. (1998). *Physical fitness and wellness* (2nd ed). Boston: Allyn and Bacon.

Hales, D. (2011). *An invitation to health* (15th ed). Pacific Grove, CA: Brooks/Cole Publishing Company.

Hoeger, W.W.K., Turner, L.W., and Hafen, B.Q. (2009). *Wellness guidelines for a healthy lifestyle* (4th ed). Belmont, CA: Thompson Wadsworth.

McCance, K. and Huether, S. (2009). *S. Pathophysiology: The biologic basis for disease in adults and children* (6th ed). St. Louis, MO: Mosby-Year Book, Inc.

National Institute of Arthritis and Musculoskeletal and Skin Disease (NIA). (2015). *Osteoporosis.* Retrieved from http://www.niams.nih.gov/Health_Info/Bone/Osteoporosis/overview.asp

Otis, C.L. and Goldingjay, R. (2000). *The athletic woman's survival guide.* Champaign, IL: Human Kinetics Publishers.

Payne, W.A. and Hahn, D.B. (2000). *Understanding your health* (6th ed). St. Louis, MO: Mosby.

Rosato, F. (1994). *Fitness to wellness: The physical connection* (3rd ed). Minneapolis: West.

Satcher, D. (1996). *Surgeon General's report on physical activity and health.* Atlanta, GA: CDC.

Sesso, H.D. and Paffenbarger, R.S. (1956). The Harvard alumni health study, Harvard School of Public Health. Boston, MA.

Texas A&M University Human Nutrition Conference. (1998). College Station, TX.

U.S. Department of Health and Human Services (DHHS). (2004). *Surgeon General's report on bone health and osteoporosis: What it means to you.* Washington, DC: U.S. DHHS.

U.S. Department of Health and Human Services (DHHS). (2016). *Surgeon General's family health history initiative*. Washington, DC: U.S. DHHS.

Whelton PK, Carey RM, Aronow WS, Casey Jr DE, Collins KJ, Dennison Himmelfarb C, DePalma SM, Gidding S, Jamerson KA, Jones DW, MacLaughlin EJ, Muntner P, Ovbiagele B, Smith Jr SC, Spencer CC, Stafford RS, Taler SJ, Thomas RJ, Williams Sr KA, Williamson JD, Wright Jr JT. (2017). ACC/AHA/AAPA/ABC/ACPM/AGS/APhA/ASH/ASPC/NMA/PCNA Guideline for the Prevention, Detection, Evaluation, and Management of High Blood Pressure in Adults: Executive Summary, *Journal of the American College of Cardiology*, doi: 10.1016/j.jacc.2017.11.005.

World Health Organization (WHO). (2008). *Controlling the obesity epidemic*. Geneva: Author.

CREDITS

Chapter 10
Safety Awareness +

OBJECTIVES

Students will be able to:

- Identify risks association with unintentional injuries
- Discuss the risks associated with drowsy driving and the factors that contribute towards it.
- Identify the steps for creating a disaster plan and actually create one
- Discuss factors contributing to family violence
- Identify actions that may reduce the risk of sexual assault.

© pockygallery/shutterstock.com

PRE-ASSESSMENT

1. Do you have an escape plan in place where you live if for some reason you would have to evacuate quickly? If so, what is it? Does it include your entire family including your pet(s)?

2. Do you have a first aid kit? Home and car? What are mandatory items in each?

3. Do you walk, jog, or run outdoors? If so, do you wear headphones? List 3 reasons why that might not be a good idea.

4. If you play sports or are involved in outside activities, do you use the safety gear required? Why or why not? Identify a few things you do where protective gear should be used and note what that would include.

Did you know . . .

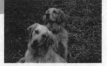

Courtesy of Shelley Hamill

According to the Center for Disease Control (CDC, 2022):

In 2018 there were:

- 130 million visits to the emergency room

- 35 million were injury related

- For persons aged 1-44 the leading causes of death were unintentional injury

- Unintentional deaths due to falls: 42,114

- Deaths due to motor vehicles: 40,698

- Deaths due to unintentional poisoning: 87,404

This chapter is designed to provide students with information to both inform and help you make the best choices. Often, being aware of potential hazards and hazardous situations can help reduce the likelihood that an injury will occur. According to the National Safety Council (NSC) accidents are defined as "the occurrence in a sequence of events that produces unintended injury, death or property damage. Accident refers to the event, not the result of the event." The term "accident" has largely been replaced with the term "incident" (NSC, 2019).

In 2020, accidents were the fourth leading cause of death in the United States after heart disease, cancer, and COVID 19 (CDC). For people ages 1-44, the leading cause of death in 2017 from 1981–2020 was unintentional injuries. Persons 10-24 accounted for 40.6% of the total deaths from unintentional injuries in that age range (CDC).

MOTOR VEHICLE SAFETY

For the first time since the Great Recession, the U.S. has experienced three straight years of at least 40,000 roadway **deaths**, according to preliminary estimates released Feb. 13 by the National Safety Council. In **2018**, an estimated 40,000 people lost their lives to **car** crashes – a 1% decline from 2017 (40,231 **deaths**) and 2016 (40,327 **deaths**) (NSC, 2019).

While the NSC does not specify what caused the specific incidents, it does note that in 2017 there was a spike in pedestrian deaths. Distracted driving accounted for 8% of crashes and drowsy driving a little over 2% NSC, 2019).

Life changed in many ways because of the COVID-19pandemic in 2020. In addition to the 350,831 COVID-19 deaths, preventable injury related deaths also experienced a dramatic increase in 2020. One component of this increase was motor-vehicle deaths. Roads became less safe in 2020 for a variety of reasons, including an increase in non-restrained occupant deaths, speeding, and alcohol impaired fatal crashes. After three consecutive years of decreases, deaths increased 8.3%; 42,338 people died in motor-vehicle crashes in 2020 compared to 39,107 in 2019.

Distracted Driving

Distracted driving is any activity that could divert a person's attention away from the primary task of driving. All distractions endanger driver, passenger, and bystander safety. These types of distractions include:

- Texting
- Using a cell phone or smartphone
- Eating and drinking
- Talking to passengers
- Grooming
- Reading, including maps
- Using a navigation system
- Watching a video
- Adjusting a radio, CD player, or MP3 player

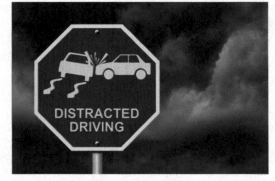

© karen roach/Shutterstock.com

According to NSC (2019), 53% of drivers believe that the new technology in cars, such as interactive dash boards and hands-free technology, are safe. The reality, is they can be very distracting. Imagine driving down the interstate at 70 miles per hour and all of sudden a coffee cup icon pops up in the middle of your dashboard with a caption that says, "consider taking a break". Distracting? And, just because hands-free is available for talking or even texting on your cell phone (and by the way, some states now require that you can only use hands free when driving), it doesn't mean you are not still distracted. Where is your attention? Is it on the road or on the conversation? Have you ever been chatting and driving and missed a turn or couldn't remember how you got there? Remember, multitasking technology is about convenience, not safety (NCS).

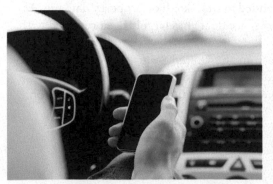

© Syda Productions/Shutterstock.com

"Operating a motor vehicle is the single most dangerous activity that we do on a daily basis and yet we feel confident that we can drive and do others things at the same time. We pride ourselves in our ability to multitask. We have been conditioned to think that we are more productive and successful if able to focus on more than one thing at a time. But can we truly multitask? John Medina, author of 'Brain Rules' says, 'Research shows that we can't multitask. We are biologically incapable of processing attention-rich inputs simultaneously.' The brain focuses on ideas and concepts one after another instead of both at the same time. The brain must let go of one activity to go to another, taking several seconds. According to Professor Clifford Nass at Stanford University, the more that you multitask, the less productive you become. When we operate a motor vehicle, many things can be considered distractions. Any secondary activity like texting, talking on a cell phone, putting on make-up, eating and drinking, adjusting your music or even your GPS can all cause problems while driving. Taking your eyes off the road for as little as two seconds can be dangerous. We have added more distractions by using our smart phones for Facebook, Twitter, Snapchat, and other social media."[1]

Drowsy Driving

The risk, danger, and often tragic results of drowsy driving are alarming. Drowsy driving is the dangerous combination of driving and sleepiness or fatigue. This usually happens when a driver has not slept enough, but it can also happen due to untreated sleep disorders, medications, drinking alcohol, or shift work (CDC). This has become such a problem, the National Sleep Foundation declared November 3—10, 2019 as "Drowsy Driving Prevention Week." Drive alert and stay unhurt.

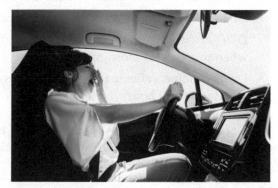

© chombosan/Shutterstock.com

No one knows the exact moment when sleep comes over their body. Falling asleep at the wheel is clearly dangerous, but being sleepy affects your ability to drive safely even if you do not fall asleep. Drowsiness:

- Makes drivers less able to pay attention to the road.
- Slows reaction time if you have to brake or steer suddenly.
- Affects a driver's ability to make good decisions.

People who do not get enough sleep and get behind the wheel are more prone to sleep related crashes. College students often fall into this category. Think about it. How many times have you gotten drowsy while driving? According to the National Sleep Foundation (NSF), it's not always easy to determine if you are too tired to drive. Here are some things to look for:

- Difficulty focusing, frequent blinking, or heavy eyelids
- Daydreaming; wandering/disconnected thoughts
- Trouble remembering the last few miles driven; missing exits or traffic signs
- Yawning repeatedly or rubbing your eyes
- Trouble keeping your head up
- Drifting from your lane, tailgating, or hitting a shoulder rumble strip
- Feeling restless and irritable

In order to make sure you are rested for that drive consider these ideas:

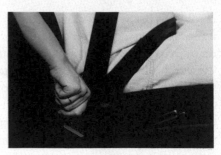

© Konstantin Kolosov/Shutterstock.com

- First, make sure you are getting a good nights sleep before hand (7-8 hours).
- The pre-drive nap: taking a short nap before a road trip can help make up for a short night's sleep.
- The mid-drive nap: if you find yourself drowsy while driving, pull over to take a short nap of 20 minutes. Make sure you are in a safe location and remember you'll be groggy for 15 minutes or so after waking up.
- The Buddy system: It's safest to drive with a partner on long trips. Pull over every two hours and switch drivers, while the other takes a nap if possible.
- Don't rush. Better to arrive at your destination safe than on time.
- Do not drink alcohol. Even very small amounts of alcohol will enhance drowsiness.
- Don't drive between midnight and 6 a.m. Because of your body's biological rhythm, this is a time when sleepiness is most intense.
- Drink caffeine: caffeine improves alertness, although be aware that the effects of caffeine will wear off after several hours (NSF. 2019).

Of course, all of the above are great ideas. But don't forget, seatbelts are a must each and every time no matter if you are in the front seat or back. Buckle up, stay focused, and safe travels.

Motorcycles

There were 5,014 fatalities for motorcycle riders and passengers in 2019 which has more than doubled since 1997 (NSC, 2019).

- Motorcycles make up 3% of all registered vehicles and only .6% of all vehicle miles traveled in the U.S.
- Motorcyclists accounted for 14% of all traffic fatalities in 2019
- 28% of riders who died in a motorcycle crash in 2019 were alcohol-impaired
- 91% of riders who died in a motorcycle crash in 2019 were male (NSC).

As a rider, it is important to make sure you not only obey the traffic laws, but also pay particular attention to other drivers. Drivers may not always see motorcycles in the mirrors or beside them, especially if riders are in their blind spot. Riders should also make sure to wear the proper safety gear required by law and consider wearing colors that stand out. While some states do not require helmets, they are the most essential part of the equipment a rider can have. In 2019, 1862 motorcyclists who died were not wearing a helmet. Helmets are estimated to be 37% effective in preventing fatal injuries (NSC). Also remember that you should never buy a used helmet as you may not know if they have ever been in a crash and if so, they have lost their protective abilities. Consider a helmet that has a face shield for full protection as bugs, rocks, even small ones, can have a

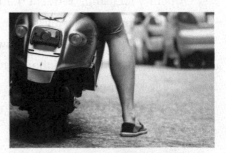

© Ekaterina Iatcenko/Shutterstock.com

strong impact when you are traveling at highway speeds. The National Safety Council (2019) notes that motorcycle crashes are considered violent events. More than 80% of all reported crashes involving motorcycles result in injury or death. For more information on how you can be a safe rider and on courses specific to motorcycle safety, check out https://www.nsc.org/road-safety/safety-topics/motorcycle-safety.

Drivers of both motorcycles and automobiles must be attentive to those around them. Making sure to check lanes before changing and not riding in a driver's blind spot can help reduce crashes. During warmer weather, people who ride motorcycles are more likely to be on the road. May is Motorcycle Safety Awareness month and motorists are reminded to "share the road" and to be extra alert to help keep motorcyclists safe.

Bicycle Safety

According to the National Highway Traffic Safety Administration (NHTSA), 857 bicyclists were kill in traffic accidents in the United States in 2018 (NHTSA, 2019). Obviously, car verses bike is never going to turn out well for the biker and it is especially important that cyclists be vigilant when riding. Never assume a driver sees you. Make sure to ride with traffic, in bike lanes if available, and follow all traffic laws. Wear bright colors or a safety vest so that you stand out when riding.

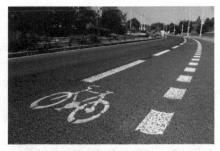

© Marsan/Shutterstock.com

Most bicycle deaths occurred between 6 pm and 9 pm, regardless of the season. They are more likely to occur in urban areas and in 2019, deaths for male cyclists were 8 times higher than for females (NHSTA). For further information on bicycle safety, visit https:// www.nhtsa.gov/road-safety/bicycle-safety

Additionally, just like motorcycle riders, it is important for cyclists to wear proper safety gear including and especially approved helmets.

Helmet Laws

Helmet laws affect both motorcyclists and bicyclists alike. "There is no federal law requiring bike or motorcycle riders to wear helmets. This causes a mix of legislation regarding helmets across all 50 states. Whether or not it is a law to wear a helmet when riding, doing so is always a good idea. Studies show that wearing a helmet can reduce one's risk of serious brain injury or death. A proper helmet absorbs the impact energy during a collision or fall, protecting the head and brain. Head trauma can lead to permanent cognitive and behavioral problems such as sleep disorders, trouble concentrating, memory loss, and disability.

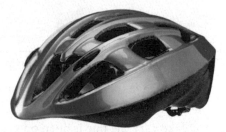

© Ljupco Smokovski/Shutterstock.com

Motorcycle helmet laws are usually written to apply to all riders or riders under a specified age. Additionally, some states' motorcycle helmet laws do not cover certain motorcycle-type vehicles, such as mopeds or motorized bicycles. There are only three states that do not have motorcycle helmet laws: Illinois, Iowa, and New Hampshire.

Nineteen states require that all riders wear a helmet. Eighteen states require riders 17 and younger to wear helmets, and nine states require riders 20 and younger to wear helmets. Delaware requires riders 18 and younger to wear helmets, and Missouri sets the age as 25." If you are planning an out of state tour, remember, they vary by state. Do your homework!

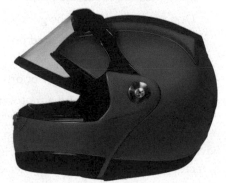

© AleksandrN/Shutterstock.com

HOME SAFETY

Poisoning

Chemicals in and around the home can poison people or pets and can cause long-term health effects. Every 13 seconds, a poison control center in the United States answers a call about a possible poisoning. More than 90% of these exposures occur in the home. Poisoning can result from medicines, pesticides, household cleaning products, carbon monoxide, and lead (CDC).

© Tribalium/Shutterstock.com

The most common causes of poisoning among young children are cosmetics and personal care products, household cleaning products, and pain relievers. Common causes among adults are pain relievers, prescription drugs, sedatives, cleaning products, and antidepressants.

Pesticides are used in about three out of four U.S. homes. They are used to prevent or kill bugs or rodents. They can also poison people or pets. Children can swallow detergents, bleaches, and other cleaning products. Remember the Tide Pods challenge? Breathing fumes from these products can also harm people and pets.

Carbon monoxide (CO) is a poison gas that is a by-product of appliances, heaters, and automobiles that burn gasoline, natural gas, wood, oil, kerosene, or propane. It has no color, no taste, and no odor (Healthy Children, 2019).

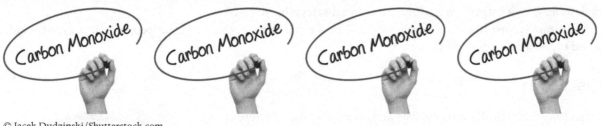

© Jacek Dudzinski/Shutterstock.com

To reduce the risk of carbon monoxide exposure consider the following:

- If you have fuel-burning appliances make sure they are in good working order and serviced regularly.
- Make sure the flue is open on gas fireplaces during operation and that they are also checked by a professional annually.
- Space heaters should be properly vented during use.
- Don't run your car in the garage.
- Generators should be vented properly as well. Make sure to follow the directions from the manufacture.
- Never use grills indoors or poorly vented spaces (like garages)
- If you are in a boat with a motor, remember, carbon monoxide can mimic sea sickness.

Of course, many people live in apartments or condominiums where units are connected. Though you have followed all of the rules your neighbors inadvertently may not have. Make sure to have a working CO detector in your residence and check it at least once a year to make sure it is working and change the batteries.

The symptoms of carbon monoxide poisoning may include dull headaches, weakness, dizziness, nausea or vomiting, confusion, and shortness of breath (Mayo Clinic, 2019). If you experience any of these symptoms, get to fresh air immediately and call 911. Remember, it is odorless and tasteless and can be life threatening.

Falls

According to the National Safety Council (NSC) falls are the leading cause of non-fatal preventable injures treated in hospital emergency rooms in 2020.

The CDC notes that death from unintentional injuries are the seventh leading cause of death among adults ages 65 or older and falls account for the largest percentage of those deaths. More than 6.8 million people were treated in an emergency department for fall related injuries in 2020.

Though some age groups may be more prone to falls, anyone can fall and there are a variety of contributing factors including:

- Walking while texting or reading texting (especially while using the stairs)
- Throw rugs or clutter
- Alcohol or drug use
- Slippery surfaces

If you have pets, make sure they are not underfoot when you are walking and also note where their toys are. Pay attention to where you are stepping and be aware of the conditions around you.

Spotlight on . . .

According to the CDC:

- Each year, at least 300,00 older people are hospitalized for hip fractures.
- More than 95% of hip fractures are caused by falling, usually sideways.
- Difficulties with walking and balance increase the risk for falls
- Vision problems increase the risk, not uncommon in the elderly.
- Medications can also play a role in falls.
- Women experience three quarters of all hip fractures.

Fires and Burns

Fire departments in the United States responded to an average of 355,400 home structure fires per year during 2012-2016. There were 11,070 civilian fire injuries and $7.3 billion in direct property damage. More than one-quarter of reported fires in 2015-2019 occurred in homes. Three-quarters of civilian fire deaths and almost three-quarters of all reported injuries were caused by home fires (NFPA, 2021).

According to the NFPA, the top five leading causes of fires are: cooking, heating, electrical, smoking and candles. Remember, other than electrical, you may play a role in preventing these types of fires by never leaving cooking unattended, not placing heaters next to flammable items, not smoking in bed (and making sure your cigarettes are out), and not leaving candles unattended.

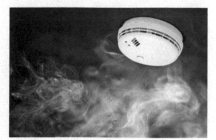

© nikkytok/Shutterstock.com

Having a working smoke alarm is imperative. Working smoke alarms cut the risk of dying in reported home fires in half. When smoke alarms fail to operate, it is usually because batteries are missing, disconnected, or dead. Additionally, having an appropriate fire extinguisher for home and auto is a good idea.

Everyone needs to have an escape plan in case of an emergency. You should know multiple exit possibilities, how to "get below" the smoke so you can get out, and where to you will meet the rest of your household once you have escaped. You should also practice the plan with everyone to minimize confusion and if you have pets, make sure to include them in your plans!

Weather Related Concerns

Depending on what part of the country, or other country, you are from, Mother Nature can create situations that require people to take cover or evacuate. Extreme heat or cold, tornados, or thunderstorms are just a few of the weather events that can cause injury or death.

According to weather.gov in 2020 there were:

- 17 fatalities due to lightning strikes
- 57 deaths due to floods
- 51 fatalities due to heat
- 76 for tornados
- 13 fatalities due to cold
- 55 fatalities due to wind

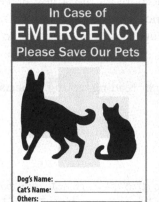

© strawberrytiger / Shutterstock.com

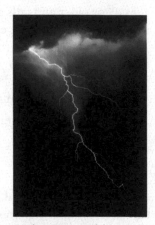

© Johan Swanepoel / Shutterstock.com

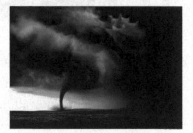

© solarseven/Shutterstock.com

These are just a few examples of how serious the threat can be. Staying informed about the weather in our surroundings, taking cover when necessary, and having a plan in case of an emergency can reduce injury and save lives.

Spotlight on . . .

Recreational Safety

There are many activities available to students, faculty and staff. Racket ball, outdoor equipment rental, even a climbing wall are just of few of the many possibilities. Your surrounding community may also offer bike trails, hiking trails, and different opportunities to participate in water sports. Let's not forget paintball, target shooting, and fencing, just to name a few. For each of these endeavors, safety needs and equipment should be addressed. Do you have the proper footwear, eye protection, head gear, or life vests needed? Have you had training on belay or can you swim? According to the CDC, there is an average of 11 drowing deaths per day; 80% of those who die from drowning are male, and 86% of people who died from boating accidents were not wearing life jackets (CDC, 2022). Nearly 30,000 sports-related eye injuries are treated in U.S. emergency rooms each year (American Academy of Opthamology, 2021). While everyone is encouraged to participate in whatever recreational activity fits your lifestyle, remember, *SAFETY* has to be included!

DISASTER PLANNING

Where will you be when disaster strikes? Hard to know, isn't it? You may have some warning but often things happen that we may not be prepared for. What would happen if you lost power or water? How long could you sustain that situation? What would happen if you were cut off from your family? What would happen if you were told to evacuate or shelter in place? You need a plan, as does your family, if an emergency or natural disaster were to take place.

Making a plan has some specific steps. First, put together a plan by talking with people in the household about the following:

1. How will your receive your emergency alerts and warning? There are many options out there.
2. What is your shelter plan (don't forget to include your pets in those plans).
3. What is your evacuation route?
4. And how will your family or household communicate during that disaster?
5. Do I need to update my emergency preparedness kit?
6. Check with the CDC and update my emergency plans due to COVID.

The second step involves considering and specific needs in the household. Are there diet issues? Medications? Food for pets or service animals? Identification?

The third step involves actually filling out a family emergency plan. There are many available on the web. And, lastly, practice the plan with the entire household. Everyone should practice so that if they are required to actually use the plan, they will know what to do!

It is also important to assemble a disaster kit. Depending on your family and pet situation, there are kits available for purchase or you can assemble one yourself. These kits are designed to help keep you safe and a bit more comfortable should you have the need to use them. Figure 10.1 contains a list of common items found in these kits. You should also have a first aid kit both in your home and car to tend to any minor injuries should that arise. First aid kits should be available in where you live, in your car, even a small kit might be useful in your backpack to deal with cuts or scrapes. There are many you can purchase commercially or put together your own.

Do you have pets? If so, they need a plan as well. You should have a copy of their vaccination records, pictures of you with them in case you are separated and you need to reclaim them. They also need something for food and water as well as small amounts of food to get through a few days. And, don't forget that there are pet first aid kits available also!

Lastly, make sure you check your kits annually to see if any items need to be replaced or added to. Has something expired? Also, make sure to check the batteries in smoke detectors, flashlights and radios. It would also be a good idea to make sure you have a charger station for your cell phone that can be used in the event of power loss.

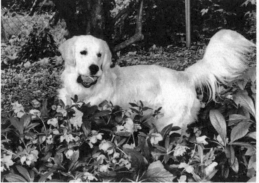

© Source: Shelley Hamill

Recommended Items to Include in a Basic Emergency Supply Kit:

- ☐ Water, one gallon of water per person per day for at least 3 days, for drinking and sanitation
- ☐ Food, at least a three-day supply of non-perishable food
- ☐ Battery-powered or hand crank radio and a NOAA Weather Radio with tone alert and extra batteries for both
- ☐ Flashlight and extra batteries
- ☐ First aid kit
- ☐ Whistle to signal for help
- ☐ Dust mask, to help filter contaminated air and plastic sheeting and duct tape to shelter-in-place
- ☐ Moist towelettes, garbage bags and plastic ties for personal sanitation
- ☐ Wrench or pliers to turn off utilities
- ☐ Can opener for food (if kit contains canned food)
- ☐ Local Maps

Courtesy of FEMA.

Figure 10.1

PERSONAL SAFETY

We often take our personal safety for granted. Yet, a crime or violent act can happen to anyone. In 2018, violet crimes were down 3.3 percent compared to 2017 and property crimes also dropped marking the 16th year in a row. That said, as previously stated, something can happen at any time.

An attacker looks for essentially three things when picking a victim:

1. Vulnerability
2. Accessibility
3. Availability

Practicing the following personal safety tips as you go about your daily activities may make you less attractive to a would be criminal.

- BE ALERT!! Know who is near you and what activities are going on around you.
- Walk with authority, look ahead and scan your surroundings
- Do not walk in poorly lit areas.
- Avoid standing at a bus stop alone, especially at night.
- If approached by someone in a car, change your direction and enter a crowded store or business.

- Carry a cell phone and some type of safety device (i.e.: flashlight, whistle, pepper spray and etc.) when walking at night.
- Be alert to someone who asks for directions and/or continues to engage you in conversation.
- If someone attempts to rob you and has a weapon, hand over the items. No material item is worth injury or your life.
- Be identification conscious. Observe your attacker's personal appearance, type of weapon used, and type of vehicle so you can accurately describe them to police.
- Immediately report the incident to the police and do not hang up until the police arrive.

Car

- Keep doors and windows locked.
- Always park in well-lighted areas.
- If being followed, do not go home. Go to a police station or well populated area.
- Be aware of your surroundings at all times.

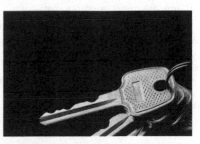

© Garsya/Shutterstock.com

Campus

- Avoid walking alone.
- Do not leave personal possessions unattended.
- Always notice other people—make eye contact.
- Avoid taking shortcuts through campus.
- Do not walk like a victim. Walk like you are on a mission.
- Always be aware of your surroundings.
- Trust your instincts. If someone or something makes you feel uncomfortable, get out of the situation.
- Use well-lighted stops if taking a bus.
- Have key in hand before reaching your room or car.
- Avoid jogging or walking alone.
- Hang up immediately once you realize the nature of a harassing call.
- Call a campus escort when on campus late at night.

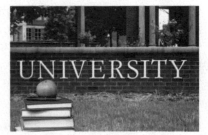

© AN NGUYEN/Shutterstock.com

College Campuses

While campus police do an excellent job of keeping the community safe, "many of the crimes on college campuses are crimes of opportunity. Theft is the most frequent crime on campus, yet it is the toughest challenge to convince students that their property can be taken. College students are typically very trusting, leaving their belongings unattended or inside vehicles in open view. Properly identifying your personal property such as backpacks, laptops, phones, and textbooks becomes extremely important. If you consider the amount of valuables you carry with you in a backpack, including wallet, cell phones, and possibly credit cards, the need for protection against theft becomes crucial. Reducing the opportunity and using common sense is the key to most crime prevention on college campuses."[1]

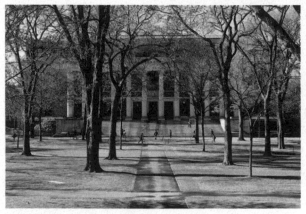

© Jorge Salcedo/Shutterstock.com

"It is also important to be cautious with the amount of personal information that you make available to the public whether it is on campus or over the Internet. Social networking sites like Facebook, Twitter, and Snapchat have become very popular, but they are not without safety concerns. With over 4 billion active users on Facebook and Instagram alone, the risk of being victimized is very real. Choose the sites you post on carefully. Two main crimes can occur by using these types of sites: identity theft and unwanted attention/stalking.

Selecting strong passwords is really important. Never use your name, your pets name or any dates that can be easily guessed, such as your birthday. Consider phrases that you can remember but only you would know and make sure to use upper and lower case lettering as well as a symbol. Always type the address directly into your browser or use personal bookmarks instead of accessing the site through an email or other Web page; you might be inadvertently typing your password into a fake site. Protect your personal information: your name, birthdate, and/or social security number can be used to create numerous kinds of accounts in your name.

Remember, anything you post on the web can be retrieved. And, those posts your friends share that ask all kinds of questions about your behaviors or things you like, don't answer! They can be another way to gain information about you. on the web can be retrieved. Never post anything to any platform that could harm you in the future. Even if you remove it, the possibility exists that someone else has copied it to another location. Be careful what you put in your profile, especially if you make it public. It could be used to create a fake account. And remember to change your passwords often. Information that can be used to locate you, such as your address, phone number, work, or class schedule, may be found and used by someone you don't want to see. And always use the privacy settings available with any site you choose to use. The less information given out, the less likely it will be used to harm you.

Stalking

Stalking refers to harassing or threatening behavior that an individual engages in repeatedly such as following a person, appearing at a person's home or place of business, making harassing phone calls, leaving written messages or objects, or vandalizing a person's property.

Stalking is not a one-time event, but rather a series of threatening incidents that, if not responded to, may end in violence. Stalking often causes pervasive, intense fear and can be extremely disruptive for the victim.

Online stalkers (cyber stalkers) can easily disguise themselves by adopting several false identities

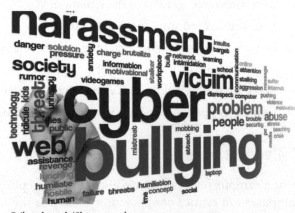

© ibreakstock/Shutterstock.com

and then harass the target through unsolicited emails, disturbing private or public messages on bulletin boards or in chat rooms, and communiqués of actual threats of harm. In addition, stalkers may pose as the victim online in order to incite others to harass and threaten the victim. Online stalking may lead to other forms of stalking.

Chapter 10 + Safety Awareness 281

Did you know . . .

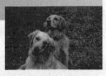

Courtesy of Shelley Hamill

- 1 in 6 women and 1 in 17 men will be victims of stalking in their lifetimes
- 15% of college women report some kind of stalking
- Can involve repeated texts and phone calls, unwanted visits, being flashed, or being sent pornography
- Young women ages 18–19 experience the highest rates of stalking.
- 75% of stalkers are individuals that the victim knows (partner, former partner, or classmate)
- 61% of female victims and 44% of male victims were stalked by a current or former intimate partner
- 7.5 million people were stalked in one year in the U.S

Remember: You have the right to break off a relationship at any time

What You Can Do

- **Once you have communicated** your disinterest, cut off all interaction and document any attempted contact.
- **Change your schedule and habits to avoid being alone.** Avoid being alone until the stalking ends, especially at night and when going from one place to another. Let others in your life know what is going on.
- **Contact** campus police and local authorities, or the Office of Victims Assistance.

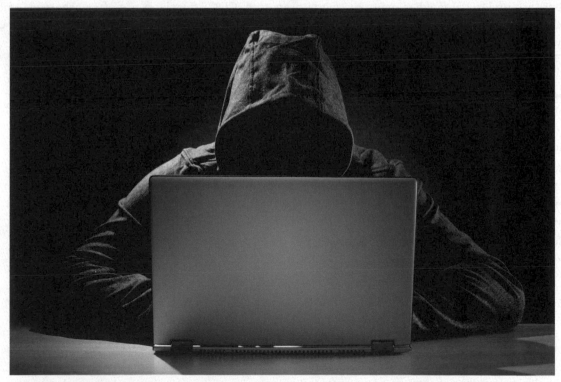

© Brian A Jackson/Shutterstock.com

Did you know . . .

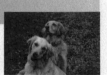

According to the Rape, Abuse, Incest Network (RAINN)

Courtesy of Shelley Hamill

- Women ages 18-24 are at an elevated risk of sexual violence.
- College women are 3x more likely to be assaulted and non college women in this age group are 4x more likely;
- Anytime a person is forced physically or verbally to have sex against her or his own will, it is rape.
- Contrary to popular thought, the majority of all sexual assaults (73%) are committed by someone known to the victim. A relative, friend, or acquaintance.
- Despite what others might say, you **DO** have recourse and **CAN** get help after an assault.
- If you are raped, not matter what the circumstances; remember that it is **NOT** your fault.
- Rape is **NOT** sex. It is an act of violence motivated by the rapist's need to dominate, control, and humiliate.
- Sexual assault can happen to anyone regardless of their race, class, age, appearance, or sexual orientation.
- Sexual trauma can be caused by rape, attempted rape, incest, unwanted sexual contact, and sexual harassment.

Sexual Violence

Millions of people are affected by sexual violence each year in the United States. It is also believed that numbers are underestimated as many cases go unreported (CDC). Survivors are often ashamed, embarrassed, afraid to tell authorities, or even to tell family and friends. Survivors may also keep quiet as they are afraid or retaliation or they don't think anyone will help.

Of the data we do have what we know according to the CDC, 2022:

- **Sexual violence is common.** 1 in 3 women and 1 in 4 men experienced sexual violence involving physical contact during their lifetimes. Nearly 1 in 5 women and 1 in 38 men have experienced completed or attempted rape and 1 in 14 men was made to penetrate someone (completed or attempted) during his lifetime.
- **Sexual violence starts early.** 1 in 3 female rape victims experienced it for the first time between 11-17 years old and 1 in 8 reported that it occurred before age 10. Nearly 1 in 4 male rape victims experienced it for the first time between 11-17 years old and about 1 in 4 reported that it occurred before age 10.
- **Sexual violence is costly.** Recent estimates put the cost of rape at $122,461 per victim, including medical costs, lost productivity, criminal justice activities, and other costs.

Date Rape

Date rape refers to being sexually assaulted by someone you know; it doesn't necessarily have to be someone you are dating. While we have noted earlier that women 18-24 are 3 to 4 times more likely to be assaulted, it can happen at any age. While men and boys can also be victims/survivors of sexual assault, the overwhelming number of assaults occur against women.

Before engaging in sexual activity, consent must be given and it must be given in an unaltered state. If you cannot give consent, it may be considered sexual assault. And, if you do not get consent, you should not continue or proceed with any sexual activity.

While sexual assault is never the survivors "fault", there are some general recommendations you can follow to protect yourself.

- When dating someone new, go on a "double date"
- Have your own transportation to and from especially for the first date.
- If you are meeting for the first time and you are alone, make sure to tell someone where you are going and what time you expect to be home.
- Always have your cell phone with you and charged.
- At a party or a bar, never leave your drink unattended. In fact, consider drinking soda instead of alcohol.
- Trust your instincts. If something doesn't feel right, leave the situation.
- Do not invite someone in to your home you do not know well. The majority of date rapes happen in homes (Health Place).

Spotlight on . . .

Being an Active Bystander:

- If you see something, do something!
- If you are unable to intervene, draw attention to the scene and call 911
- Keep an eye out for each other when attending social gatherings or parties, especially where alcohol is being served.
- If you came to the party with friends, make sure to leave with them; don't leave a friend behind especially if they may be in an altered state

Remember, we all have a responsibility to look out for one another and to keep our community safe.

Steps to Consider Taking if You are Sexually Assaulted

- Your safety is important. Are you in a safe place? If you are not feeling safe, consider reaching out to someone you trust for support.
- What happened is not your fault. Something happened to you that you did not want to happen and that is not ok.
- Call the National Sexual Assault Hotline at 800-656-4673. You will be connected to a trained staff member from a local sexual assault service provider in your area (RAINN.org).

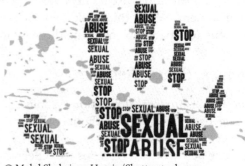

© Mohd Shahrizan Hussin/Shutterstock.com

Remember, as discussed in the chapter on healthy relationships, consent is crucial for preventing sexual coercion and unwanted sexual behavior. Consent can and should be incorporated as an essential and fun part of sexual communication.

Spotlight on . . .

Lesbian, Gay, Bisexual, Questioning, Transgender Youth

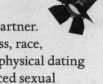

It is estimated that 1 out of 4 LGBQ/T youth will experience abuse from a dating partner. Dating abuse affects all youth, regardless of sexual orientation, gender identity, class, race, or other identity lines. According to the CDC, 17% of LGB youth had experienced physical dating violence, 16% had experience sexual dating violence, and 22% had experienced forced sexual intercourse during the past 12 months (CDC).

Among Transgender youth, 27% feel unsafe at or going to school, 35% are bullied at school, and 35% have attempted suicide (CDC).

INTIMATE PARTNER VIOLENCE

According to the CDC, intimate partner violence (IPV) is abuse or aggression that occurs in a close relationship. It can refer to current and former partners, or even ex-dating partners. There are four types of IPV: physical violence, sexual violence, stalking, and psychological aggression.

IPV affects millions of people each year. It is estimated that 1 in 4 women and 1 in 10 men have experienced some form of IPV in their lifetime. U. S. crime data suggests that 1 in 6 homicide victims are killed by an intimate partner. Further, nearly half of female homicide victims in the U. S. are killed by a current or former male intimate partner (CDC).

© arindambanerjee/Shutterstock.com

If you or a friend are dealing with IPV, seek help. Call police or go to a shelter. No one needs to stay in abusive situations.

ENVIRONMENTAL SAFETY

We have spent time discussing ways to protect people. Next we will cover suggestions on protecting our environment. While this could be a chapter by itself, thinking just a bit about things we could all do to help out and then implementing those strategies is important.

Reduce, Reuse, Recycle

The Environmental Protection Agency (EPA) defines sustainability as meeting the needs of the present without compromising the ability for future generations to meet their own needs. Easy ways to live green are to reduce, reuse, and recycle. The best way to have a positive effect on your environment is to get involved with programs through your campus or community. Simple things can make big differences. WHAT CAN YOU DO?

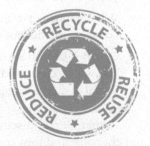

- Recycle, recycle, recycle!
- Bring your own cloth bags to the store

© graphego/Shutterstock.com

- Ride your bike, if you can
- Drive less and don't rev your engine
- Turn off the faucet when you are brushing your teeth (really, it saves water)
- Consider showering instead of taking a tub bath (though don't stay in the shower forever).
- Use both sides of the paper when printing
- Unplug your cell phone charges when not in use and turn off your computers.
- Carpool when you can.
- Make sure to dispose of old electronics properly.
- Use paper straws and reduce you use of plastics.
- Use energy efficient bulbs.

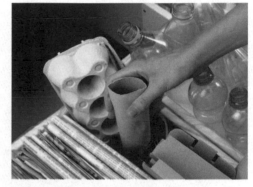

All of these, and many more are simple adjustments we can make each date to help protect our environment.

So, what can you do to reduce your carbon footprint? How are you protecting the planet for ours and future generations? Find out at www.carbonfootprint.com. Make a difference each day!

© Photographee.eu/Shutterstock.com

Are You a Wise Consumer?

There were many safety concerns addressed in this chapter. Some focused on natural occurrences and others identified activities we might chose to participate. Do you have a first aid kit? Do you wear the appropriate safety gear when participating in sport or outdoor activity? If you are engaging in outdoor activities, do you check the weather forecast before you go out? Are you being careful in your on-line communications to avoid hacking? All of these are things, among many others, that health literate people and wise consumers are aware pay attention to.

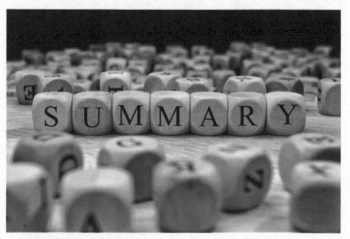

© Fabrik Bilder/Shutterstock.com

Safety is a huge topic. This chapter has only touched the surface on many of the more common safety concerns for college students. Take the time to be prepared, use proper safety equipment, know your surroundings, and plan ahead. While it is not possible to predict every possible risk, it is possible to mitigate many of them by thinking ahead.

NOTES

PERSONAL REFLECTIONS . . . SO, WHAT HAVE YOU LEARNED?

1. What do think your campus could do to improve security and why?

2. Do you recycle? Every time? Why or why not?

3. What is distracted driving? Do you drive distracted, honestly? How do we get people to understand how dangerous it is?

4. Why are young people more susceptible to driving sleepy? Why is drowsiness dangerous even if you don't fall asleep? What are steps that you will take when you are driving if you become drowsy?

NOTES

RESOURCES ON CAMPUS FOR YOU!

Services

Campus Police promotes and preserves a safe and secure campus environment by delivering quality police and community safety service in a professional and sensitive manner. The department is committed to the professional growth of its police officers, support staff, and the continual development of its relationship with faculty, staff, students, and Residence Life.

REFERENCES

American Academy of Opthamology, 2021. https://www.aao.org/eye-health/tips-prevention/injuries-sports

Bever, D.L. (1995). *Safety—A personal focus* (3rd ed). St. Louis, MO: Mosby Year Book.

Bikers Rights, *50 state helmet law review*. Retrieved 2016 from http://www.bikersrights.com/states/50state.html.

Centers for Disease Control and Prevention. *Accident or unintentional injuries*. Retrieved 2016 from

CDC, 2017. https://www.cdc.gov/violenceprevention/communicationresources/infographics/yrbs-lgb-tdv.html Retrieved March, 2022.

CDC, 2019. Retrieved from http://www.cdc.gov/nchs/fastats/accidental-injury.htm http://www.cdc.gov/nchs/fastats/accidental-injury.htm.

CDC, 2022. Injuries and violence are leading causes of death. Retrieved March, 2022. cdc.gov/injury/wisqars/animated-leading-causes.html

Center for Disease Control and Prevention. *Important facts about falls*. Retrieved 2016 from http://www.cdc.gov/HomeandRecreationalSafety/Falls/adultfalls.html.

Center for Disease Prevention and Control. Retrieved March, 2022. https://www.cdc.gov/nchs/fastats/emergency-department.htm

CDC, 2018. Ten leading cause of death by age group, United States-2018. Retrieved March, 2022. Cdc.gov/injury/images/lc-charts/leading_causes_of_death_by_age_group_2018_1100w850h.jpg

Centers for Disease Control and Prevention. *Drowsy driving: asleep at the wheel*. Retrieved January 2016 from http://www.cdc.gov/Features/dsDrowsyDriving/index.html.

CDC, 2022. Leading causes of death. Retrieved March, 2022. /nchs/fastats/leading-causes-of-deathhtm

CDC, 2018. Ten leading cause of death by age group, United States-2018. Retrieved March, 2022. Cdc.gov/injury/images/lc-charts/leading_causes_of_death_by_age_group_2018_1100w850h.jpg

Center for Disease Control and Prevention. *Unintentional drowning*. Retrieved January 2016 from http://www.cdc.gov/HomeandRecreationalSafety/Water-Safety/wathttp://www.cdc.gov/nchs/fastats/emergency-department.htmerinjuries-factsheet.html.

Center for Disease Control and Prevention. (last reviewed 2022). Accidents or unintentional injuries. Retrieved Mach, 2022. cdc.gov/nchs/fastats/accidental-injury.htm

Centers for Disease Control and Prevention. *Poisoning prevention.* Retrieved 2016 from http://www.cdc.gov/HealthyHomes/ByTopic/Poisoning.html.

CDC, 2021. Older adult fall prevention, retrieved March, 2022. cdc.gov/falls/index.html?CDC_AA_refVal=HTTPS%3A%2F%2Fwww.cdc.gov%2Fhomeandrecreational safety%2Ffalls%2Findex.html

Centers of Disease Control and Prevention. Retrieved January 2016 from (http://webappa.cdc.gov/cgi-bin/broker.exe).

CDC, 2016. Hip fractures among older adults, retrieved March, 2022. cdc.gov/falls/hip-fractures.html

CDC, 2022. Retrieved March, 2022. Drowning Facts. cdc.gov/drowning/facts/index.html

CDC, 2021. Stalking: Know it. Name it. And stop it. Retrieved March, 2022. cdc.gov/injury/features/prevent-stalking/index.html

CDC, 2021. Stalking: Know it. Name it. And stop it. Retrieved March, 2022. cdc.gov/injury/features/prevent-stalking/index.html

Charlotte Mecklenburg Police Department. Retrieved 2016 from from www.cmpd.org.

Distraction.gov. *Facts and statistics.* Retrieved 2016 from http://www.distraction.gov/stats-research-laws/facts-and-statistics.html.

Federal Bureau of Investigation Crime Report, 2015.

Federal Emergency Management Agency and American Red Cross. (2008). *Preparing for disaster. U.S Department of Homeland Security.*

Hazard Flood Report, 2020. 2020 Flash Flood/River Flood fatalities. Retreived, March, 2022. weather.gov/media/hazstat/flood20.pdf

Hazard Cold Report, 2021. 2020 Cold Related Fatalities, Retrieved, march 2022. weather.gov/media/hazstat/cold20.pdf

Hazard Wind Report, 2021. 2020 Wind Related Fatalities. Retrieved, march, 2022. weather.gov/media/hazstat/wind20.pdf.

Hazard Tornado Report, 2021. 2020 Tornado Fatalities. Retrieved, March 2022. weather.gov/media/hazstat/tornado20.pdf

Gorlick, A. (2009). *Media multitaskers pay mental price. Stanford Report.* Stanford University News.

Helmets.org.

Office of Sustainability, & Texas A&M University. (2008). *Help make sustainability an Aggie tradition.*

Mayo Clinic.org, 2019.

National Coalition Against Domestic Violence

National Highway Safety Administration , 2020. https://injuryfacts.nsc.org/motor-vehicle/overview/introduction/

National Highway Traffic Safety Administration, (2013). *Distracted driving.*

National Fire Protection Association, 2021. Home Structure Fires. Retrieved March, 2022. nfpa.org/News-and-Research-Data-research-and-tools/Building-and-Life-Safety/Home-Structure-Fires#:~:text=Most%20home%20fires%20and%20fire'fire%20setting%C%20and%20smoking%20materials

National Institute of Mental Health, & National Center for the Prevention and Control of Rape. Retrieved from www.fullpower.org

National Oceanic Atmospheric Administration, National Weather Center, & National Hurricane Center. (2012).

NSC, 2019. Retrieved from https://injuryfacts.nsc.org/glossary/National Fire Protection Agency. Retrieved 2016 from NFPA.org.

National Safety Council. (2019). Motorcycles (retrieved March, 2022), injuryfacts.nsc.org/motor-vehicle/road-users/motorcycles/

National Highway Traffic Safety Administration, 2019. Traffic Deaths in 2018, but still 36,560 people died. Retreived March, 2022. NHTSA.gov/traffic-deaths-decreased-2018-still-36,560-people-died

NHTS, 2019. Bicycle Safety. Retreived, March, 2022. nhtsa.gov/road-safety/bicycle-safety

National Safety Council, 2020. Top Ten Preventable injuries. Retrieved, March, 2022. https://injuryfacts.nsc.org/all-injuries/deaths-by-demographics/top-10-preventable-injuries/data-details/#:~:text=Falls%20are%20the%20leading%20cause,and%20the%20Consumer%20Product%20Safety

National Safety Council. (2011). *Injury facts.* 2011 Edition. Itasca, IL.

National Safety Council, n.d. Motorcycles. Retrieved, March, 2022. Injuryfacts.nsc.org/motor-vehicle/road-users/motorcycles/

National Weather Service. (2014). *Summary of natural hazard statistics for 2014 in the United States.* Retrieved from http://www.nws.noaa.gov/os/hazstats/sum14.pdf.

RAINN, n.d. Steps You Can Take After Sexual Assault . Retrieved, March, 2022. rainn.org/articles/steps-you-can-take-after-sexual-assault

Rape, Abuse and Incest Network. Retrieved January 2016 from www.RAINN.org

Ready, 2022. Make a Plan. Retrieved, March, 2022. ready.gov/plan

Sawyer, R., Desmond, S., and Gabrielle, M. (1993). Sexual communication and the college student:Implications for date rape. *Health Values: The Journal of Health Behavior, Education and Promotion.*

Sports Eye Injuries. The coalition to prevent sports eye injuries. Retrieved 2016 from http://www.sportseyeinjuries.com/fastfacts.aspx.

theNetworklaRed. *What is partner abuse.* Retrieved 2016 from http://tnlr.org/about-partner-abuse/

Transgender Identities and experinces, 2019. https://www.cdc.gov/mmwr/volumes/68/wr/mm6803a3.htm Retrieved March, 2022.

The TerraPass. Retrieved from http://terrapass.com

Weinberg, C. (1994). *The complete handbook of college women.* New York: New York University Press.

Williams, B. K. and Knight, S. M. (1997). *Healthy for life—wellness and the art of living.* Pacific Grove, CA:Brooks/Cole Publishing Company.

Hazard Lightening Report, 2020. 2020 Lightening Fatalities. Retrievied, March, 2022. weather.gov/media/hazstat/lightening20.pdf

Winthrop University. *Sexual violence: Sexual assault facts.* Retrieved January 2016 from http://www
.winthrop.edu/victimsassistance/default.aspx?id=38994

https://worldpopulationreview.com/state-rankings/helmet-law-states

CREDITS

NOTES

Glossary

Chapter 1

Health   state of complete physical, mental, and social well-being and not merely the absense of disease or infirmity

Health disparities   social determinates that play a role in the health status of individuals

Primary Prevention   behaviors to avoid the development of disease

Secondary Prevention   aimed at early detection of disease

Tertiary Prevention   works to improve the quality of life for individuals with various diseases by limiting complications and disabilities, restoring function, and slowing or stopping the progression of a disease.

Wellness   life philosophy about making informed healthy choices

Chapter 2

Adrenaline   hormone secreted by the adrenal glands that increases rates of blood circulation and breathing, prepaing muscles for exertion

Alarm stage   immediate response to the stressor

Cortisol   released in response to stress, and helps control blood sugar levels and influence blood pressure

Disordered eating   when individuals use eating habits to cope with the stress they are feeling, leading to extreme leves of caloric restriction or consumption

Distress   negative stress

Eating disorders   characterized by unhealthy eating pattersn that lead to diagnosable conditions that are life-threatening

Eustress   positive stress

exhaustion stage   the body's response to the stressor is weakening

GAS (General Adaptation Syndrome)   a three-stage response to stress imposed on the nervous and hormonal systems of the body

Insomnia   the inability to have a regular sleep practice, which can lead to negative health outcomes

Mindfulness   when we are aware of where our energy and thoughts are directed

resistance stage   the body reacts to the stressor, the adaptation stage

Stress   non-specific response to the demands placed on the body

Stressor   any real or perceived event that pressures us to cope

Chapter 3

Amenorrhea   loss of menstrual cycle

Anorexia nervosa   state of starvation and emaciation, resulting from severe dieting and excessive exercise in an effort to control body size

Autonomy   a level of input that is valued in the group

Cognition   refers to our processes of perception, learning, and reasoning and problem solving

Competence   level of confidence you have that you can contribute to the community in a positive way

Courage   quality of spirit that enables a person to face the uknown or new ideas without fear of imlications or repercussions

Critical thinking   mental process of reaching an answer or conclusion through conceptualizing, analyzing, synthesizing, and evaluating the information

Curiosity   desire to learn more about something

Emotional Intelligence   the abililty to monitor one's own and others' feelings and emotions, to discriminate among them, and to use this information to guide one's thinking and action

Emotions   positive, negative, or neutral alerts to something important in ourselves or our environment

Empathy   ability to understand and share the feelings of others

Extrovert   someone who finds energy from interactions and time spent with others

Feelings   experiential state that builds within us in response to sensations, sentiments, or desires we encounter

Female Athlete Triad   consists or disordered eating that leads to amenorrhea that leads to osteoporosis

Happiness   stable state of positivity and contentedness

Health literacy   ability that an individual can find, understand, and use health related information, resources, and services that affect their decisions and actions on health

Humility   modest view of one's own importance

Integrity   quality of being honest and upholidng moral principles

Intellectual/Mental   refers to the dimension of thinking or being rational

Introvert   someone who mentally "turns in", shy away from large crowds or awkward situations

Joy   dynamic, excitable moment

Learned Helplessness   anticipation or action that the individual has no control over a situatio n and can see no positive outcome

Learning   refers to the process of taking the cues that you perceived and applying them to previous ones to store as memory

Learning discipline   intake of new information

Learning style   way in which an individual can learn

Meditation   practice that allows you to calm your thoughts and achieve greater mental and emotional clarity

Osteoporosis   loss of bone mass

Patience   ability to wait and pause on a final judgement until all facts and information are considered

Perception   refers to interpreting data that you sense (hear, see, smell, feel, taste, etc.)

Persistence   continual search for information

Reasoning/Problem Solving   refer the ability to rationalize a plan to solve a problem

Relatedness   level of relation you have to the community

Religion   a specific system of beliefs, practices, rituals, and symbols for a purpose

Resiliency   having the ability to bounce back from obstacles and adversity within our daily lives by having the ability to cope with the life stressors we face

self-confidence   confidence or trust that you have in your abilities, qualities, or judgements

Self-efficacy   having the confidence in yourself to make things happen and believing in your ability to succeed in all or most of the situations that you face in your life.

Self-esteem   a feeling of self-worth, how you view yourself, happiness within your spirit, and the ability to meet life's challegnes each day

Self-reflection   serious thought about one's character, actions, motives, life, behavior, and beliefs

Sensibility   refers to our responsiveness toward other things or persons, such as feelings of another person or changes in the environment

Spiritual Health   refers to the state of harmony within yourself and with others, focusing on a balance of self needs and world demands

Spiritual intelligence   refers to an ability to access higher meanings values, abiding purposes, and unconscious aspects of the self

Spirituality   based on your personal beliefs and following your inner path, still maintaining a belief in something larger

Systematic thinking   application of an organized set of concepts, ideas, or principles into real life situations

Willingness to learn   discipline that includes a teachable spirit

Chapter 4

Activities of daily living   encompasses all the different movements that an individual would do each day to support independent living

aerobic   "in the presence of oxygen" and can be used with cardiovascular when describing a type of exercise

anaerobic exercise   "in the absence of oxygen" exercise performed at intensity levels so great that the body's demand for oxygen exceeds its ability to supply it.

Angina Pectoris   a condition caused by insufficient blood flow to the heart muscle that results in severe chest pain

Atherosclerosis   a build-up of fatty deposits causing blockage within the blood vessel

Blood pressure   pressure in the heart to move blood through the body

Body composition   ratio of body fat to lean body mass

Cardiovascular endurance   the ability of the body to perofrm prolonged, large-muscle, dynamic exercise at modertate to high levels of intensity

Cardiovascular fitness   refers to the ability of the heart, lungs, circulatory system to perform at optimum level for extended periods of time

Circulator System   the function and efficiency of the heart

complete fitness   comprised of health-related fitness and skill related fitness

Diastolic Blood Pressure   lowest arterial pressure attained during the heart cycle

Exercise   considered a structured type of physical activity; has a specific purpose or goal to a type of exercise

flexibility   range of motion around a joint

Frequency (FITT)   refers to the number of exercise sessions per week

Functional exercise   exercises that mimim everyday movements

health-related fitness   cardiovascular fitness, muscular strength, muscular endurance, flexibility, and optimal body composition affect the body's ability to function efficiently and effectively

Heat cramps   bodily cramps due to prolonged exposure to the heat and dehydration

Heat exhaustion   more common, primarily individuals suffereing from dehydration.

heat stroke   life threateninng condition, requires hospitalization with prolonged exposure to heat

Individual differences   individuals will respond differently to the same training programs

Intensity (FITT)   refers to how hard one is working

mobility   used to describe how effecient we are with functional and sport-specific movement

Moderate Activities   activities you can still speak while doing them (line dancing, biking with no hills, gardening, tennis doubles)

msucular power   explosive ability of muscles

muscular endurance   ability of a muscle to perform sustained contractions over time

muscular fitness   important because of its effect of efficiency of human movement and basal metabolic rate

muscular hypertrophy   increase in the size of muscle fibers

muscular strength   maximum amount of weight a muscle can lift at one time

Myocardial Infarction   heart attack

Overload   for the body to beocme more efficient or stronger, it must be stressed beyond its normal working capacity

Overtraining   lack of enough recovery time

Physical activity   body movement, performed over a period of time

Rate of Perceived Exertion(RPE)   a numbered scaled technique used to measure how hard someone is working

Resting heart rate   rate of heartbeat at rest, and is an indicator of cardiovascular fitness

Reversibility   the reversal of fitness adaptations due to reduced or no activity

RICE   used in most injuries. (Rest, Ice, Compression, and Elevation)

Sedentary lifestyle   includes little to no physical activity; a leading factor of chronic disease and death

skill-related fitness   includes agility, balance, coordination, reaction time, speed, and power

Stroke Volume   the amount of blood pumped from the heart in each heartbeat

Systolic Blood Pressure   highest arterial blood pressure attained during the heart cycle

Target heart rate range   is the intensity of training necessary to achieve cardiovascular improvement

Time(FITT)   duration of exercise

Type(FITT)   the mode or type of exercise

Vigorous Activities   difficult to carry on a conversation due to the intensity of the exercise (running, basketball, soccer, swimming laps)

Chapter 5

antioxidants   compounds that aid each cell inthe body facing an ongoing barrage of damage resulting from daily oxygen exposure, environmental pollution, chemicals and pesticides, additives in processed foods, stress hormones, and sun radiation.

Carbohydrates   the body's main source of fuel

Celiac disease   chronic digestive condition from the protein gluten, found in wheat and other grains

complex carbohydrates   relatively low in calories, nutritionally dense, and are a rich source of vitamins, mninerals, and water

dehydration   loss of bodily fluid, can be mild to very dangerous

dietary fiber   a type of complex carbohydrate that is present mainly in leaves, roots, skins, and seeds.

essential amoino acids   the body cannot produce these, therefore, it must be supplied through the diet

fat soluble vitamins   vitamins A,D,E, and K are transported by the body's fat cells

food allergy   directly affects the immune system, and can cuase severe or life-threatening symptoms

food intolerance   often affects only the digestive system and causes less serious symptoms

French Paradox   includes bread, cheese, and wine; high in saturated fats, but limited in terms of portions

insoluble fiber   does not dissolve in water; therefore, it cannnot be digested by the body

lactovegetarians   eat dairy products, fruits, and vegetables but do not consume any other animal products

macrominerals   seven minerals the body needs in relatively large quantities

Macronutrients   provide energy in the form of calories. Carbohydrates, fats, and proteins make up the sources of macronutrients

Mediterranean Diet   consists of traditional foods from countries bordering the Mediterranean Sea; encourages furits, vegetables, whole grains, legumes, nuts, seeds, and heart-healthy fats, while processed foods, added sugar, and refined grains should be restricted

microminerals   essential to healthy living, needed in smaller quantities

Micronutrients   regulate bodily functions such as metabolism, growth, and cellular development (vitamins and minerals)

minerals   inorganic substances that are critial to many enzyme functions in the body

monosaturated fats   found in foods such as olives, peanuts, canola oil, and peanut oil)

non-essential amino acids   manufactured in the body if food proteins in a person's diet provide enough nitrogen

Nordic Diet   way of eating that focuses on locally sourced foods in the Nordic countries; contains less surgar and fat but twice the fiber and seafood than average Western diet

ovolactovegetarians   eat eggs as well as dairy products, fruits, and vegetables, but still do not consume meat, poultry of fish

polyunsaturated fats   found in margarine, pecans, corn oil, cottonseed oil, sunflower oil, and soybean oil

Prebiotics   foods that fuel probiotics, and provide energy for probiotics

Probiotics   live microorganisms intended to confer a health benefit on the host; help digest food, destroy disease-causing cells, or produce vitamins

saturated fats   found primarily in animal products (meats, lard, butter, cream, cheese, and whole milk) do not melt at room temperature

semivegetarian   eats fruits, vegetables, dairy products, eggs, and a small selection of poultry, fish, and other seafood, but does not consumer any beef or pork

simple carbohydrates   carbohydrates that do not provide a rich source of other nutrients, providing empty calories

soluble fiber   dissolves in water. Assists the body with the excretion of fats

Traditional Okinawa Diet   reflects the traditional eating patterns of those living on Okinawa; low in overall calories and fat, but high in carbs

trans fat   does not occur naturally in plant or animal products, but rather is formed when liquid oils are made into solid fats

unsaturated fats   derived from plant products (vegetable oils, avocados, and most nuts)

vegans   diets are completely void of meat, chicken, fish, eggs, or milk products. Primary source of protein are vegetables, fruits, and grains

vitamins   necessary for normal body metabolism, growth, and development.

water   a substance essential to life

water soluble vitamins   include the vitamin B and vitamin C. They are not stored in the body for significant amount of time

West African   includes lean meat, vegetables, and cereal staples; low in calories and nearly devoid of processed foods

Whole grains   food made from the entire grain seed, usually called the kernel, which consists of bran, germ, and endosperm

Chapter 6

Left-brain thinkers   more logical, analytical, and objective

Right-brain thinkers   more intuitive, thoughtful, and subjective

Chapter 7

Anal canal   contains two sphincter muscles, which open and close like valves

Birth control   broad term encompassing all methods designed to prevent pregnancy and birth

Clitoral hood   consists of inner lips, which join to form a soft fold of skin, or hood, covering and connecting to the clitoris

Clitoris   usually the most sensitive part of the female genitalia and consists of erectile tissue, which becomes engorged with blood, resulting in swelling during sexual arousal that enables it to double in size

Contraception   refers to all methods designed to prevent contraception or fertilization

Contraceptive Implant   soft capsules, about 1.5 inches long, placed under the skin in a woman's upper inner arm. The capsules release progestin which usually prevents ovulation from occuring, preventing pregnancy.

Contraceptive Patch   the female will place a thin plastic patch on the skin of the buttocks, stomach, upper outer arm, or upper torso once a week for three weeks in a row. Do not use the fourth week. The patch releases combined hormones that protect against pregnancy for one month.

Cowper's glands   repsonsible for depositing a lubricating fluid for sperm and a coating for the urethra

Depo-Provera   a hormone shot injected into the arm or buttocks every twelve weeks preventing ovulation, which prevents pregnancy.

Diaphragm and Femcap   latex cup (diaphragm) or silicone cup (Femcap) requires fitting by a clinician. It is coated with spermicide before placement in the vagina.

Epididymis   tightly coiled tube on top of each testis

Fallopian tubes   located on each side of the uterus, extend from the ovaries to the uterus, and transport mature ovum

Family planning   implies the desire to have children at some point in time

Fertility Awareness-based Methods (FAMs)   a woman must chart her menstrual cycle and must be able to detect certain physical signs in order to predict unsafe days

Foreskin   loose portion of tissue covering the glans penis

Glans penis   end of the penis and covered by foreskin

Hymen   small membrane around the vaginal opening and it's function is to protect the vaginal tissues early in life

IUD   Intrauterine device requires a health care professional to insert a small plastic device through the cervix and into the uterus. The IUD contains copper or hormones that impede conception.

Labia Majora   two longitudinal folds of skin that extend on both sides of the vulva and serve as protection for the inner parts of the vulva

Labia Minora   delicate inner folds of skin that enclose the urethral opening and the vagina

Male condom   a latex sheath, placed over the penis prior to intercourse

Mons Pubis   soft fatty tissue covering the pubic symphysis

Ovaries   where eggs are produced and released, usually once a month

Penis   organ through which semen and urine passm and is structured into three main sections: the root, the shaft, and the glans penis

Perineum   smooth skin located between labia minora and anus

Scrotum   pouch of skin, which hangs from the root of the penis and holds the two testicles

Sterilization   operation performed on the female (tubal ligation) or male (vasectomy)

Testes   reproductive ball-shaped glands inside the scrotum, also known as the testicles

The pill   a prescription medication containing the hormones estrogen and/or progesterone

Theoretical effectiveness   estimates how any fertility control method should work if it is used consistently and correctly

Urethra   opening for urine to be excreted from the bladder

Vagina   located between the urethral opening and the anus

Vaginal Ring   the female will insert a small, flexible ring deep into the vagina for three weeks and take it out for the fourth week. It releases combined hormones that protect against pregnancy for one month.

Vas deferens   long tube through which sperm travel during ejaculation

Vulva   female visible external genitalia

Withdrawal method   the man will pull his penis out of the vagina before he ejaculates to keep sperm from joining an egg

Chapter 8

2C-B   psychadelic drug and similar to MDMA.

Adderall   stimulant used to treat ADHD

Alcoholism   alcohol dependence

Amphetamines   drugs that speed up the nervous system

Bidis   small, thin, hand-rolled cigarettes imported to the United States, primarily from India and other Southeast Asian countries.

Binge drinking   pattern of drinking that brings a person's blood alcohol concentration to .08 or above.

Caffeine   a stimulant as well as a psychotropic drug

Cigarette Smoking   greatly impairs the respiratory system and is a major cuase of chronic obstructive pulmonary diseases (COPD)

Cocaine   addictive stimulant drug made from the leaves of coca plant

Codeine   natural derivative of opium

Depressants   sedatives or anxiolytic drugs that depress the central nervous system

Driving while intoxicated   (DWI) now having normal use of your mental or physical faculties because of alcohol or other drugs; or a blood alcohol concentration of .08 or more.

Ethyl alcohol   also known as ethanol

Eugenol   active ingredient of clove. Deadens sensations in the throat, allowing smokers to inhale more deeply and hold smoke longer in the lungs.

Gamma Hydrozybutyrate (GHB)   fast acting, powerful drug that depresses the nervous system

Hallucinogens   also known as "psychedelics", are drugs that affect perception, sensation, awareness, and emotion

Hashish   a form of marijuana that can be smoked in a pipe

Heroin   derived from a naturally occuring substance in the Oriental poppy plant called opium

Hookahs   water pipes that are used to smoke specifically made tobacco that is usually flavored

Hydrocodone   narcotic used to relieve paine and suppress cough

Inhalants   poisonous chemical gases, fumes, or vapors that produce psychoactive effects when sniffed.

Intoxication   transient state of physical and mental disruption due to the presence of a toxic substance

Kretekes   known as clove cigarettes that contain eugenol

Marijuana   naturally occuring plant called Cannabis sativa, whose leaves and stems can be dried, crushed, and rolled in cigarettes (joints) to be smoked.

MDMA   "ecstacy", chemical structure similar to methamphetamines and mescaline

Methamphetamines   extremely addictive and powerful drug that stimulates the central nervous system, commonly known as "meth"

Nicotene   colorless, oily compound that is extrememly poisonous in concentrated amounts

Opium   derived from the poppy seed, is the base compound used for all narcotics

Oxycodone   drug used for moderate to severe pain relief, has a high potential for abuse

Ritalin   drug more powerful than caffeine but not as potent as amphetamines. Prescribed for individuals with ADHD.

Rohypnol   tranquilizer, similar to Valium but ten times more potent

Smokeless tobacco   not a safe alternative to cigarette smoking. Includes chewing tobacco, snuff, and dissolvables

Tar   by-product of burning tobacco

The Good Samaritan Law   protects individuals who offer assistance to someone in danger from prosecution.

Tolerance   when an individual adapts to the a mount consumed so that larger quantities are needed to achieve the same effect

Chapter 9

aneurysm   artery loses its integrity ad balloons out under the pressure created by the pumping heart

arteriosclerosis   thickening and hardening of the arteries.

atherosclerosis   build up of fatty deposits and other substances such as cholesterol, cellular waste products, calcium, and fribin

coronary artery disease   gradual narrowing of the coronary arteries to the myocardium, the heart muscle

hypertension   high blood pressure

myocardial infarction   occurs when an artery that provides the heart muscle with oxygen becomes blocked or flow is decreased.

peripheral vascular disease   partial or total blockage in a vessel outside of the brain or heart that may cause high blood pressure

systolic   arterial pressure when the heart is contracting and forcing the blood through the arteries

"Stroke"/brain attack   vessels that supply the brain with nutrients become damaged or occluded and the brain tissue dies because of insufficient oxygen

Chapter 10

carbon monoxide   poinson gas that is a by-product of appliances, heaters, and automobiles that burn natural gas, wood, oil, kerosene, or propane

date rape   sexual assault by someone you know

distracted driving   any activity that could divert a person's attention away from the primary task of driving

drowsy driving   combination of driving with sleepiness or fatigue

intimiate partner violence   abuse or aggression that occurs in a close relationship

pesticides   used to prevent or kill bugs, rodents or other "pests"

stalking   harrassing or threatening behavior that an individual engages in repeatedly

Index

prevention, 248
risk factors, 247–248
skin, 250
testicular, 252
Cannabinoids, 215–216
synthetic, 216
Car, 279
Carbohydrates, 100–101
Carbon monoxide (CO), 204
poisoning, 274
Carcinoma cancers, 247
Cardiorespiratory endurance, 73
Cardiovascular disease (CVD)
exercise and, 238–239
person at risk for, 238–239
risk factors of, 236–237
types of
arteriosclerosis, 239
atherosclerosis, 239
hypertension, 239–240
Cardiovascular fitness, 73
Casual friendships, 135
Celiac disease, 116
Center for Disease Control (CDC),
265, 269, 274, 275
Cervical cancer, 251
Cervix, 154
Chemotherapy, 248
Childhood obesity, 246
Chlamydia, 177–178, 183
Chlamydia trachomati, 177
Cholesterol, 237
ChooseMyPlate.gov, 108
Chronic disease, effect of physical
activity on, 71
Chronic Hepatitis B, 183
Chronic lower respiratory diseases
(CLRD), 8
Cigar smoking, 206
Cigarette smoking, 236
Circulatory system, 71
Circumcision, 157
Clitoral hood, 154
Clitoris, 154
Close friendships, 135–136
Club drugs, 220
Cocaine, 199, 219
Codeine, 218
Cognition, 51
Cognitive dissonance theory, 12
College campuses, 279–280
College, stress in, 26
Colon cancer, 252

Commitment, 138
Common cold, 28, 260
flu vs., 261
Communicable diseases
common cold, 260
hepatitis, 260
HIV/AIDS, 259
influenza, 260–261
meningitis, 260
mononucleosis, 259–260
Communication, 128–129
in age of technology, 129
open, 128
styles, 130–131
Competence, 50
Complete fitness, 78
Complex carbohydrates, 100
Compromise, 132
Condom
female, 165
male, 164, 173
Consent, 128
Contemplation, 10–11
Contraception, 160–161
emergency
abortion, 176
adoption, 175
male contraceptives, 175
parenthood, 175
unplanned pregnancy, 175
Contraceptive implant, 171, 174
Contraceptive patch, 168–169, 174
Cooldown, 86
Coping strategies, stress, 31–35
Corona, 157
Coronary artery disease, 239
Corpus cavernosa, 158
Corpus spongiosum, 158
Corticosteroids, 225
Cortisol, 24
Courage, 53
Cowper's glands, 157
Crack, 219
Craft beer, 209
Critical thinking, 53
Curiosity, 53
Cutaneous lupus erythematosus
(CLE), 258
Cyber stalkers, 280

D

Date rape, 137–138, 282–283
drug, 221

Dating in age of technology, 136–137
Death, 213
causes of, 8
roadway, 270
Depo-Provera, 169–170, 174
Depressants, 224
Depression, 30, 58
Diabetes, 237, 253–255
exercise and, 255
people get, 255
prevention, 255
symptoms of, 254
Diagnostic and Statistical Manual of
Mental Disorders (DSM-5), 214
Diaphragm, 165, 173
Diastolic, 240
DiClemente, Carlo, 10
Diet plans, 121
Dietary alternatives
food allergies and sensitivities,
115–116
vegetarianism, 114–115
Western diet, alternatives to,
117–118
Dietary fiber, 100
Dietary Guidelines for Americans,
98–99
antioxidants, 107
carbohydrates, 100–101
fats, 102–103
macronutrients, 99–105
micronutrients, 105–108
minerals, 105–106
protein, 104–105
vitamins, 105
water, 107–108
Disaster planning, 277–278
campus, 279
car, 279
college campuses, 279–280
personal safety, 278–279
stalking, 280–281
things can do, 281–282
Dissociative drugs
hallucinogens, 222
ketamine hydrochloride, 222
lysergic acid diethylamide, 223
magic mushrooms, 222
phencyclidine hydrochloride, 222
Distracted driving, 270–271
Distress, 24–25
Division of Student Life mission, 20
Dopamine, 220